BECOME AN

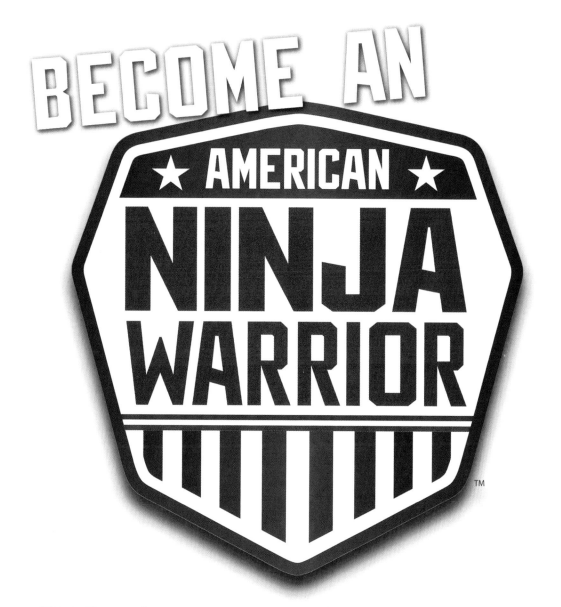

★ AMERICAN ★

NINJA
WARRIOR

™

THE ULTIMATE INSIDER'S GUIDE

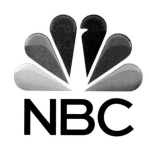

NBC

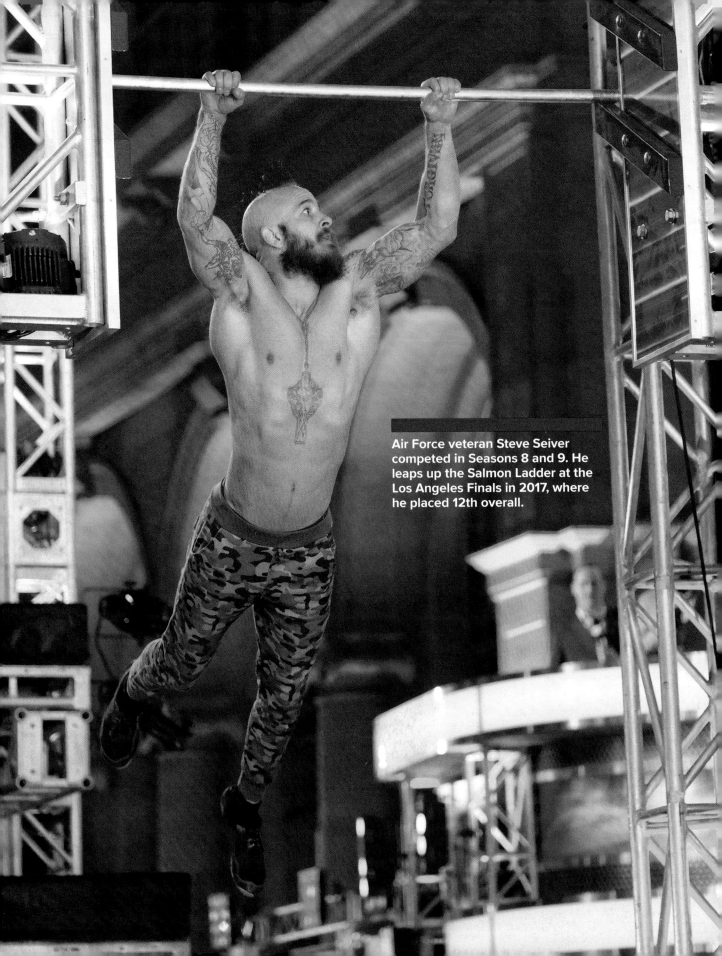

Air Force veteran Steve Seiver competed in Seasons 8 and 9. He leaps up the Salmon Ladder at the Los Angeles Finals in 2017, where he placed 12th overall.

BECOME AN

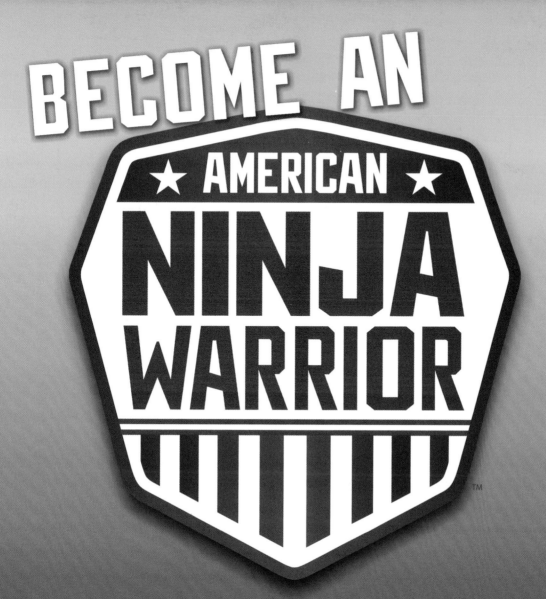

★ AMERICAN ★

NINJA WARRIOR

™

THE ULTIMATE INSIDER'S GUIDE

THE EXPERTS AND COMPETITORS OF *AMERICAN NINJA WARRIOR*

St. Martin's Griffin
New York

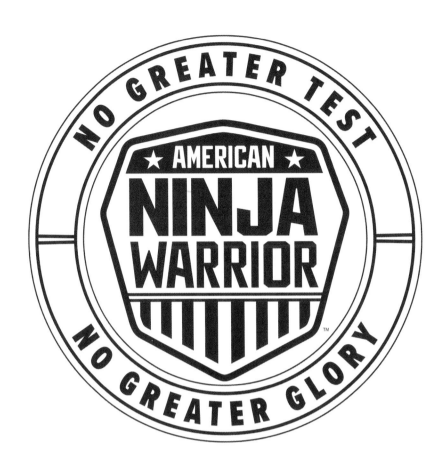

www.stmartins.com

The Library of Congress Cataloging-in-Publication Data is available upon request.

ISBN 978-1-250-18330-9 (paper over board)
ISBN 978-1-250-30366-0 (Barnes & Noble edition)
ISBN 978-1-250-18331-6 (ebook)

Our books may be purchased in bulk for promotional, educational, or business use. Please contact your local bookseller or the Macmillan Corporate and Premium Sales Department at 1-800-221-7945, extension 5442, or by email at MacmillanSpecialMarkets@macmillan.com.

First Edition: June 2018

10 9 8 7 6 5 4 3 2 1

"Kingdom Ninja" Daniel Gil uses his agility and speed to get across the Striding Steps in 2017.

ACKNOWLEDGMENTS

NBC Entertainment

Chairman NBC Entertainment: Bob Greenblatt

President, NBC Entertainment, Marketing and Digital: Len Fogge

Executive Vice President, Digital: Rob Hayes

Senior Vice President, Digital and Print Creative: Gerry Logue

Senior Vice President, Digital Business Development & Strategy: Ann McGowan

Executive Vice President, Chief Financial Officer: Brad Melnick

Vice President, Brand Development & Marketing: Joni Camacho

President, Alternative & Reality Group: Paul Telegdy

Executive Vice President, Business Affairs, Alternative & Specials: Lee Straus

Vice President, Alternative Programming: Steve Ridgeway

Vice President, Business Affairs: Corey Fitelson

Executive Vice President, Communications: Chip Sullivan

Executive Vice President, Entertainment Publicity: Rebecca Marks

Vice President, Entertainment Publicity: Traci Saulsberry

Press Director: Leslie Schwartz

Press Manager: Kevin Castech

American Ninja Warrior

Host: Matt Iseman

Host: Akbar Gbajabiamila

Co-host: Kristine Leahy

Executive Producer: Arthur Smith

Executive Producer: Kent Weed

Executive Producer: Brian Richardson

Executive Producer: Anthony Storm

Executive Producer: Kristen Stabile

Director: Patrick McManus

President, Bellon Entertainment: Greg Bellon

Macmillan/St. Martin's Press

Publisher: Jennifer Enderlin

Executive Editor: Marc Resnick

Editorial Assistant: Hannah O'Grady

Managing Editor: Amelie Littell

Manufacturing Coordinator: Eric Gladstone

Produced by The Stonesong Press, LLC

Project Director: Ellen Scordato

Text and Editorial: Dina Santorelli, Alyssa Jennette

Special thanks to Nikki Lee

Designed by studio2pt0

Art Director, Designer: Stan Madaloni

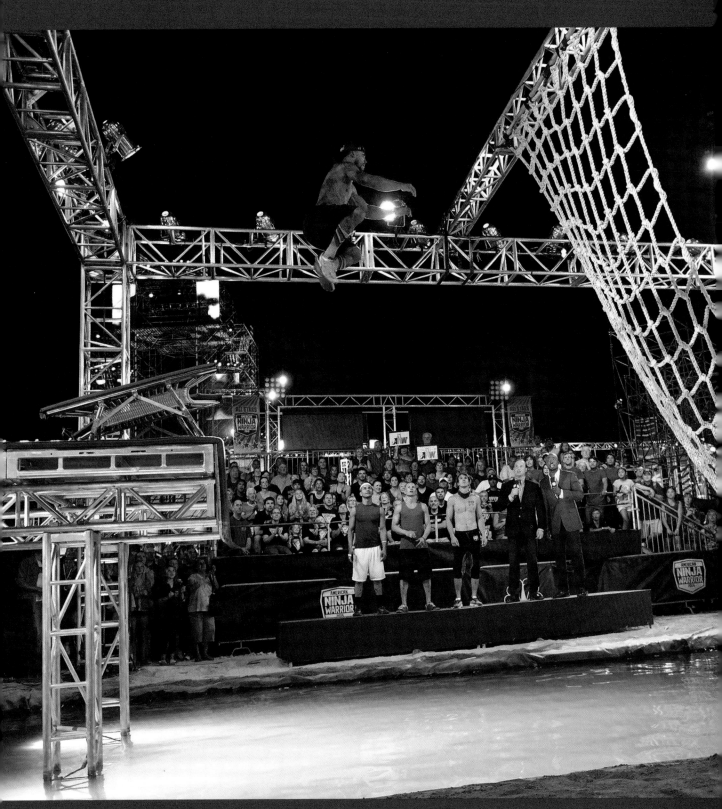

JJ Woods competes in the 2016 *American Ninja Warrior All-Star Special: Skills Challenge.*

BECOME AN AMERICAN NINJA WARRIOR: THE ULTIMATE INSIDER'S GUIDE

CONTENTS

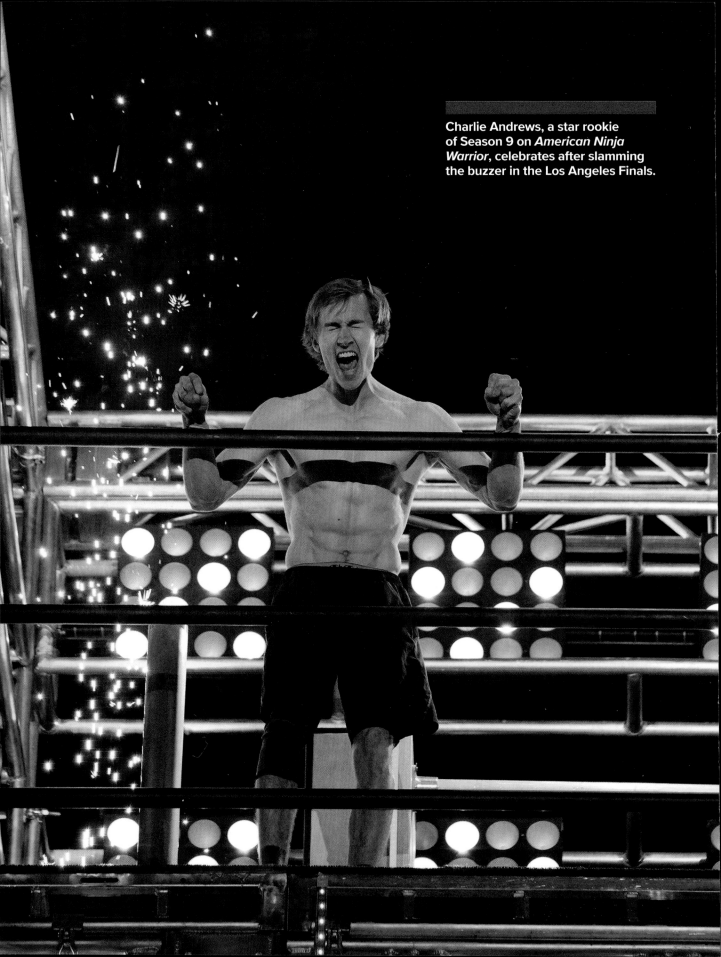

Charlie Andrews, a star rookie of Season 9 on *American Ninja Warrior*, celebrates after slamming the buzzer in the Los Angeles Finals.

INTRODUCTION

"Welcome to *American Ninja Warrior*!" roars host Matt Iseman, and so begins the next installment of the action-packed Emmy-nominated NBC competition series that has become a television summer sensation and an athletic phenomenon.

Now in its tenth season, *American Ninja Warrior* is based on the hit *SASUKE*–known worldwide as *Ninja Warrior*–from the Tokyo Broadcasting System Television (TBS). *American Ninja Warrior* follows hundreds of athletes each season who inspire millions by testing their skills on one of the world's toughest obstacle courses. Ninjas from across the United States train year-round in order to dominate a series of obstacles that challenge their agility, balance, endurance, and, in particular, upper-body and grip strength. If they've got what it takes in both the Qualifying and City Finals rounds, they move on to Las Vegas, Nevada, for the National Finals, where they have a chance to take home $1 million in prize money.

However, standing between them and a big payday is the infamous Mt. Midoriyama, a demanding final obstacle course modeled after the famed course located at the Midoriyama outdoor studio lot in Yokohama, Japan. Ninjas have to clear three increasingly difficult stages of obstacles (and beat the clock in two of them) leading up to Stage Four–a

taxing 75-foot rope climb that they need to scale in 30 seconds to hit that final buzzer and be crowned the new American Ninja Warrior.

As if that weren't challenging enough, competitors have only one chance–a single run–to do it. That means with one misjudged swing or missed grip they risk a potentially season-ending fall. While in the early rounds of *American Ninja Warrior* it is possible to stumble and still go through to the National Finals in Vegas–provided ninjas go far enough and fast enough–the Finals are a nail-biting single elimination. One slip-up, and they're out.

In nine seasons, only two competitors have made it all the way, achieving "Total Victory." Who could forget the historic climb of cameraman Geoff Britten up Stage Four of Mount Midoriyama, becoming the first-ever American Ninja Warrior in Season 7? Or, moments later, busboy Isaac Caldiero's epic ascent up the massive summit–in 26.14 seconds–narrowly beating Britten's time to take home the million-dollar prize?

WARRIOR WORDS

TOTAL VICTORY: Completing Stage Four of the *American Ninja Warrior* National Finals. In nine seasons of *American Ninja Warrior*, only two competitors—Geoff Britten and Isaac Caldiero, both in Season 7—were able to achieve this remarkable feat. (Throughout the decades of *Ninja Warrior* series broadcast globally, fewer than 10 athletes have achieved Total Victory, known as *Kanzenseiha* in the original Japanese version and among many competitors around the world.)

MMA ATHLETES, MOMS & MORE

In nine years, tens of thousands of athletes have answered *American Ninja Warrior*'s call to compete. Climbers. Track stars. MMA fighters. Olympians. Gymnasts. Pole vaulters. NASCAR drivers. Military members. Moms. Dads. Grandparents. Teachers. Doctors. Students. Hair stylists. Entrepreneurs. *American Ninja Warrior* has seen them all!

And fans have seen many of them again and again. They are the veteran ninjas we've come to know and love. Like "Island Ninja" Grant McCartney, the flight attendant for Hawaiian Airlines, who first danced his way into our hearts in Season 7. Or stunt woman Jessie Graff who, in Season 8, became the first woman in *American Ninja Warrior* history to conquer Stage One of the National Finals. Or fan favorites stunt man Flip Rodriguez and gym owner

"Real Life Ninja" Drew Drechsel, two of the most consistent competitors to run the course. Time and time again, they come back. To finish what they started. To beat the obstacle that took them down. To show the world—and themselves—that they're not done yet.

Will they find redemption? Or will they get wet? There's no telling who will clear an obstacle or hit a buzzer on any given day. Who could have predicted "Mighty" Kacy Catanzaro, at 5 feet tall, would go on to make two record-breaking runs in Dallas during Season 6, cementing her place in *American Ninja Warrior* history as the first woman to complete a Qualifying course as well as the first woman to qualify for Vegas's Mount Midoriyama?

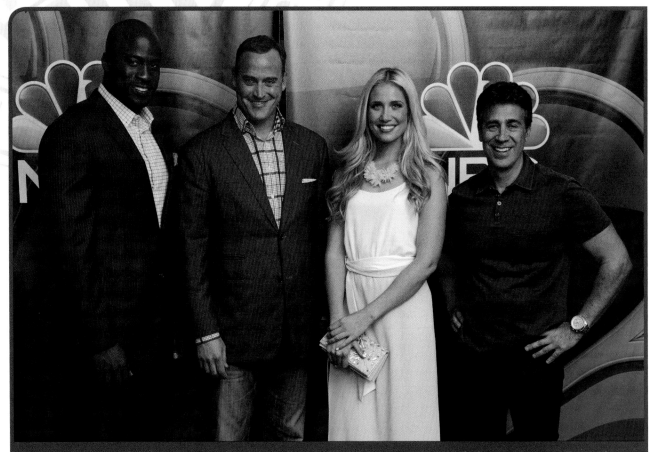

Pictured (left to right): Hosts Akbar Gbajabiamila and Matt Iseman, cohost Kristine Leahy, and Executive Producer Arthur Smith.

It just goes to show: Never judge a ninja by their cover.

And then there are the rookies, the fresh faces among the familiar, the ninja stars of tomorrow. Every season, they walk up to that starting line ready to defy gravity as well as expectations in their quest for victory, which, as any fan of the show knows, is about more than just slamming down a buzzer. Victory on *American Ninja Warrior* is about getting to the starting line as much as the finish line. It's about perseverance through adversity, about digging deep and rising up, and about celebrating what our bodies and minds can do when they work together. While most competition shows have winners and losers, every ninja who appears on *American Ninja Warrior* is already a winner, has already trained and often beaten incredible odds just to be there—whether or not they go on to crush the course.

Like 33-year-old Zach Gowen who lost a leg to cancer when he was only eight years old and competed without his prosthetic in the Indianapolis Qualifying round of Season 8, making it halfway through the course. And 41-year-old Jimmy Choi, of Season 9, a tech consultant from Illinois who was diagnosed at age 27 with young-onset Parkinson's Disease. Although Choi's inspirational run in the Kansas City Qualifiers ended on the Broken Pipes obstacle, he became a hands-down winner of the night. These athletes are the crux of what *American Ninja Warrior* is about—making the impossible possible. As cohost Akbar Gbajabiamila said the night of Choi's run: "Just because you have a disability doesn't mean you don't have the ability."

WARRIOR WORDS

GETTING WET: Failing to clear an obstacle, resulting in an anguishing fall into a pool of water below.

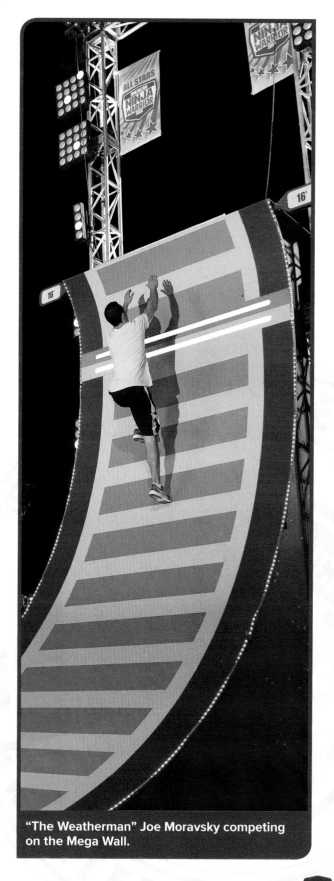

"The Weatherman" Joe Moravsky competing on the Mega Wall.

ALL-ACCESS PASS

Whether you're a longtime fan of *American Ninja Warrior* or new to the show, this book will take you behind the cameras for a rare glimpse at what goes into putting together each and every episode. You'll hear from hosts Matt Iseman and Akbar Gbajabiamila, the voices of *American Ninja Warrior*, whose commentary not only brings the competition to life but also brings smiles to our faces. You'll read how Iseman's famous "American Ninja Warrior" growl came to be and why Gbajabiamila likes to shout his familiar "I see you!" to ninjas running the course.

You'll find out how the show executives and production teams work throughout the year and all night long during shooting to capture the best of America's cities in order to showcase the best of America's ninja athletes. You'll learn about the ATS Team, the organization that crafts those famously daunting obstacles. And you'll also hear from the ninjas themselves on what it's like to stand before the course for the first time, the training it took to get them there, and how *American Ninja Warrior* has changed their lives—and our lives—forever.

For nearly a decade, *American Ninja Warrior* has spawned a pop culture movement that has made athleticism not only accessible but also fun. Across the United States, ninja gyms are sprouting up in city after city, giving all of us the opportunity to experience—firsthand—the level of difficulty of an *American Ninja Warrior* course and what it takes to master it.

And that's exactly the point. To train hard. To fall down and get up. To find a way when all the odds seem to be against you. *American Ninja Warrior* reminds us all that superheroes require perseverance as much as tremendous body strength and training and that if at first they don't succeed, they come back and try again.

At its core, *American Ninja Warrior* celebrates the journey of an athlete and invites us all to come along and share in the triumphs and tragedies that arise when you have the courage to push beyond your reach. Will this be the season that your favorite ninja achieves Total Victory? Will a rookie take the course by storm? Will an extra swing on the Floating Steps' hanging rope cost an athlete valuable seconds that will keep him or her from advancing to the next round? Will a ninja glide across the Broken Bridge or another agility obstacle with ease? Will another female competitor join the elite club of women to make it up the Warped Wall?

Anything can happen on *American Ninja Warrior*. That's because anything can happen when athletes don't accept their limitations and choose, instead, to ignore them.

> " I have a saying that to be good is not good enough if you dream of being great. Everyone has a certain ambition and can persevere, but I think there's a certain threshold. The ones that really go beyond that are the ones who have the ability to dream, and dream big.
> —Host Akbar Gbajabiamila "

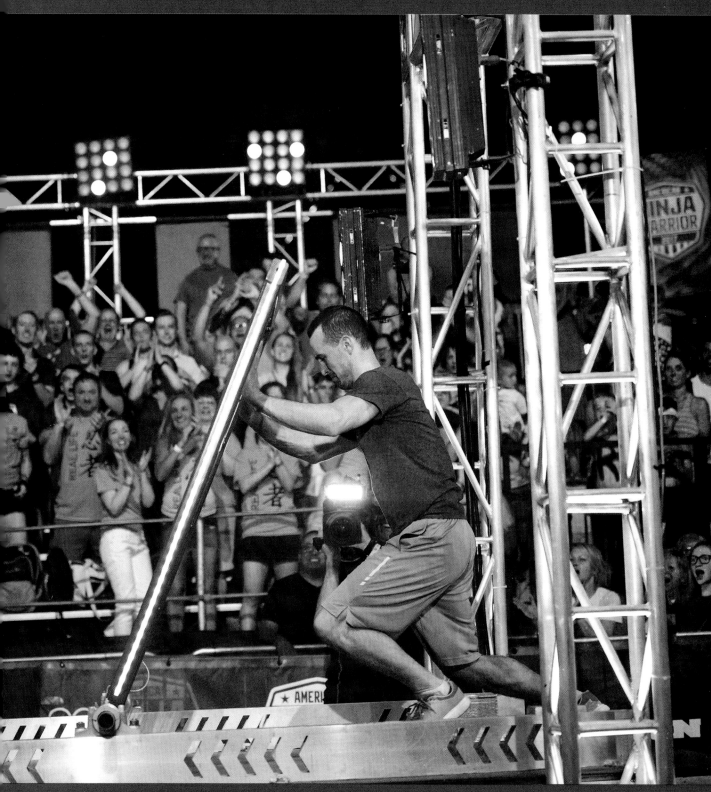
"The Weatherman" Joe Moravsky competes on the Las Vegas Finals course in Season 9. He made it farther than any other ninja, falling only at Time Bomb in Stage 3.

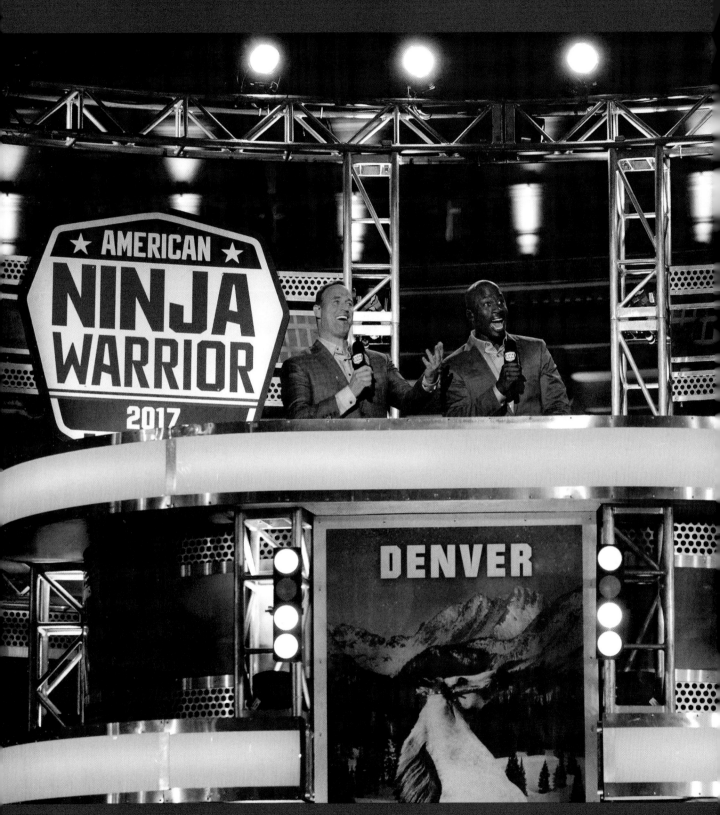

Hosts Matt Iseman and Akbar Gbajabiamila at the Denver Finals in Season 9, 2017.

CHAPTER 1

THE SHOW

In 1997, a new show called *SASUKE* premiered on Japanese television as a special to the regular primetime show *Muscle Ranking* and would go on to become one of the premier sports entertainment shows of the Tokyo Broadcasting System Television (TBS). The concept—pitting 100 competitors against a daunting four-stage obstacle course—caught on with viewers and over the years grew wildly popular around the world.

In the United States, the G4 television network—a fledgling digital cable and satellite television channel owned by G4 Media—began airing *SASUKE*, known as *Ninja Warrior*, which started to gain traction with American audiences. "It was quite unusual for a US network to air a Japanese show in Japanese—we didn't dub the dialogue—and it was a gamble putting it on the air," says former G4 executive Laura Civiello, who acquired the show from TBS agent Bellon Entertainment. "Despite the fact that it first started at the past-midnight slot in October 2006, it quickly moved up to prime time by March 2007."

In May 2007, G4 held its first "*Ninja Warrior* Marathon" broadcast in an effort to grow the audience for the new show. The event lasted 53 hours straight and brought the biggest ratings success for G4 since the network launched its broadcast.

AMERICAN NINJA CHALLENGE

While it's true that *Ninja Warrior* was quickly gaining in popularity, the show didn't have any American competitors beyond athletes who were given an invitational status, such as former Olympic medalist Paul Hamm, for example. In 2007, the G4 Network started *American Ninja Challenge*, a predecessor to *American Ninja Warrior* that was intended to be a nationwide selection event to

send Americans to Japan to compete in *SASUKE*. (*SASUKE* legend Makoto Nagano made an appearance on *American Ninja Challenge* as a special guest.) The show reaffirmed the popularity of obstacle-course-style competition with American audiences and, when it ended its run in 2009, provided a solid foundation for *American Ninja Warrior*, which premiered the same year.

AMERICAN NINJA WARRIOR, SEASONS 1 & 2

The inaugural season of *American Ninja Warrior* was based on a three-day event G4 held in California in August 2009 in order to select the 10 best competitors for *SASUKE*, which was in its 23rd season. Some 250 athletes competed, and the televised event was turned into an eight-episode run that became another smash hit for G4, scoring the highest male 18-to-34 rating among all G4 programs at the time.

Following that success, G4 upped the ante for Season 2. In August 2010, the network set up a course and held a large-scale event in Venice Beach, Los Angeles (which later grew into the host location of the Los Angeles Qualifiers until it moved to the Universal Studios lot in 2015). The top 15 competitors were selected out of approximately 300 who took on the obstacle course and were brought to a four-day Ninja Boot Camp in the remote California mountains. There, they vied for the top 10 spots and the right to travel to Japan in order to compete in *SASUKE 26* (there had been no American participation via G4 in *SASUKE 24* and only three Americans competed in *SASUKE 25*).

Among the 10 American competitors to represent the United States, five of them—Paul Kasemir, Brent Steffensen, Travis Furlanic, "The Godfather" David Campbell, and Brian Orosco—made it to Stage Two, and all, with the exception of Furlanic, made it to Stage Three. *American Ninja Warrior*'s Season 2 became yet another smash hit for G4, marking the new highest rating in G4 history.

A. SMITH & CO. PRODUCTIONS

Audiences for *American Ninja Warrior* continued to grow, and in an effort to step up production and boost the excitement factor, G4 brought in A. Smith & Co. Productions, a successful California-based production company. Since its founding in 2000, A. Smith & Co. has become one of the largest production companies in North America, creating over 4,000 hours of programming and producing more than 175 television shows for more than 47 networks, including *Hell's Kitchen*, *Spartan: Ultimate Team Challenge* and *Team Ninja Warrior*, among many others. Currently, three of *American Ninja Warrior*'s four executive producers hold positions with A. Smith & Co.: Arthur Smith serves as chief executive officer, Kent Weed is president, and Anthony Storm is vice president and executive producer. Storm and Brian Richardson, who was hired by A. Smith & Co., serve as the showrunners of *American Ninja Warrior* and oversee the day-to-day operations.

"We watched the Japanese show. We knew there was something special there," says Smith. "There was this very niche kind of thing where we realized there were these Americans who were familiar with *SASUKE*, who had been exposed to it either through the internet or through G4, and they were saying they wanted to take on *SASUKE*."

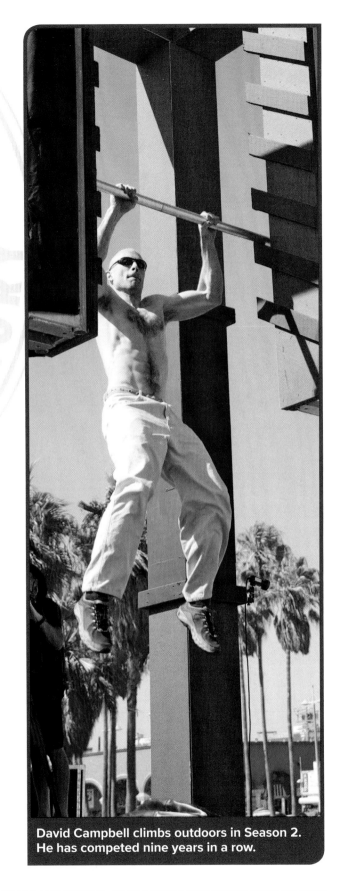

David Campbell climbs outdoors in Season 2. He has competed nine years in a row.

HOSTS OF AMERICAN NINJA WARRIOR

	Host	Cohost	Sideline Reporter
2009/Season 1	Blair Herter	Alison Haislip	n/a
2010/Season 2	Matt Iseman	Jimmy Smith	Alison Haislip
2011/Season 3	Matt Iseman	Jimmy Smith	Alison Haislip
2012/Season 4	Matt Iseman	Jonny Moseley	Angela Sun
2013/Season 5	Matt Iseman	Akbar Gbajabiamila	Jenn Brown
2014/Season 6	Matt Iseman	Akbar Gbajabiamila	Jenn Brown
2015/Season 7	Matt Iseman	Akbar Gbajabiamila	Kristine Leahy
2016/Season 8	Matt Iseman	Akbar Gbajabiamila	Kristine Leahy
2017/Season 9	Matt Iseman	Akbar Gbajabiamila	Kristine Leahy

> G4 was a cable channel targeted at young males—video gamers—and it ran several Japanese programs, including *SASUKE*. G4 decided to try an American version of *SASUKE* to build on the popularity. In the first few seasons, small courses were built for the early rounds, but for the finale, building all four stages of Mount Midoriyama was too expensive for a small cable channel's budget. It was much easier to just take the finalists to Japan where the course was built. However by Season 4, the ratings success of the show meant it was economically feasible to build an American version of Mount Midoriyama in Las Vegas for the finale, and it has been rebuilt there every year.
>
> —Executive Producer Brian Richardson

SUMMER SURPRISE

With every new season, *American Ninja Warrior* continued to perform well for G4. However, the show was still relatively unknown to mainstream audiences, since G4 was a relatively unknown network. G4 and A. Smith & Co. all wanted to find a bigger audience. "Getting the finale on NBC would create more exposure for the show and really benefit the brand, benefit G4," executive producer

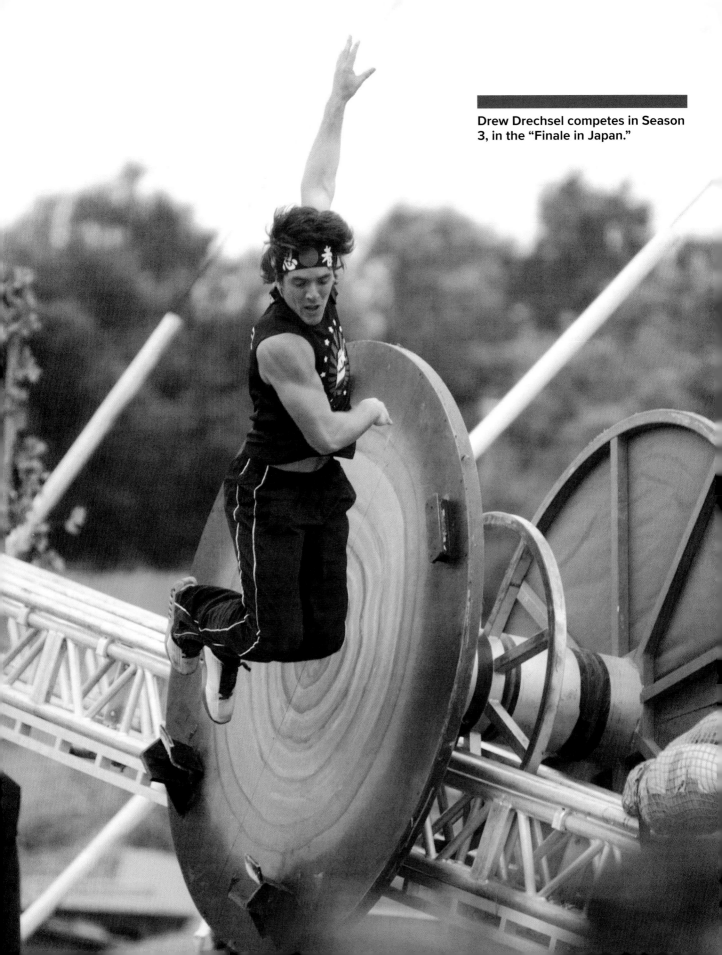

Drew Drechsel competes in Season 3, in the "Finale in Japan."

Arthur Smith says. "This was a little cable show that was doing well, and we made a pitch to NBC to get it on."

NBC took a chance, and *American Ninja Warrior* aired on NBC as a two-hour prime-time special in 2011. It was a Monday night in August—historically not a ratings bonanza—and preseason football had begun, but the show surprised the network. Not only did it hold its own against some stiff competition, but ratings were up 400 percent in comparison to the same time slot the previous year.

RISING TO THE OCCASION

In its early days, *American Ninja Warrior* appealed mostly to hardcore athletes—cross-fitters, gymnasts, fitness buffs, and parkour athletes who wanted a shot to compete on Mount Midoriyama, the grueling final obstacle course of *SASUKE*. This made casting somewhat limited.

"It wasn't broad like it is today," says *American Ninja Warrior* executive producer Kent Weed. "It didn't reach out to every American. We were very challenged with a lot of these athletes—a lot of them didn't have stories. They were just gym rats. And all the obstacles were derivative directly from *SASUKE*."

"We really thought *American Ninja Warrior* was going to be a one-off on NBC and we were going to go back and continue what we were doing with G4," adds executive producer Arthur Smith. "That's the truth. We never thought we were going to be on NBC for good, but it was kind of a test for us, and we all rose to the occasion and surprised a lot of people, so everything changed the day after it first aired on NBC."

After *American Ninja Warrior*'s surprise showing on NBC, conversations began between the network and show executives about how to do more the following season, which would wind up having split coverage between G4 and NBC. "For Season 4, we did 25 hours total—15 exclusively for G4 and 10 for NBC," Smith says. "And the following year it changed. It

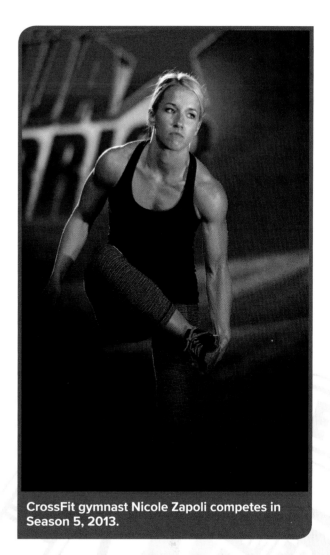

CrossFit gymnast Nicole Zapoli competes in Season 5, 2013.

became 14 for NBC and G4 had been transitioned to a new network called Esquire [which is now defunct], and we did eight hours on Esquire."

Season 6 brought even more *American Ninja Warrior*—a total of 32 hours, all on NBC, Smith says, with Esquire airing reruns. "The growth of the show kind of parallels our journey through the Comcast NBC family," he says. "It started off as the show on G4, which had this groundswell of support, and then we had this kind of experimental synergy in Season 3, and as a result of that, in Season 4 and Season 5 the hours were split. By Season 6, NBC said, 'Hey, we really have something here, and we're going to do it all!'"

In Season 6, *American Ninja Warrior* premiered on NBC as part of its summer lineup, and the grand prize, which had been $500,000, was increased to $1 million in Season 7. (Beginning in Season 8, if multiple competitors complete Stage Four, they split the prize money.) "It went from a niche network to a broad-based network, and it went from a niche sport to a broad-based sport," says executive producer Arthur Smith.

> With *American Ninja Warrior*, you look at these athletes, and they're not your NFL, NBA major league guys. These are ordinary people doing extraordinary things, and they're so relatable to the everyday person. No matter where I go, people always tell me, 'Man, I know that person' or 'I am that person.' Competition is in the DNA of everyone—everyone's competitive in some form. When you see it displayed on TV in such a positive environment, it's compelling.
>
> —Host Akbar Gbajabiamila

GOING REGIONAL

In the beginning, *American Ninja Warrior* was essentially a smaller-scale and smaller-scope version of the show that's known today. For example, the competition of Season 2 took place in Venice Beach—and *only* Venice Beach.

"When we got to Season 3, even for a small cable network, there were thousands of people who wanted to be on the show," says executive producer Arthur Smith. "We realized that the movement needed to be broadened in Season 4. We're grateful that NBC saw the vision of that, too."

The result of that vision? Beginning in Season 4, *American Ninja Warrior* hit the road—traveling to two cities, Miami and Dallas, in addition to Los Angeles in order to enlist competitors. The geographical scope widened as the series progressed, with a total of four cities in Season 5, five cities in Seasons 6 and 8, and six cities in Seasons 7 and 9.

As *American Ninja Warrior* toured the country, its familiar format took shape: regional Qualifiers narrowed the competitor field for the regional City Finals; those who made the cut, plus a group of Wildcards, would punch their ticket to the National Finals in Vegas. (Wildcards would be eliminated in Season 9.) The competitors who completed Stage Four would become the *American Ninja Warrior*.

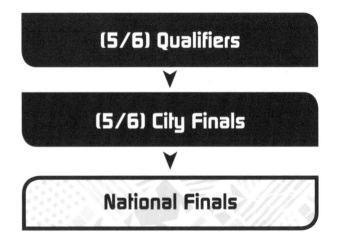

(5/6) Qualifiers

▼

(5/6) City Finals

▼

National Finals

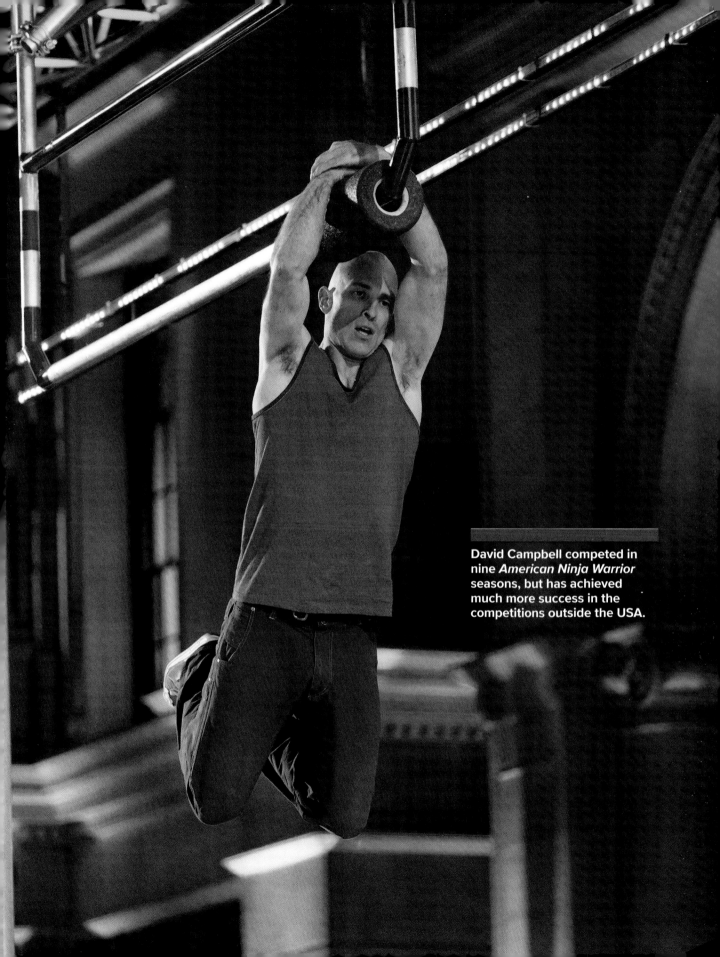

David Campbell competed in nine *American Ninja Warrior* seasons, but has achieved much more success in the competitions outside the USA.

NATIONAL FINALS ON AMERICAN SOIL

In Season 4, with regional Qualifying rounds now taking place and *American Ninja Warrior*'s scope, competitor pools, and audiences growing, show executives felt they needed to pay off that growth—and culminate the competition—at the national level. "It was time to bring the Finals to American soil," says executive producer Kent Weed.

Indeed, for the first time, *American Ninja Warrior*'s season finale would be held in Las Vegas, where *SASUKE*'s Mount Midoriyama would be recreated—with over 1,000 feet of structural steel, matching the exact specs that made it famous in Japan—before a backdrop of the Las Vegas Strip.

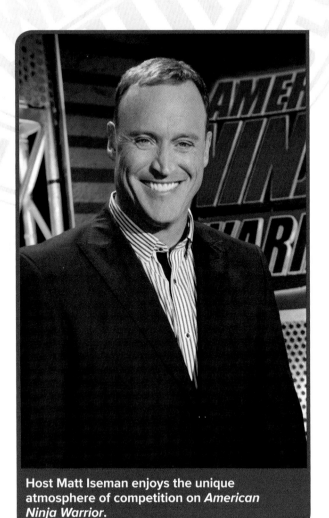

Host Matt Iseman enjoys the unique atmosphere of competition on *American Ninja Warrior*.

> Everyone has a story to tell, and in those few moments we have competitors on the show, whether it's for one obstacle or 10, we try to bring that person into your living room and engage the viewer to his or her unique story.
>
> —Director Patrick McManus

> Competition shows have become so popular because they always have stakes, but what makes *American Ninja Warrior* so unique is that it's a competition show where the athletes don't really compete against each other—they compete against themselves.
>
> —Host Matt Iseman

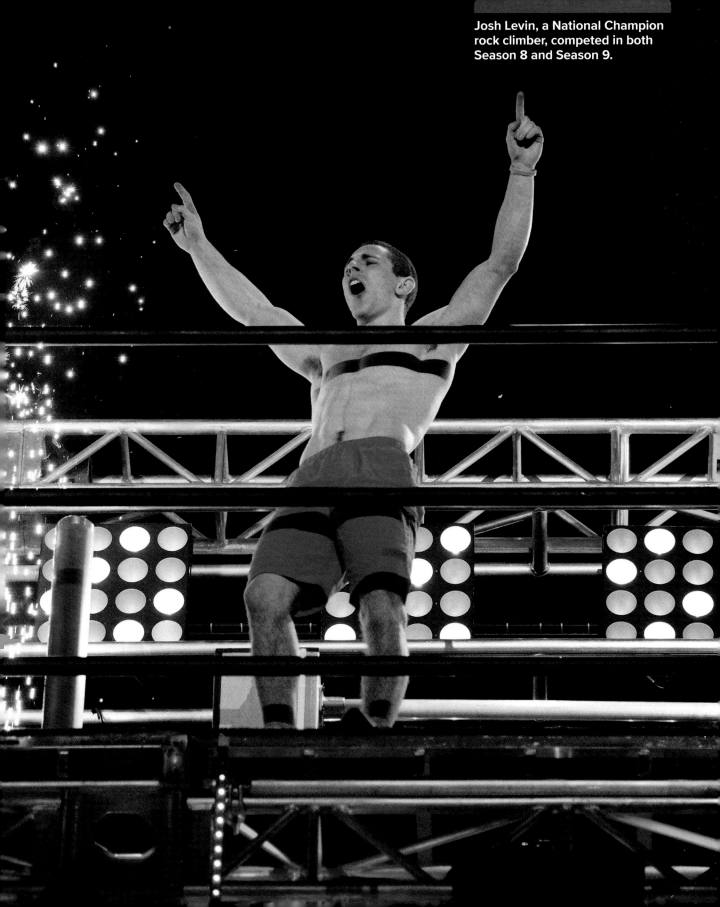

Josh Levin, a National Champion rock climber, competed in both Season 8 and Season 9.

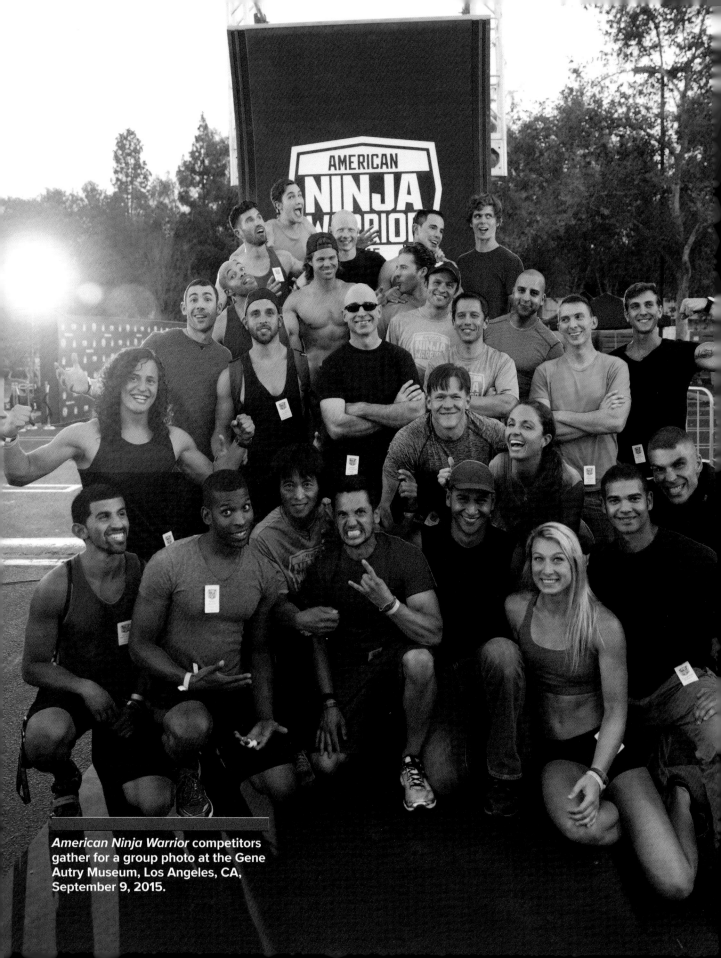

American Ninja Warrior competitors gather for a group photo at the Gene Autry Museum, Los Angeles, CA, September 9, 2015.

> The show's positive messages are a large reason for its popularity. It's a program about the power of community, support, and empathy. It's inspirational to watch the ninjas root for each other and help each other improve. It's motivating to see people overcome their personal hardships and use ninja training as a way to improve their lives. And it appeals to all races, genders, and generations.
>
> —Executive producer Anthony Storm

A COMPETITION SHOW WITHOUT COMPETITION

The big question, when *American Ninja Warrior* first aired in the United States, was whether American audiences would accept a competition show without winners and where the athletes were not aggressive among one another: rather than exhibiting cutthroat competition, ninjas lifted up each other and got better together.

"The idea of not having a winner at the end of the season was unthinkable and unacceptable to Western broadcasters, and it took years for me to get this fundamental concept of *SASUKE* understood and accepted," says Makito Sugiyama, chief, global business, of TBS, who is in charge of *SASUKE*'s global distribution. "In fact, *SASUKE* didn't sell at least the first three to four years after TBS started offering this show internationally. I believe *SASUKE* is still the only noncomedy physical reality series that doesn't necessarily have a winner at the end of each season, which makes it unique from other reality series.

"It was a gamble for any producer to adopt this concept," continues Sugiyama. "However, the concept showed how tough the obstacles were and changed viewer expectations from routinely having a winner at the end to wondering whether there *would* be a winner at the end."

FAMILY SHOW

Audiences took to the format in droves. *American Ninja Warrior* wasn't just about winning, that was true, but it was jam-packed with camaraderie and positive messaging—working hard, following goals, adopting healthy lifestyles, being kind and supportive to one another. Suddenly, that narrow audience of male CrossFitters and parkour athletes that had watched the first few seasons had broadened to a demographic that included not only women but a wide variety of age brackets and income and fitness levels. It had become a show for everyone, particularly families.

"*American Ninja Warrior* sends out such a great message," says executive producer Arthur Smith. "We're very in touch with our ninja fans and ninja community out there, and we hear time and time again that *American Ninja Warrior* is a show that people watch with their family."

"If you fall, get up and try again," adds executive producer Kent Weed. "We watch a lot of sports with our kids, but very rarely is there a sport that you can watch and then go out in the backyard and play with them the next minute. I coach soccer and Little League, but it's just not the same as being side by side with them."

DID YOU KNOW?

American Ninja Warrior is only one of the versions of *SASUKE* or *Ninja Warrior*, which has been broadcast in various languages in 165 countries and territories around the world (the productions in Asia are branded under *SASUKE*, while the rest are *Ninja Warrior*). There are nearly 20 different local versions of the show:

American Ninja Warrior (USA)
SASUKE MALAYSIA (Malaysia)
SASUKE SINGAPORE (Singapore)
Ninja Warrior Türkiye (Turkey)
Ninja Warrior Sverige (Sweden)
SASUKE VIETNAM (Vietnam)
Ninja Warrior UK (UK)
SASUKE CHINA (China)
SASUKE NINJA WARRIOR INDONESIA
   (Indonesia)
Danmarks Ninja Warrior (Denmark)
Ninja Warrior France (France)
Ninja Warrior Germany (Germany)
Ninja Warrior Italy (Italy)
Ninja Warrior Netherlands (Holland)
Arabian Ninja Warrior (Middle East)
Australian Ninja Warrior (Australia)
Ninja Warrior España (Spain)
Ninja Warrior Hungary (Hungary)
Ninja Warrior Austria (Austria)

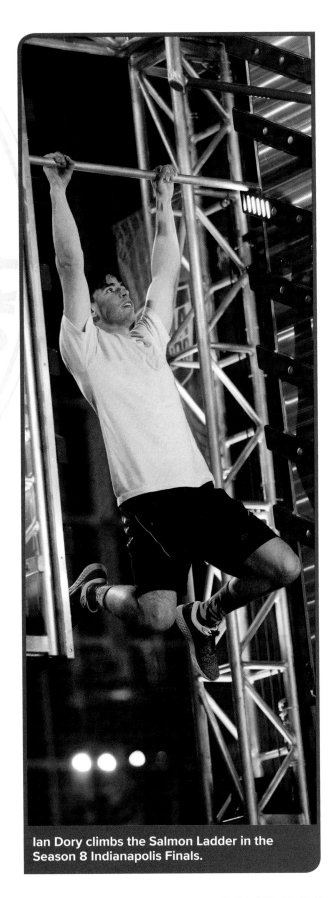

Ian Dory climbs the Salmon Ladder in the Season 8 Indianapolis Finals.

BACKSTAGE NINJAS

Today, millions of viewers tune in each season to watch their favorite ninjas tackle the *American Ninja Warrior* obstacle course. But what those viewers may not know is that there are legions of backstage ninjas working together, behind the scenes, to produce everything they see—from the lights to the course to the ninja background stories. Leading the charge are *American Ninja Warrior*'s four executive producers: Arthur Smith, Kent Weed, Anthony Storm, and Brian Richardson, who oversee the production, which incorporates hundreds of people operating massive amounts of equipment. These include approximately:

- 30 editors and post staff in Los Angeles
- 28 lighting technicians/grips
- 25 production assistants
- 23 cameramen and women
- 18 security handlers
- 14 obstacle course build crew
- 13 semi truck drivers
- 12 field producers
- 9 tech crew members
- 9 production staffers
- 8 transportation team members
- 6 casting team members
- 6 audio engineers/producers
- 5 catering crew members: Crews eat a lot.
- 3 accountants
- 3 medics/EMT
- 2 makeup/hair
- 2 wardrobe people
- 2 assistant directors
- 1 director

That's more than 200 people to produce a single episode!

SCOUTING CITIES

Each season, the *American Ninja Warrior* production team is on the move—some six to eight trucks haul equipment from city to city for the Qualifying and City Finals rounds. But how are these cities chosen?

> We arrive on location with a dozen big semitrailers. Five days later, the course is up and running. Then it's all packed away and trucked off to the next city.
>
> –Adam Biggs, director of photography/ lighting designer

The decision begins with the show executives, who scout all over the country for suitable locations. "We're always looking for new, exciting cities that offer an interesting backdrop behind the course," says Brian Richardson, executive producer. "We also try to spread them out geographically—a city in the Southeast, a city in the Midwest, etc. And we always have to think of what the weather will be like there when shooting in the spring."

Typically, *American Ninja Warrior* show executives start scouting for the new season in the fall. In deciding whether a particular city is a good fit for the show, many aspects are taken into consideration, such as:

- Is there an interesting cityscape? Think the Las Vegas Strip. Or the Carrie Furnace outside of Pittsburgh, Pennsylvania.
- Does the city have a good energy? City centers—with their lights and sounds—often provide just the right juice to fuel the ninjas.
- Can the city accommodate the *American Ninja Warrior* obstacle course's large footprint? It is

longer than a football field including the end zones—about 370 feet long—with additional space needed, width-wise, for the production crews and audience.

"We need a big space for the course and all the equipment," Richardson says. "We are there for two or three weeks as we build, film the competition, and then break down the course, so sometimes cities just can't accommodate us on the dates we need. It's kind of a jigsaw puzzle to find the right city at the right time."

TECH TALK

During the Qualifying and City Finals rounds, *American Ninja Warrior* employs approximately 40 cameras—a mix of Technocranes, Steadicams, drones, handheld cameras, robotic cameras, and POV cameras. There was even a Goodyear blimp shooting for the show on a few occasions! In Las Vegas, production uses a helicopter camera for all aerial shots along with a couple of cable cameras that produce the dynamic shots from above.

IF THE CITY FITS

Once locations are chosen, the production team must determine how to adapt the ninja course into each unique city setting. This involves numerous planning designs to decide where and how the obstacle course will navigate. For example, in Season 8's Indianapolis location, the course was adapted into a crescent shape to fit into the unique circular downtown location of Monument Circle. In

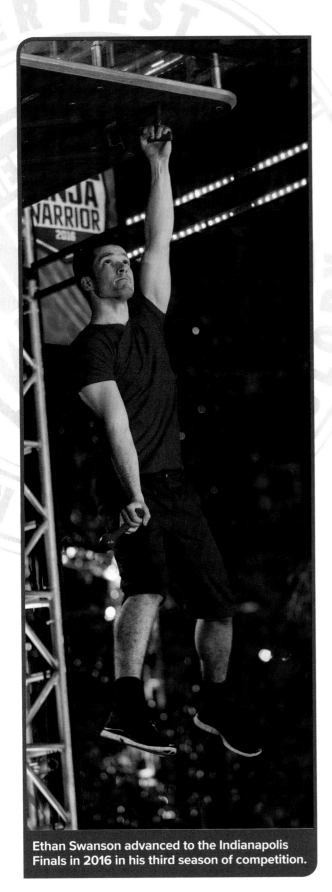

Ethan Swanson advanced to the Indianapolis Finals in 2016 in his third season of competition.

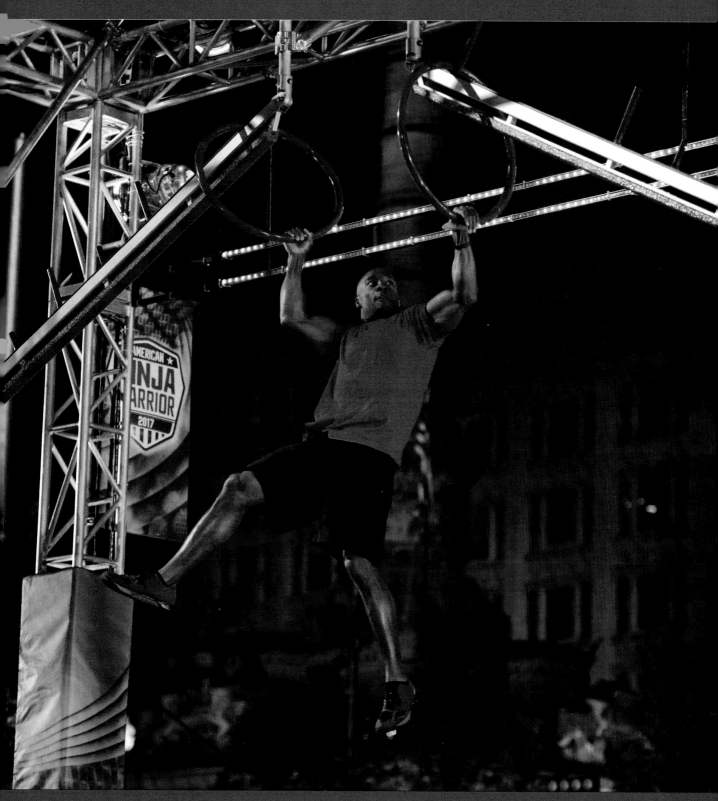

Naeem Mulkey made it through the Ring Jump at the Cleveland Finals in July 2017, but the next obstacle, the I-Beam Gap, stopped him, along with more than half the ninjas who attempted it.

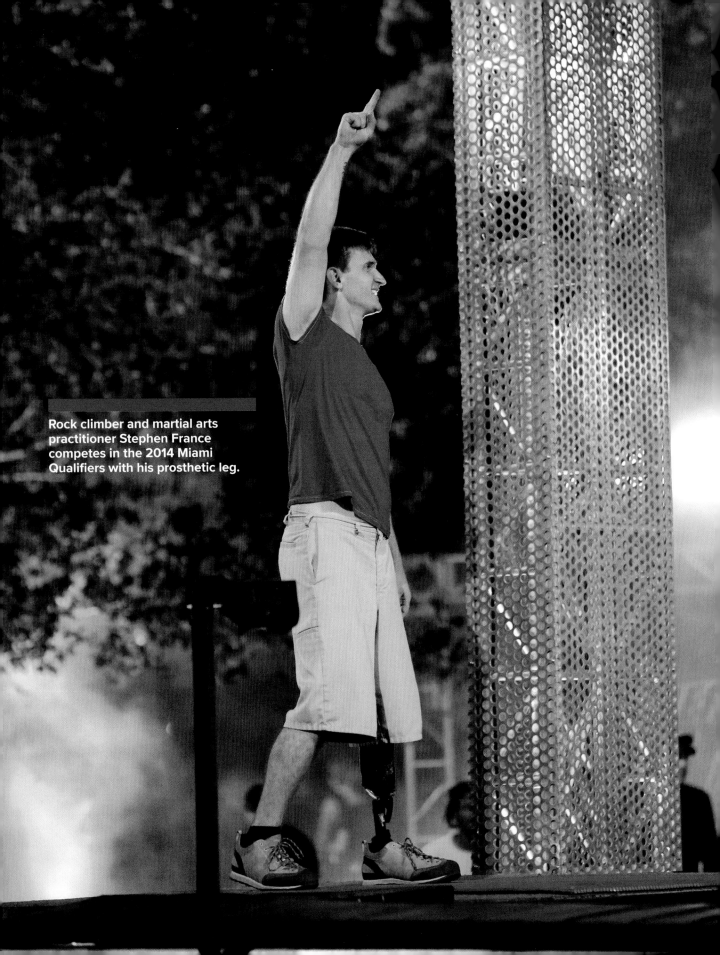

Rock climber and martial arts practitioner Stephen France competes in the 2014 Miami Qualifiers with his prosthetic leg.

Pittsburgh, the course weaves its way around an old steel mill. In Los Angeles, it snakes through the back lot of Universal Studios.

"No location is the same," says Adam Biggs, director of photography/lighting designer, who has been with the show since Season 2. "Each one gets a different look and feel. Each one has its own unique challenge. Giving life and color to every location is constantly changing. It's one of the things I love about the show."

A TALE OF NINJA CITIES

CITY TIMELINE	Season 1	2	3	4	5	6	7	8	9
City									
Los Angeles, California	★	★	★	★	★	★	★	★	★
Miami, Florida				★	★	★			
Dallas, Texas				★		★			
Denver, Colorado					★	★		★	
Baltimore, Maryland					★				
St. Louis, Missouri						★			
Kansas City, Missouri							★		★
Houston, Texas							★		
Orlando, Florida							★		
Pittsburgh, Pennsylvania							★		
San Pedro, California							★		
Atlanta, Georgia								★	
Indianapolis, Indiana								★	
Oklahoma City, Oklahoma								★	
Philadelphia, Pennsylvania								★	
San Antonio, Texas									★
Daytona Beach, Florida									★
Cleveland, Ohio									★

SETTING UP

Streetlights, trees, fire department access, traffic patterns—these are aspects that production needs to take into consideration when setting up the course. "Generally, when we go scout a place, we'll know there will possibly be some issues to work around, and we have such a limited amount of time in each place that I just document everything with pictures and videos," says Michael Carney, *American Ninja Warrior*'s production designer. "I'll take a rolling tape and go up and down the street. The production team doesn't even know what the approved obstacles are going to be at this point. They just know roughly the course size and the obstacle box size."

Carney's team is in charge of how the show "looks" and how the obstacles are dressed and treated, and, along with the director of photography (DP), decides how a city works for the show and what it takes to fit it in the space. "We know the Warped Wall is our hero shot—that's the most important thing, from a set standpoint—and it's in both nights of shooting. It's got to look the best," Carney says.

DIFFERENT CITIES, DIFFERENT COURSES

Fans of *American Ninja Warrior* know that in each of the Qualifying and City Finals rounds of any given season, the obstacle course is not the same for each city—for example, in Season 9, ninjas running the course in San Antonio encountered a somewhat different course than those running in Denver. This disparity is a conscious decision on the part of show executives.

"There are a couple reasons why," says executive producer Kent Weed. "The number one reason was just diversity and for the audience to see something new and fresh every week. Secondly, every time we did a new obstacle, the ninjas would take pictures and video of it and start building the obstacle and practicing, literally the next day. So if we were to keep those same obstacles in every city, by the time we go to our fourth or fifth city, they would have

had a lot of practice on these obstacles, which are supposed to be new."

"David Campbell was the first notable person to actually build a course in his backyard. This was in Season 2," notes executive producer Arthur Smith. "Now it happens all the time. Ninjas build courses in Alaska. They build them on their ranch. They're in gymnasiums, they're in backyards. In their homes. They're building variations of them at work. We have to stay one step ahead."

THE HEAT OF THE NIGHT

Starting in Season 5, *American Ninja Warrior* production began shooting all episodes at night. (The Las Vegas National Finals of Season 4 and occasionally other regional Qualifiers were shot at night prior to Season 5.) There are essentially two nights of back-to-back shooting in each city—the

> "Most people are just waking up and getting in the shower when we're wrapping up for the night and heading home to bed. This leads to the mental challenge of staying awake and functioning at peak capacity at 3 A.M.—but if the ninjas can do it, so can the crew!
>
> —Adam Biggs, director of photography/ lighting designer

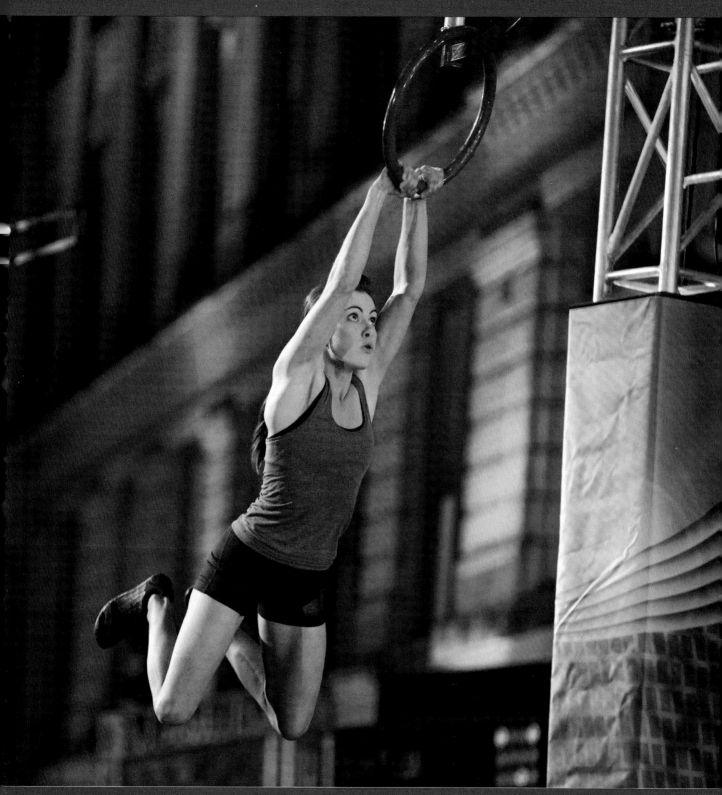

Although the Sky Hooks took her out in Season 9's San Antonio Qualifiers, "Mighty" Kacy Catanzaro got her revenge on the obstacle in the City Finals.

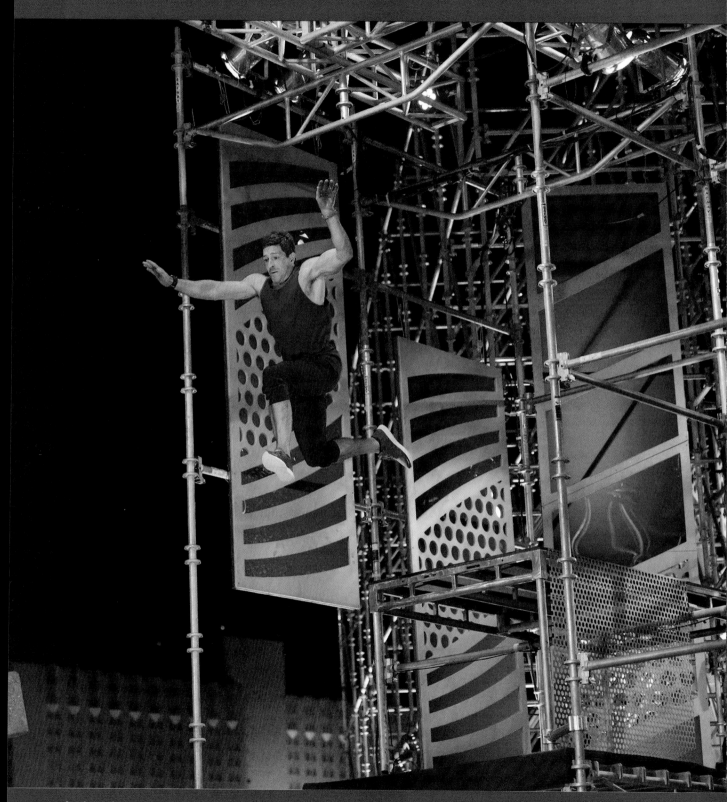

Andrew Lowes makes a dramatic jump in the 2017 National Finals.

first night is for the Qualifiers, the second night is for the City Finals. This may come as a surprise to fans of the show, since a city's Qualifiers and City Finals rounds often air more than a month apart; in reality, these rounds are shot over two consecutive nights.

That means that ninjas aren't the only ones who have to race against the clock. So does the production crew, which has to make sure all of the night's competitors—including a limited number of walk-ons—get their turn at the course so they can wrap up shooting about 45 minutes before sunrise. "The biggest single challenge shooting at night is time—getting everything done before the sun comes up," says Adam Biggs, director of photography/lighting designer. "This means all departments have to operate at 100 percent. *All night.*"

> Years ago, I saw the original *Ninja Warrior* on TV and thought it looked like a fun challenge. I would tell people, 'I can do that stuff!' Time went on, and I forgot about it. My wife was watching TV one day, showed me *American Ninja Warrior*, and told me that I should try it. I found a local ninja gym, did fairly well, and the rest is history.
>
> —Geoff Britten

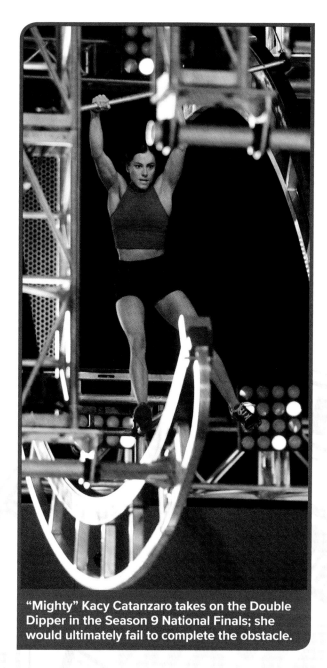

"Mighty" Kacy Catanzaro takes on the Double Dipper in the Season 9 National Finals; she would ultimately fail to complete the obstacle.

He adds, "*Ninja Warrior* really is like a highly choreographed camera dance. Everyone has a specific and important job, and our camera team has to be in excellent physical/mental condition—from the drones that are giving us a sense of geography and showing a grand scale of where the course fits into the location to the tireless camera operators who have to run along the side of the course and follow every move the ninjas make."

LIGHTS OUT!

In Season 5, some design changes were afoot as well, relating to what's called the obstacle course's "truss"—the framework of rafters, posts, and struts that provide the support structure. (Think of that tall Mount Midoriyama configuration.) In earlier seasons, the truss was covered, or hidden, creating a more "literal" design sense, according to Michael Carney, production designer. Production relied on the natural light of the sun to highlight the course.

However, when production moved to nights, the decision was made to go "sportier" with the truss, whose framework provided a nice contrast with the night sky, enhancing the production design. Show executives did away with the truss cover. "We started minimizing the architecture, and we were saying that what really looked good was the truss lighting," Carney says. "It really became a show more about the lighting than large architectural pieces on the set."

TECH TALK

The technical challenge of shooting a show like *American Ninja Warrior* at night is the massive amount of lighting needed to light the obstacle course and the surrounding environment. Over 25 miles of electrical and data cable are installed each time production rolls into a city and sets up the course. More than 1,000 lights are designed and placed into each location.

WORKING WITH MOTHER NATURE

American Ninja Warrior's shooting schedule begins in March, and the production crew travels through six cities until the end of May or June, when the National Finals take place. That means that shooting is taking place outdoors in the spring, which can be temperamental, weather-wise.

The *American Ninja Warrior* crew has seen it all! Light, cold rain. Torrential downpours. Hail. Ice. A stifling 120-degree heat. "Sometimes we have to hunker down and wait out the worst of it," says Adam Biggs, lighting designer/director of photography. "Sometimes we can work through it, but no matter what we survive and get it done. Season 9 was by far the worst! We got hit with massive rain in every city. Even Vegas!"

"You know how you come out in the morning and your car got wet and you left your towels outside and they're soaking wet? It's the same thing on the course," says Patrick McManus, who serves as director of *American Ninja Warrior*. "The dew point hits at certain times, in certain cities, on certain dates. Moisture starts to condense on the metal, and you can't hold on. So we do a lot of different things to try to keep that course dry. We have big blowers that you don't really notice on TV—big fans that keep everything dry. If the Warped Wall is wet, you're not going to go up!"

> " I think there's a photo floating around of a snowman we built and put at the top of the Warped Wall in Denver. Snowball fights in May while we were in Denver? Crazy!
>
> –Adam Biggs, director of photography/ lighting designer "

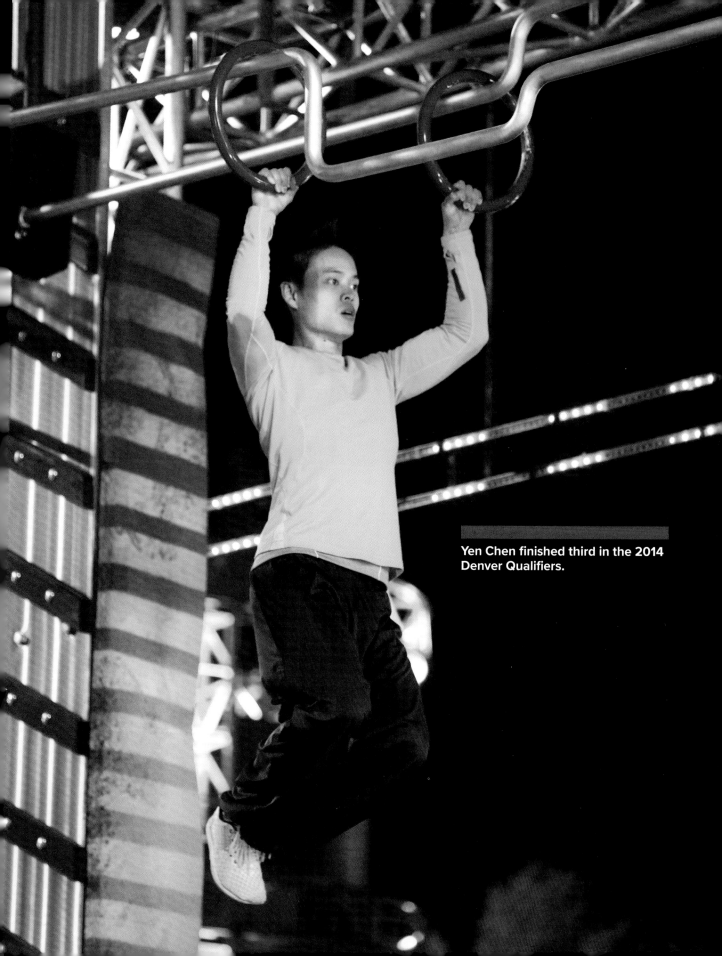

Yen Chen finished third in the 2014 Denver Qualifiers.

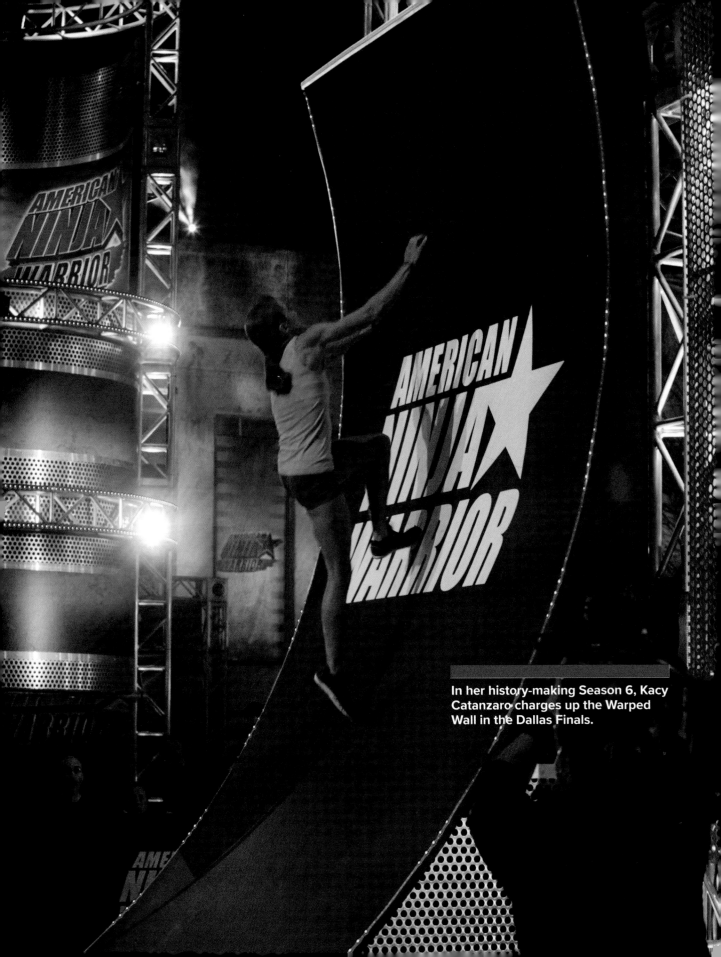

In her history-making Season 6, Kacy Catanzaro charges up the Warped Wall in the Dallas Finals.

> *American Ninja Warrior* is one of the only truly family-friendly shows left on television. It's something you can sit down and watch with your mom, dad, grandmother, two-year-old brother, teenage sister, and you never have to worry that something will be said that you have to explain or cover someone's eyes. I think a lot of families use *American Ninja Warrior* as family time, so it doesn't surprise me that kids who have been watching the show for eight years have started training and becoming competitors on the show. We have people from all types of backgrounds with different struggles, body types, and ages who are able to take on the obstacles, and I think it gives the viewers at home the idea that they too can be an American Ninja Warrior.
>
> —Cohost Kristine Leahy

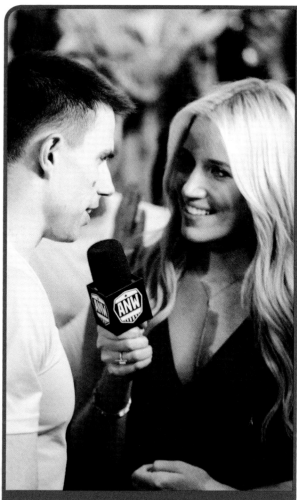

Cohost Kristine Leahy interviews Sean Bryan at the Los Angeles Finals in Season 9.

SAFETY FIRST

With so much unpredictability with the weather, *American Ninja Warrior* executives have to make sure the course is safe and fair for the athletes, since not all the obstacles react well with water. When you're dealing with grip strength, in particular, rain and dew can make for slippery conditions. Therefore, executives will stop the action if it's too wet or if there's lightning. Still, since production has to keep to a specific schedule, if the weather isn't cooperating for a prolonged period of time, show executives have to find a way to shoot, even if it means combining the Qualifying and City Finals rounds into the same night!

THE HOSTS

Who could imagine *American Ninja Warrior* without the play-by-play, playful banter, and wordplay of its intrepid hosts? Hosts Matt Iseman and Akbar Gbajabiamila and cohost/sideline reporter Kristine Leahy bring the action to viewers, not only providing ninja histories and obstacle course stats but also interaction with the ninjas themselves, cheering them on when they slam down a buzzer and howling in agony when they take a swim. Let's learn more about our fearless ninja hosts.

MATT ISEMAN

It is the booming voice of Matt Iseman that heralds each new episode of *American Ninja Warrior*. How did Iseman, who has served as host since 2010, create that famous roar?

"It actually kind of started as a joke," he says. "Those moments coming in and out of commercial breaks are called 'wraps,' and we were shooting one, and my voice was a bit hoarse. It came out gravelly, like Bruce Springsteen after a bad cold. But the producer, Holly Wofford, loved it. She said, 'Try that again, only put some effort into it.' And my signature growl was born."

FAN FARE

Matt Iseman and Akbar Gbajabiamila's colorful commentary is a big part of the appeal of *American Ninja Warrior*. Gbajabiamila, in particular, is known for his enthusiastic off-the-cuff verbal word play. In fact, a Twitter account, @ANWAkbarism, is dedicated to making those of-the-moment phrasings immortal. Run by an anonymous fan beginning in March 2015, the Twitter account catches every inspiration and fun quote. @ANWAkbarism sees you, Akbar!

Many fans know Iseman as the *American Ninja Warrior* host or perhaps as the winner of NBC's *New Celebrity Apprentice* in 2017. (His ongoing battle with rheumatoid arthritis transformed him into a strong supporter of the Arthritis Foundation, the charity he represented while on *Celebrity Apprentice*.) However, long before he donned a suit, Iseman was wearing scrubs. He attended Princeton University (he pitched for the school's baseball team for four years) and earned his medical degree from the Columbia College of Physicians and Surgeons. Iseman quickly realized he preferred stand-up comedy to stethoscopes. Encouraged by his father who told him, "Life is short, do what makes you happy," Iseman quit medicine to pursue stand-up comedy and has headlined clubs all around the country, proving that, in the end, laughter may be the best medicine.

Iseman began his hosting career on *Scream Play* for E! and on Casino Night for GSN, and shortly thereafter started a five-year run as the "go-to guy" on Style's *Clean House*, which was number one on the network during that time. That led to work as host of the spin-off *Clean House Comes Clean* and a multi-episode special *Clean House: The Messiest Home in the Country*, which earned him a Daytime Emmy Award.

How does he approach his hosting duties for *American Ninja Warrior*? "For me, it's all about getting as much rest as possible," he says. "I'm a very enthusiastic guy, and when we tape *American Ninja Warrior* we go all night long. A lot of it is doing my homework. Watching the submission videos, reading about the ninjas, getting to know them, but once the night starts, it's all a blur. I'm really just a fan, sitting in the host tower with the best seats in the house."

Iseman also brings his wit and humor to the *American Ninja Warrior* spinoff *Team Ninja Warrior*.

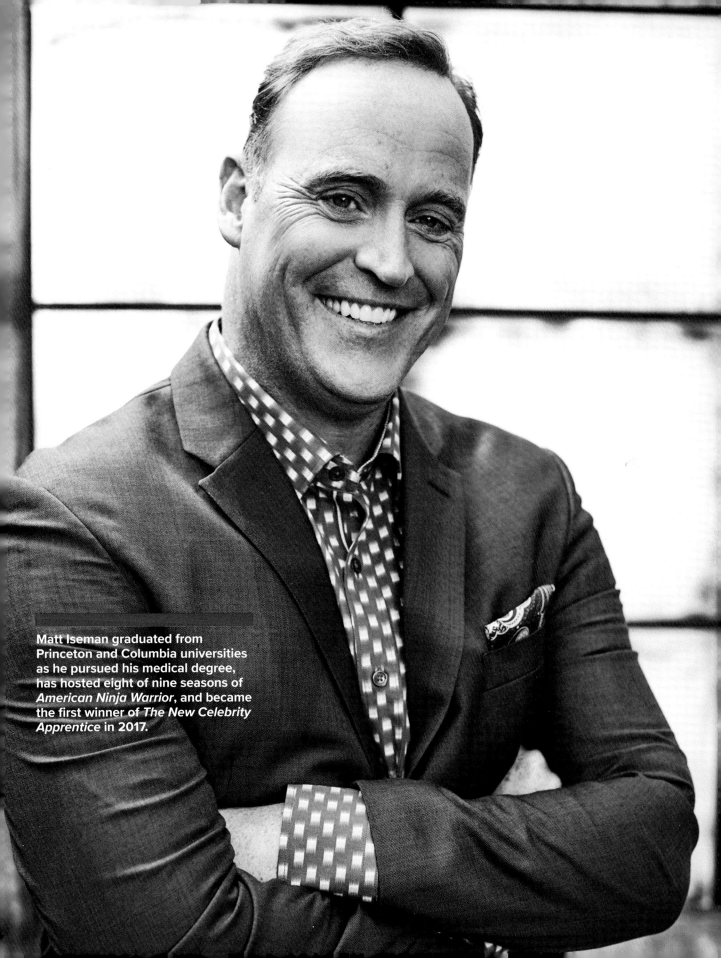

Matt Iseman graduated from Princeton and Columbia universities as he pursued his medical degree, has hosted eight of nine seasons of *American Ninja Warrior*, and became the first winner of *The New Celebrity Apprentice* in 2017.

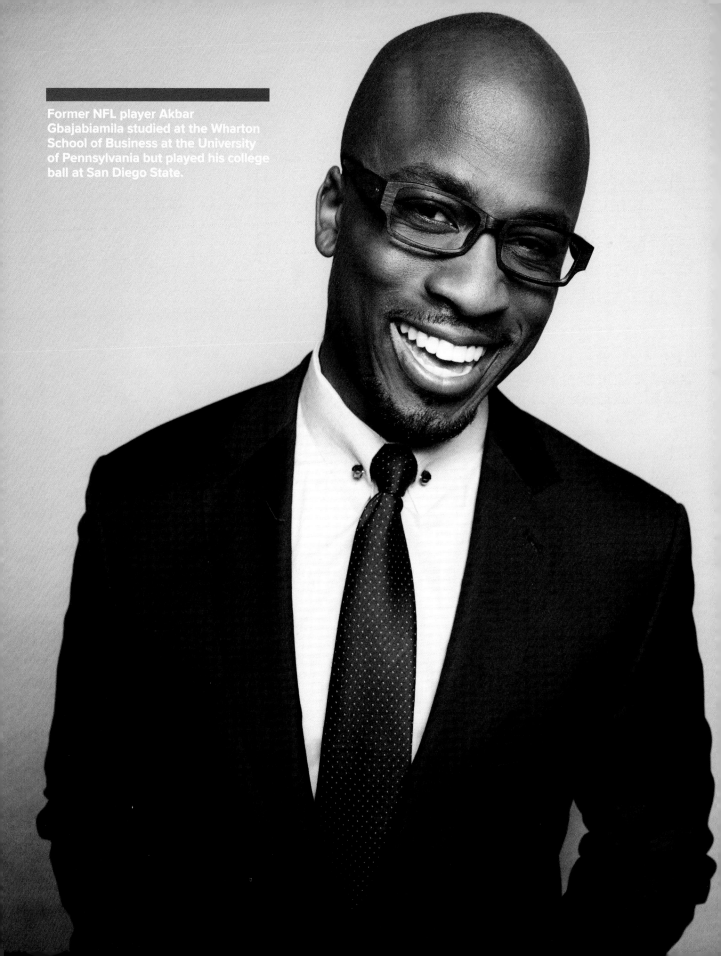

Former NFL player Akbar Gbajabiamila studied at the Wharton School of Business at the University of Pennsylvania but played his college ball at San Diego State.

> It really is awesome working with Akbar—someone who knows what it's like to perform at the highest level—and he's also got that workman's mentality packed in his lunchbox. He's one of the hardest workers I've ever met, and he has an unbridled enthusiasm that matches mine. We really are both fans up there. I feel like we're Statler and Waldorf from the Muppets. Only better looking.
>
> —Host Matt Iseman

AKBAR GBAJABIAMILA

Akbar Gbajabiamila, one of seven children of Nigerian immigrants, was born in Los Angeles and played college football for San Diego State University. He graduated with a bachelor's degree in Communication and New Media Studies, and completed a certified entrepreneurship program at the Wharton School of Business in 2005. The Southern California native played five years in the NFL as a linebacker and defensive end with the Oakland Raiders, San Diego Chargers, and Miami Dolphins before retiring in 2008.

Throughout his NFL career, Gbajabiamila had an interest in broadcasting, and in 2005, he was selected as one of the NFL's first athletes to attend their Broadcast Boot Camp, an intense workshop aimed at training athletes for potential careers in broadcasting and journalism.

While playing for the San Diego Chargers, Gbajabiamila contributed to KSWB, an NBC radio affiliate in San Diego, and cohosted *Football Night in San Diego* from 2006 to 2008. He went on to serve as an analyst for the Mountain Network and CBS Sports before joining the NFL Network in 2012. Gbajabiamila's ability to connect with everyone from viewers to competitors to professional athletes has made him one of the most relatable television

personalities in sports and entertainment. That knack for commentating actually began at a young age, Gbajabiamila says. His dad, his coaches, and even his 11th grade math teacher, Ms. Kay Briscoe, would tell him he talks "too much." "I wonder what Ms. Briscoe would say now," Gbajabiamila says with a laugh. *"Boy, you deserve what you're doing right now, fella!"*

A fan of the World Wrestling Federation (now World Wrestling Entertainment), Gbajabiamila used to watch Friday night wrestling with his mother and father as a kid. "I remember them sitting on the couch, because even though my mom would say Hulk Hogan was her boyfriend, I don't think they were into it. Yet it was something they could at least watch for entertainment," he says.

Gbajabiamila used to love the verbal gymnastics that the wrestling commentators would use. "I always found the hyperbolic language that they would use to describe certain things amusing," he says. "I don't know if anyone else did, but I did, and I try to bring that same energy and color to *American Ninja Warrior*. If my mom was alive, I'm pretty sure she'd be excited. She was always telling me, 'You're gonna be a lawyer,' and I'm, like, *Mom, I don't know* . . . I remember taking communication law at San Diego

State, and it was one of the last classes I had to take to graduate. It kind of solidified the idea that I would never become an attorney. The amount of stuff that they have to know, and all of the laws . . . it's beyond me."

> It really is such a dream to work with Matt. You know we get asked all the time about our chemistry and how we feed off each other so well, and I think it goes back to us both genuinely wanting to see these ninjas succeed. We both truly want to cheer for each and every ninja that runs the course.
>
> —Host Akbar Gbajabiamila

KRISTINE LEAHY

While hosts Matt Iseman and Akbar Gbajabiamila spend most of their time in the host tower on *American Ninja Warrior*, sideline reporter Kristine Leahy is down in the trenches with the ninjas. With a microphone in hand, she's right next to the course for an on-the-spot interview, capturing the emotion of a run, whether it ended with a buzzer or a swim, and is often the one to inform ninjas that they've made it to the next round.

"My goal in the postrun interview is to bring out whatever that competitor is feeling in the moment,"

Leahy says. "Sometimes that's pure joy, and sometimes it's disappointment and sadness. I am there to capture those pure feelings. Sometimes it's very easy, and sometimes I have to pull a bit, but I always want the person to feel like they were genuinely represented and able to share whatever it is they were feeling in the moment. Then there are some interviews that are just pure comedy, and I let that happen naturally as well."

Throughout Leahy's career, she has displayed a passion for bringing out the human side of athletes

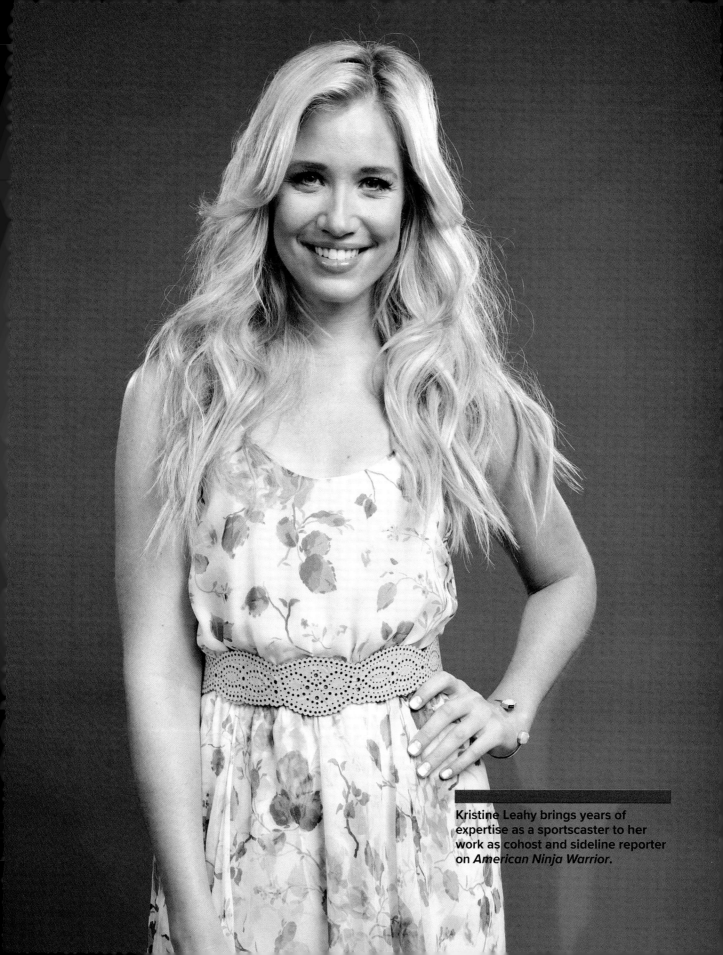

Kristine Leahy brings years of expertise as a sportscaster to her work as cohost and sideline reporter on *American Ninja Warrior*.

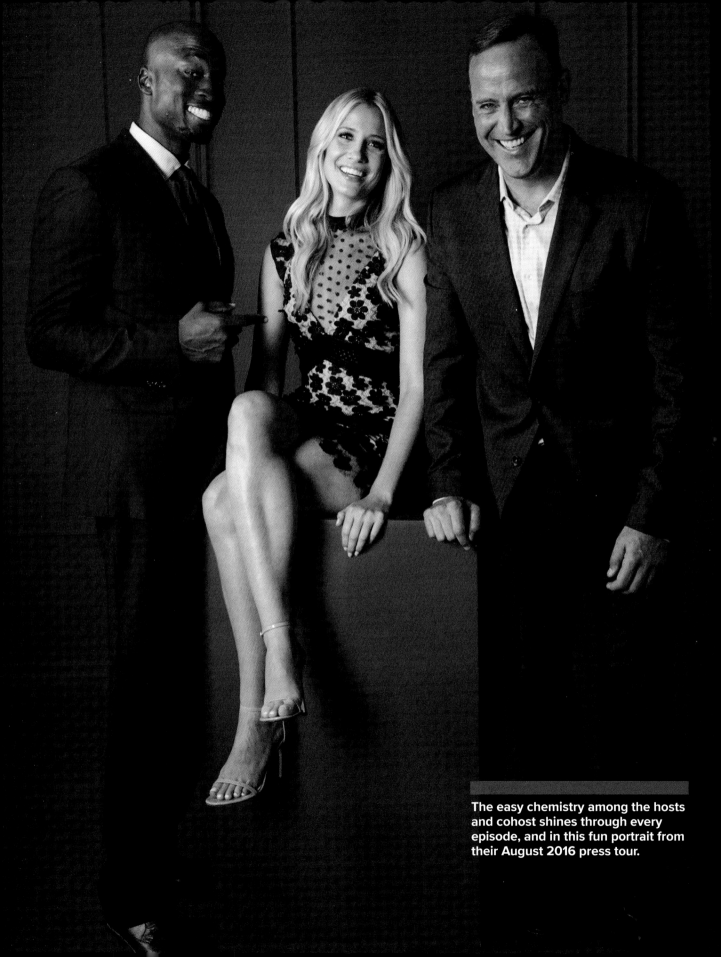

The easy chemistry among the hosts and cohost shines through every episode, and in this fun portrait from their August 2016 press tour.

and portraying their stories through one-on-one interviews and features. Before joining *American Ninja Warrior*, Leahy spent two and a half years working across various platforms in the CBS and Turner Sports family. She worked the college basketball sidelines for March Madness and was also a sideline reporter for CBS Sports Network's college football and basketball packages. In addition, she filled in as a host on CBS Sports Network's show *Lead Off*, contributed to KCAL's Dodgers pregame show *Think Blue*, anchored CBS-LA's Sports Central, and covered the NBA playoffs, MLB playoffs, and the Los Angeles Kings' run to the Stanley Cup. She even made a bit of history by becoming the first woman in California to call a horse race at Hollywood Park!

Leahy, who currently is the cohost of sports talk show *The Herd with Colin Cowherd*, grew up in Chicago during the height of Michael Jordan's basketball reign and got hooked on sports and competition. After high school, she moved east and earned a bachelor of science in Journalism from Boston University, where she was part of the team that created BUTV's first sports talk show, a program she coanchored for three years. From there, she worked as a reporter and host for New England sports radio station WEEI before moving on to work for the 17-time world champion Boston Celtics, where she spent two years as a host and in-house team reporter at TD Garden and for Celtics.com. Leahy then spent a year as the lead sports anchor for Fox Boston, where she covered both a Stanley Cup and a Super Bowl, before moving out west. She currently lives in Los Angeles and is on the board of the Variety Boys and Girls Club of Boyle Heights.

Leahy says talking with the ninjas postrun is much different than interviews she's done in traditional sports, because she doesn't have to be unbiased. "I can be happy or sad for the ninjas, which makes it easier to do the interview," she says.

" Matt and Akbar and I have become really great friends. We play jokes on each other and talk, go to dinners, you name it. We all happened to be at the 2017 Super Bowl so we met up for lunch and, oddly enough, shopping. We helped Akbar pick out a purse for his wife, Matt football gear for his girlfriend, and me engagement rings for whenever that day happens.

—Cohost Kristine Leahy "

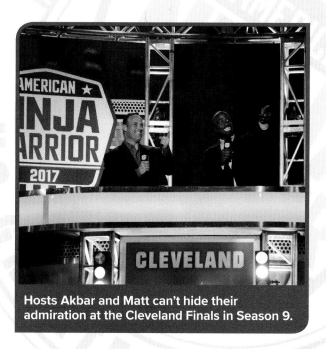

Hosts Akbar and Matt can't hide their admiration at the Cleveland Finals in Season 9.

FIERCE, BUT FUN

Although the obstacle course work can be intense on *American Ninja Warrior*, the hosts and the ninjas always seem to be having a good time. The show executives also have a sense of humor—how else can you explain a Tyrannosaurus rex or streaker crashing the course?

"It's amazing that the guy in the T. rex costume was able to compete with all of that extra stuff on him. It was funny," says host Akbar Gbajabiamila. "The streaker was *classic*. Matt and I were totally thrown off by it, and I think the producers had to

go with it. Everything you heard us calling with the streaker was as-is, right there and then. That was a one-take wonder."

The T. rex actually showed some impressive agility on the first three obstacles when he made his appearance during the Atlanta Qualifier in 2016, but extinction loomed as the dinosaur got taken out by the Spin Cycle. The streaker made it all the way to the Warped Wall, but before he could make his second attempt up the wall he was carted away by security.

EVEN MORE NINJA WARRIOR!

If you want to catch more of your favorite ninjas doing what they do best, there's plenty of ninja action out there with these *American Ninja Warrior* spinoffs:

- **USA VS. THE WORLD:** During the Season 5 finale of *American Ninja Warrior*, it was announced that the first-ever team competition in *American Ninja Warrior* history would take place, a special matchup titled *USA vs. Japan*. The success of that special led to the team ninja concept widening its scope, and *USA vs. The World* was born, which features teams of elite ninjas from different regions of the globe facing off against one another.

- **TEAM NINJA WARRIOR:** Premiering in 2015, this show features teams of your favorite ninjas competing head-to-head as they run the famous *American Ninja Warrior* obstacle course. (An inaugural college edition saw ninjas from MIT and the University of Wisconsin square off in an intense final round, with the University of Wisconsin ninjas crowned the show's first ninja college champions.) If you think one ninja running the course is exciting, two ninjas is twice the fun!

- **AMERICAN NINJA WARRIOR ALL-STAR SPECIAL: SKILLS CHALLENGE:** Much like any sports franchise's all-star game celebrates the best of the best in its field, so does this installment of *American Ninja Warrior*, which brings together elite and fan-favorite ninjas to compete in both team events and supersized skills challenges. Upping the fun quotient is the involvement of the *American Ninja Warrior* hosts, who pick teams to face off against one another in the team events.

- **CELEBRITY NINJA WARRIOR:** Celebrities can be ninjas too, after all, and in 2017, the first celebrity edition of *American Ninja Warrior* premiered as part of a three-hour block of programming commemorating Red Nose Day, a charitable movement to help stop child poverty. Celebrities, who were coached by some of the fans' favorite ninjas, took a turn on the show's iconic obstacle course, earning $5,000 for Red Nose charities with each obstacle they completed. Participating celebs included *Arrow* star Stephen Amell, who crushed the course like a good superhero should, and *World of Dance* judge Derek Hough, who lost his grip on the Fly Wheels and got wet, but, ever the champion, rose from the water, whipped off his shirt, cleared the Fly Wheels the second time around, and completed the course.

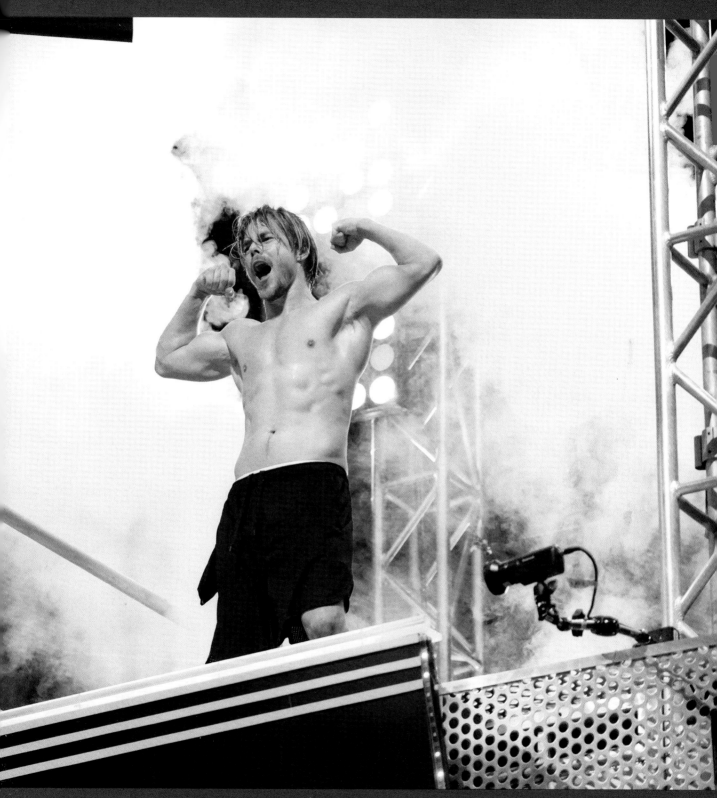

Derek Hough rises triumphant in his second try on the Fly Wheels on the 2017 Red Nose Day special of *American Ninja Warrior*.

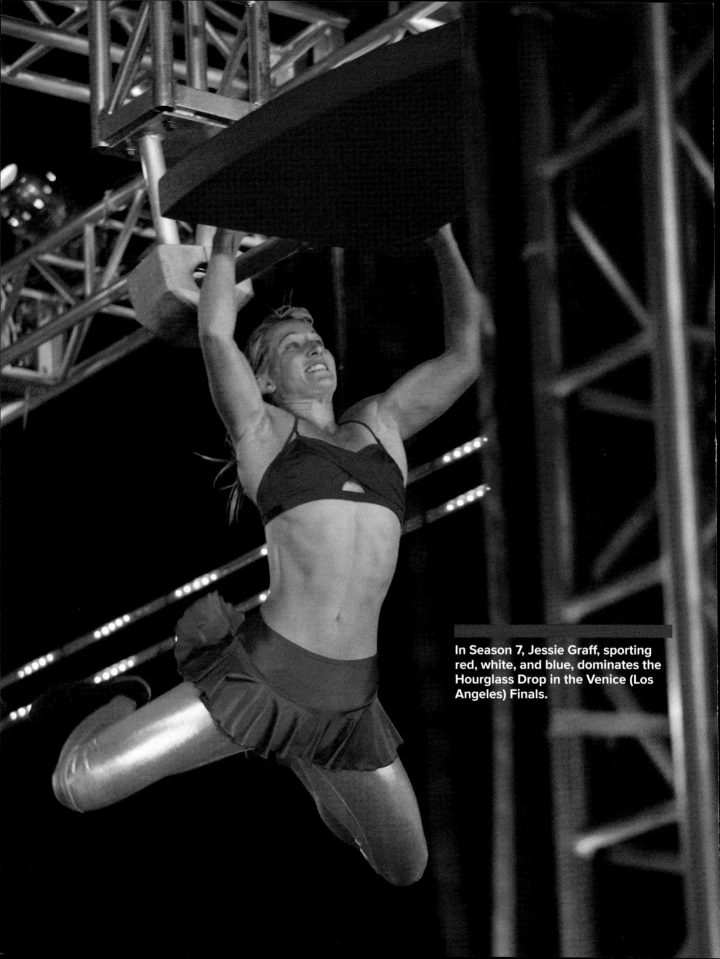

In Season 7, Jessie Graff, sporting red, white, and blue, dominates the Hourglass Drop in the Venice (Los Angeles) Finals.

CHAPTER 2

THE COURSE

The Warped Wall. The Salmon Ladder. The Hourglass Drop. These are just a few of the obstacles that fans have come to know and love on *American Ninja Warrior*. The obstacles are the lifeblood of the show and are as creative as they are daunting. From season to season, there's no telling what's in store for the ninjas, who have to be prepared for anything and everything on the obstacle course. That's because there's no warm-up. There's no practice round beforehand. All the obstacles that are new to the show are also new to the ninjas. And because every year the ninjas get stronger and smarter and evolve, so, too, must the course evolve, which means that the only thing to be expected on each new season of *American Ninja Warrior* is the unexpected.

> One of the rare times that ninjas got to practice on obstacles was in the first two seasons when we did the Boot Camp, which was designed to basically get them in shape to go to Mount Midoriyama in Japan. There was an obstacle from *SASUKE* called the Floating Boards—four panels that were 3 feet wide and 5 feet long and were hanging by chains in between each other. You had to transfer from one to the next. Nobody could do it. For three days, practicing this obstacle, nobody could do it. Now, everybody does it. There's a technique. They figured it out, but it's fascinating, and ninjas love that challenge. They appreciate it. I can't say how many ninjas come up to me and say thank you for this amazing course. It's so much fun. I love it.
>
> —Executive Producer Kent Weed

MOUNT MIDORIYAMA

In order to become an American Ninja Warrior, athletes must move through the Qualifying and City Finals rounds, which have 6 and 10 obstacles, respectively. Then it's on to the four stages of Mount Midoriyama, the National Finals course in Las Vegas. Ninjas must complete four stages in the time allotted (except Stage Three, which is untimed) in order to move on:

- **Stage One** is mostly about speed and agility. Ninjas must successfully complete eight obstacles within a time limit that changes from season to season—depending upon the obstacle lineup—in order to advance to Stage Two.
- **Stage Two**, built entirely over water, tests strength and endurance, and ninjas must complete all six obstacles within a specific time limit.
- **Stage Three**, also over water, is the ultimate test, with seven or eight obstacles that challenge mostly upper-body strength, but also lower-body and leg strength. There is no time limit, so it's just the ninjas versus their own limits.
- **Stage Four**: The tower! Athletes must complete a daunting 75-foot rope climb to hit a final buzzer in under 30 seconds. That's over 2 feet per second!

DESIGNING ITS OWN OBSTACLES

When *American Ninja Warrior* became independent from *SASUKE* production in Season 4, show executives wanted to begin designing new and original obstacles. Although many of the iconic *SASUKE* obstacles—such as the Warped Wall, Jumping Spider, and Salmon Ladder—continue to be an important part of *American Ninja Warrior*, as the seasons went on more and more obstacles were derived from executives' own inspiration.

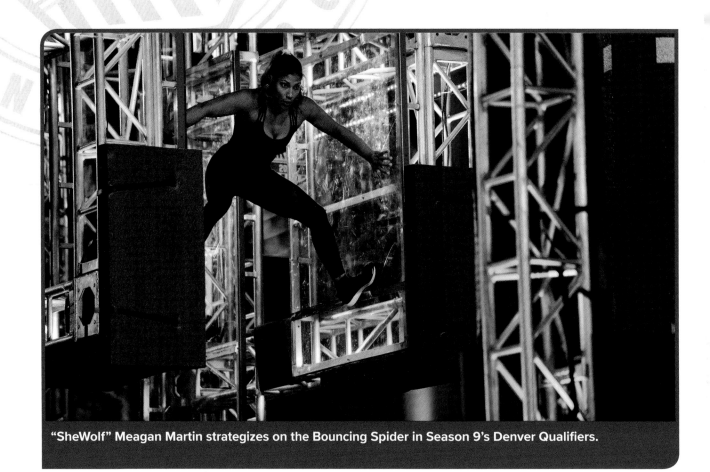

"SheWolf" Meagan Martin strategizes on the Bouncing Spider in Season 9's Denver Qualifiers.

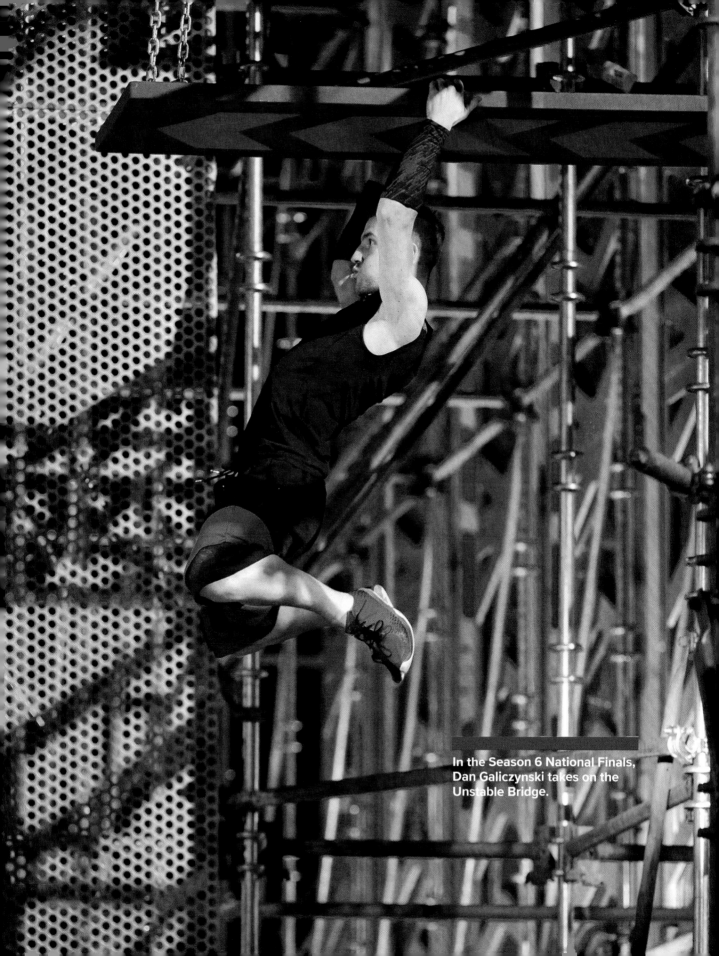

In the Season 6 National Finals, Dan Galiczynski takes on the Unstable Bridge.

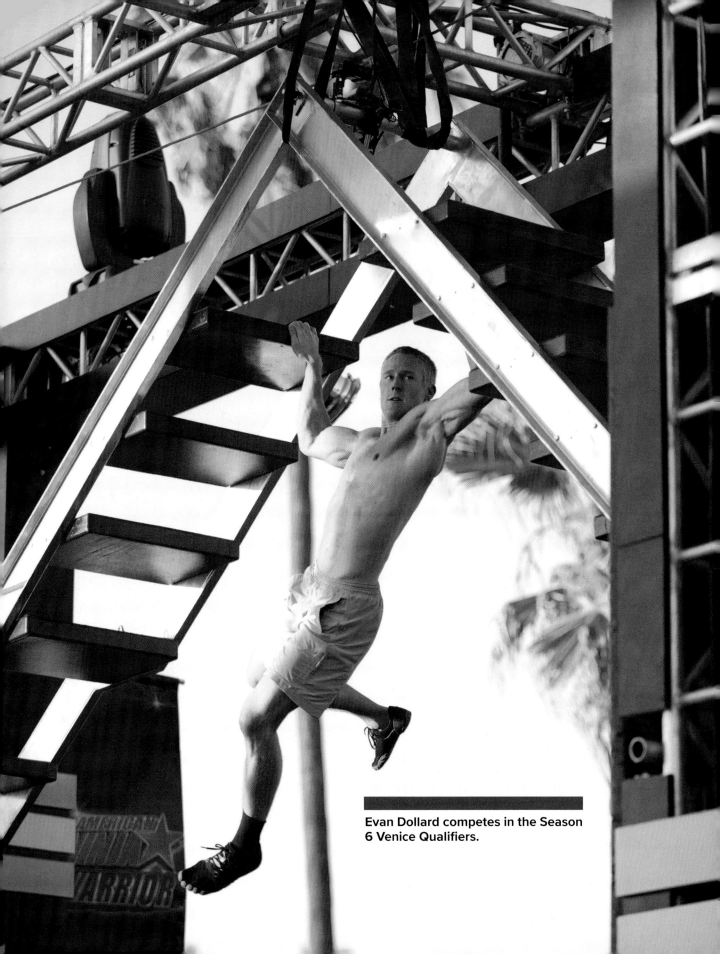

Evan Dollard competes in the Season 6 Venice Qualifiers.

THE ATS TEAM

Creating the infamous obstacles is a team effort between the executive producers at A. Smith & Co. Productions, the company behind *American Ninja Warrior,* NBC, and the ATS Team, a Los Angeles-based company that offers entertainment industry solutions, including production, rigging, challenge, art, and stunt experience.

"At the start of the season, we discuss with ATS which obstacles worked and which didn't from the year before," says *American Ninja Warrior* executive producer Brian Richardson. "We discuss how many new obstacles we want to introduce for the season. Some ideas are thrown around and drawn up by both ATS and the producers, and then we start prototyping."

ATS, which has been working with *American Ninja Warrior* executives since Season 4, builds smaller versions of obstacles in its warehouse, and testers run through them so that adjustments can be made—making them smaller, steeper, further apart, more challenging, less challenging, whatever is deemed necessary.

"We come back almost every week for testing and retesting before an obstacle is approved," Richardson says. "Then when obstacles are

built on the course, we test again. We are often tweaking an obstacle right up until we start the competition to make sure it's the right level of difficulty. We have a great relationship with ATS, but ultimately it is the producers who make final decisions on the obstacles."

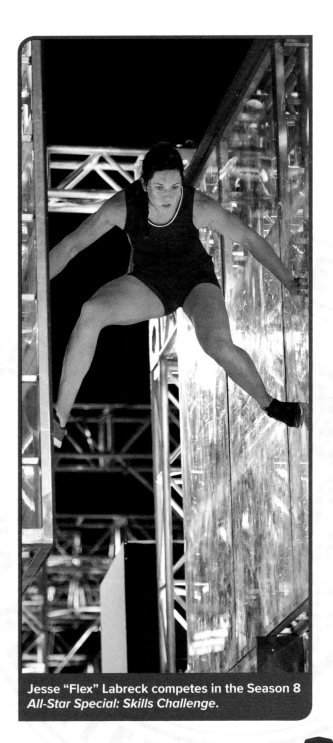

Jesse "Flex" Labreck competes in the Season 8 *All-Star Special: Skills Challenge.*

FINDING THE SWEET SPOT

Talk about a challenge! The *American Ninja Warrior* team is faced with creating a stunt obstacle course that is in the sweet spot of difficult yet achievable, safe yet adventurous, and grandiose yet mobile. "We have a very strong team of athletes who are constantly on the move, designing new challenges for the ever-growing athletes competing on *American Ninja Warrior*," says JJ Getskow, lead course designer and project manager for the ATS Team.

Obstacle inspiration comes from just about anywhere, explains executive producer Anthony Storm. He and executive producer Kent Weed are the creative and driving force behind the obstacles. "The executive producers bring ideas to the table. ATS brings ideas. Fans send in ideas," Storm says. "We're inspired by everything around us—playgrounds, obscure international sports, previously successful obstacles—and we're constantly pitching each other concepts."

Throughout the fall, the executives meet periodically with ATS and brainstorm ideas for the upcoming season. "ATS and our production designers create some sketches, and we tinker with the concepts more on paper," Storm says. "Then ATS builds some prototypes, and we start testing. Show executives ultimately make all the final decisions on the design of the obstacles and the course layouts. We test everything in the shop and in the field, oftentimes up until just minutes before the competition begins."

"Most of it comes from one small idea at the team table and grows from one small inspiration to the next," Getskow adds. "When you put talented, athletic people all in one room, imagination is abundant, and there are no limits."

By the end of December and into early January, it is time to start prototyping. Each season, the ATS Team demos the obstacles in its facility for the *American Ninja Warrior* executive producers, challenge producers, and the design/testing team. Once approval is secured, ATS starts the official build of the obstacle, and that can take days to weeks, depending on the type of fabrication and materials that are needed to make the obstacle last through hundreds of runs.

All of the obstacles are made in-house at the very hidden and secretive ATS facility. "It's kinda like Area 51," Getskow says. "In all seriousness, we do try to keep all the new obstacles behind the curtain. The only real reason for the covert operations is to keep the playing field fair for all competitors. If a potential ninja does see what we are designing to challenge them on the course, they have a leg up to train appropriately."

The Invisible Ladder had nothing on Travis Rosen in Season 8. He powered through the obstacle, completing the Atlanta Finals course.

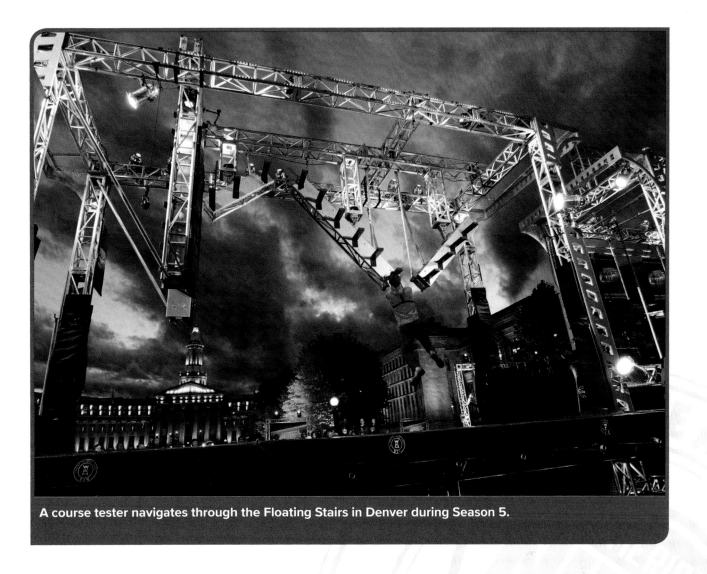

A course tester navigates through the Floating Stairs in Denver during Season 5.

WEATHER OR NOT

Because the courses are run outdoors, show executives and the ATS Team must create obstacles that perform well in various weather conditions. "Temperature is not really a concern," says executive producer Anthony Storm. "All of the obstacles can be run in extreme heat—it's always over 100 degrees in Las Vegas—and cold. We've had athletes on the course when the mercury went below freezing."

The only condition, however, that will shut down competition is moisture. "There are many skills that simply can't be tested in wet conditions," Storm says. "Balance and grip strength are very difficult to maintain when surfaces are wet. So instead of designing weatherproof obstacles, we make extensive plans to cover the course at the first sign of rain—or in a very light rain we may also add grip tape to certain obstacles to make them easier to hold on to or maintain footing. As soon as the weather clears, we are ready to go again."

"We try our best to make every obstacle play the same for each competitor in all weather conditions," adds JJ Getskow, lead course designer and project manager for the ATS Team, "but at the end of the day we sometimes have to go by the rule of golf—play it as it lays."

TESTERS

The ATS Team employs a group of full-time testers consisting of talented athletes who are well-versed in many areas of athleticism, including climbers, stunt men, gymnasts, parkour specialists, and decathletes. These testers have to be just as good as—or better than!—most of the ninjas themselves in order to determine how competitors are going to perform. JJ Getskow, lead course designer and project manager for the ATS Team, notes that testers are analyzing a wide range of aspects, from safety to difficulty, which is broken down into particulars such as precision, effect of the obstacle on certain muscle groups, dynamics, and body control.

Additionally, when the obstacles go on the road and get installed in each of the cities for the Qualifying and City Finals rounds, there is extensive field testing not only with a small, strong ATS team of testers—who are like obstacle roadies!—but with local and traveling ninjas who go to every city to support their fellow ninjas.

"We test the obstacles on the road for a number of reasons," says executive producer Anthony Storm. "First, the prototypes in the shop are often not full-size, so this is our first opportunity to see the obstacle in its proper length and scope and witness how it plays over water. Secondly, the testing in the shop is limited to the local available testers on that given day. On the road, we can run dozens of people of all shapes and sizes through the obstacles to test how

100 diverse ninjas will react during competition. Lastly, we need to see how difficult the course will play with all of the obstacles run consecutively. Until that point, we've only tested them individually in the shop. Now we get to see the cumulative effect of running them back-to-back."

While in the field, *American Ninja Warrior* executives continue dialing in the difficulty of the obstacles by changing distances, angles, holds, and materials. Then testers run the full course, and changes are made based on those results. The testers are organized by the show's challenge producer, who in Season 9 was Adam Sheldon.

"Adam has a large database of athletes in every part of the country and reaches out to them once we lock down our city," Storm notes. "He also reaches out to local gymnastics teams, climbing clubs, colleges, and ninja gyms, and he spreads the word that *American Ninja Warrior* is looking for testers. Additionally, if the walk-on line is long, we offer anyone there the chance to work as testers, but they forfeit their spot in line." (Usually, only the first 20 to 25 walk-ons get on the course to compete.)

"These on-location testers are vital in making the course difficulty appropriate for that city," Getskow adds. "The ninjas keep training and getting stronger and more talented, which pushes us to be more creative."

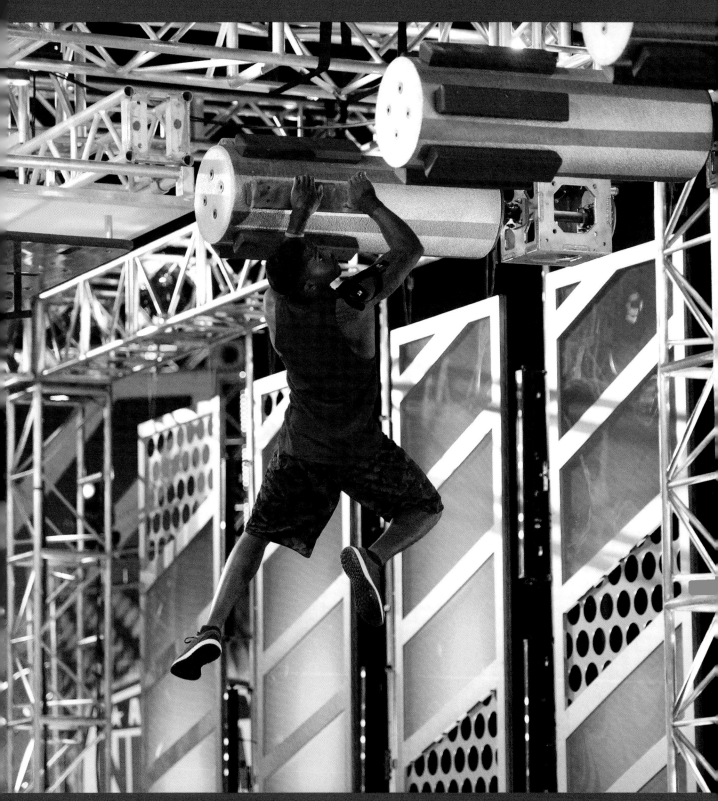

Najee Richardson, shown here on the Nail Clipper, made it all the way to Stage Three of the National Finals in Season 9.

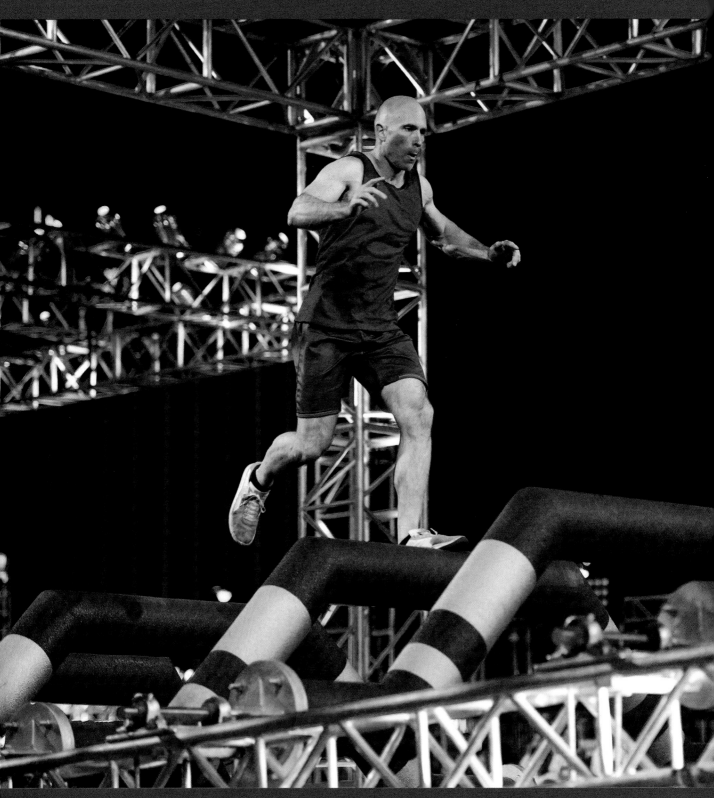

"The Godfather" David Campbell gets across the Domino Pipes in the National Finals on his way to completing Stage One in Season 9.

DID YOU KNOW?

challenge producer and I explain the competition's general rules and the individual rules for each obstacle. We provide a demonstration by a local tester or someone from ATS, and then we take questions from the competitors. It takes about 40 minutes to complete."

"Sometimes rules have to be repeated because the ninjas are competitors and they sometimes talk among themselves on strategies to complete the obstacle and miss important information," Getskow adds.

THE RULES

American Ninja Warrior executive producers determine the "rules" of each obstacle—what ninjas can and can't do in order to complete it. The ATS Team then builds these "rules" into the design during the concept phase.

"We want each obstacle to be attempted with the intent that it was designed," explains executive producer Anthony Storm. "If we allowed athletes to use their hands on all the balance obstacles, they could scoot across on their rears for many of them. That's not the challenge provided. So the rules are determined after we've asked testers to attempt every conceivable method of completing an obstacle. Once we've seen all the shortcuts, we decide if any rules are necessary to preserve the intent of the design." These rules then are enforced by the challenge producer who walks the course with every competitor during shooting to ensure successful completion of each obstacle.

The ninjas themselves are informed of the overall competition rules in each city. This is when they get their first look at the obstacles for the course. "Just a few minutes before competition begins, we walk all the athletes through the rules," Storm says. "We do it in two groups—half before competition starts and the latter half after our lunch break. The

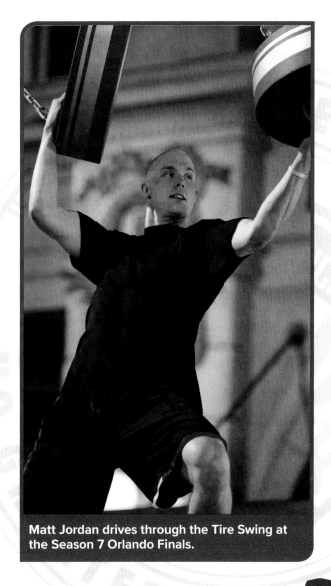

Matt Jordan drives through the Tire Swing at the Season 7 Orlando Finals.

> Everyone said, 'Oh, the women aren't big enough for the Jumping Spider. They'll never be able to get enough height. Their legs are too short.' And then Meagan Martin did it, and now other women have followed. These athletes continually rise to the occasion and surprise us. They're getting better. They're getting significantly better.
>
> —Executive Producer Arthur Smith

MEN AND WOMEN, COMPETING TOGETHER

American Ninja Warrior is one of the few sports where men and women compete on the same course—a concept that has been a part of the show since the beginning.

"We love that our show is comprised of men and women," says executive producer Arthur Smith, "and we know that so much of the popularity of the show has to do with women participating in the sport. Women's participation was there from the beginning, but it has grown exponentially."

However, according to executive producer Kent Weed, while he and Smith were on board, the network needed convincing. "We were pushed many times by the network, 'You sure you don't want to change obstacles for the women? You're sure you don't want to make it easier?'" Weed says. "We said, 'No, we love it. They'll get better.' We kept saying that they'll figure it out. I work with these obstacles. I know. A lot of it is technique, and they have a shot." (In nine seasons of *American Ninja Warrior*, only one obstacle—Body Prop—has been adjusted for competitors, and that was for height, not gender.)

Women have more than a shot. They began to dominate the *American Ninja Warrior* course. In Season 6, "Mighty" Kacy Catanzaro, who is only 5 feet tall, became the first woman to get up the Warped Wall and complete a Qualifying and City Finals round. "When Kacy Catanzaro became the first woman to complete a Qualifying course, our women submissions doubled the next season," Weed says. "She inspired a whole new generation of female athletes."

Catanzaro's run became one of *American Ninja Warrior*'s critical milestone moments that broadened the show's appeal. "No one thought it was possible for somebody who was 5 feet—let alone 98 pounds—to accomplish it," Smith says. "Kacy's technique was so perfect—she wasn't only the first woman, she was also the shortest by like 3 or 4 inches."

"It's funny, because Jessie Graff has been doing it for a long time and only made it past the fifth obstacle until Kacy did the Warped Wall," Weed notes. "Once she completed the Wall, it removed the ceiling for the women and they said, 'You know what, I can do this now.'"

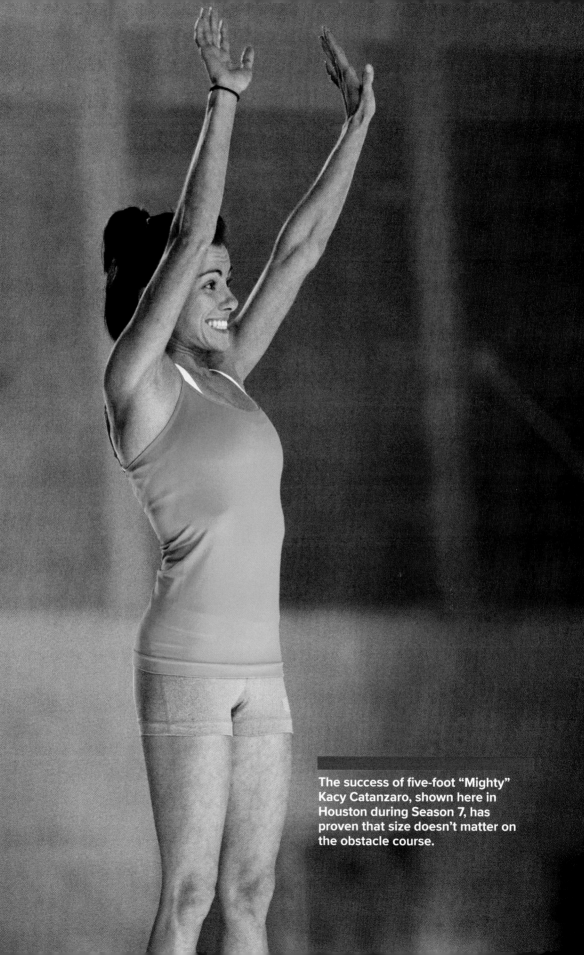

The success of five-foot "Mighty" Kacy Catanzaro, shown here in Houston during Season 7, has proven that size doesn't matter on the obstacle course.

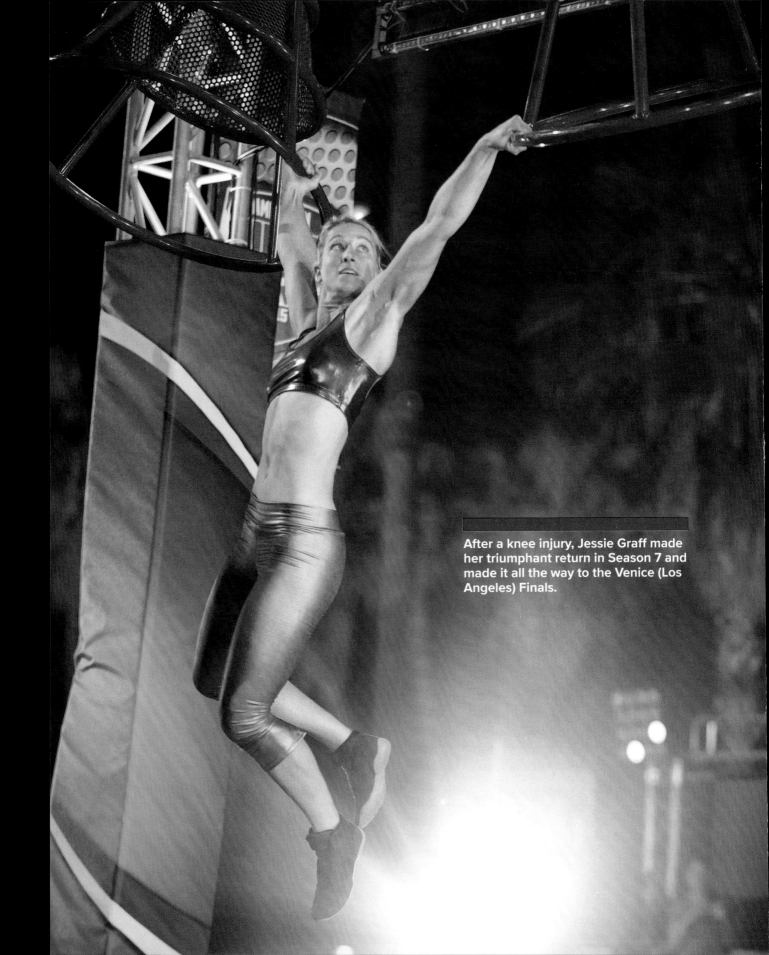

After a knee injury, Jessie Graff made her triumphant return in Season 7 and made it all the way to the Venice (Los Angeles) Finals.

NINJA KNOW-HOW

HOW DOES THE OBSTACLE COURSE DIFFER FOR MEN AND WOMEN?

JESSIE GRAFF: "I think women may have a physical advantage on the Floating Boards and possibly the Body Prop, because of hip and wrist flexibility. No woman has made it to either of those obstacles yet, as they're both on Stage Three. Other than that, the only physiological difference I see is that men build and maintain muscle more easily, giving them an advantage on almost every obstacle. We just have to be more scientific and calculated with our strength training, and more strategic on the course."

JESSE "FLEX" LABRECK: "Some of the girls who compete are much shorter—they're 5 feet or 5 foot 1 [Labreck is 5 foot 7]—so that's a lot more challenging for them, but there are some short guys out there, too."

MEAGAN MARTIN: "It really comes down to height more than gender. Generally, women are smaller than men, so some obstacles can be more challenging. For example, the Warped Wall isn't something a 6-foot-tall man really needs to think about, but for me, at 5-foot-3-3/4, there's more of a technical aspect to clearing it. I can still do it. I just have to make sure I do it in a certain way."

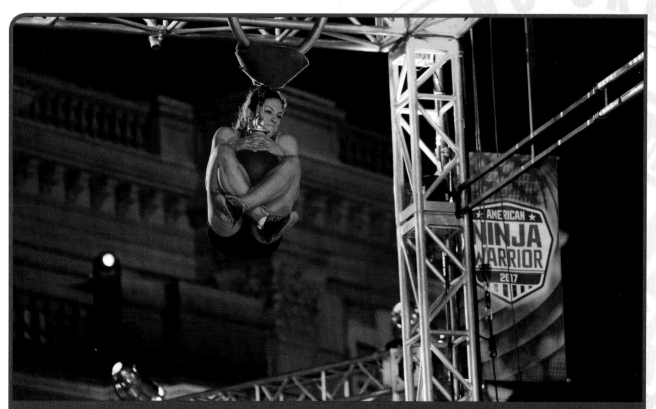

Rebekah Bonilla locks in on the Cannonball Drop during the Los Angeles Finals in Season 9.

THE OBSTACLES

In nine seasons of *American Ninja Warrior*, approximately 200 obstacles have appeared. Some come directly from *SASUKE*. Others are brand new to the show. Some come back season after season. Others make an appearance only once and are never seen again. Some return with modifications or in different course positions, but all have gone through rigorous testing. What follows is a short description of each obstacle, listed alphabetically, that has appeared on *American Ninja Warrior*, followed by a season guide.

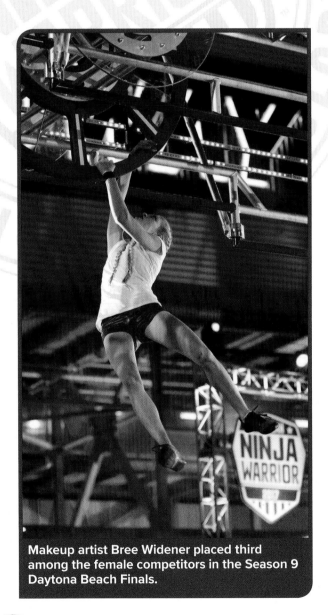

Makeup artist Bree Widener placed third among the female competitors in the Season 9 Daytona Beach Finals.

AREA 51

Area 51 held the seventh position in Stage Three of the National Finals of Season 7, replacing the Spider Flip of Season 6. To clear this obstacle, competitors use their arms and legs to navigate through six suspended rotating disks until they reach a resting bar. Area 51 was replaced by the Walking Bar the next season and, much like an Unidentified Flying Object, has yet to be seen again.

ARM BIKE

Most bicycles don't require incredible upper-body strength. This one does. The Arm Bike premiered as the first obstacle in Stage Three of Season 3. To complete the obstacle, athletes have to use their arms, instead of their feet, to pedal a bike along a suspended track.

ARM RINGS

The Arm Rings appeared as the eighth obstacle on the Southwest and Northwest Finals courses in Season 4 and also in Season 6 at the Denver Finals. Athletes are challenged to hang from two rings and maneuver them across differently shaped horizontal poles with various rises and dips. Fans may remember 52-year-old Jon Stewart fighting his way through the Arm Rings in Season 6, completing a long dismount and inspiring host Akbar Gbajabiamila to say, "Tough times don't last, but tough people do."

BALANCE BRIDGE
(SEE TILTING TABLE)

BALANCE TANK

Appearing in Stage Two of Seasons 4 and 5, the Balance Tank challenges ninjas to balance on top of

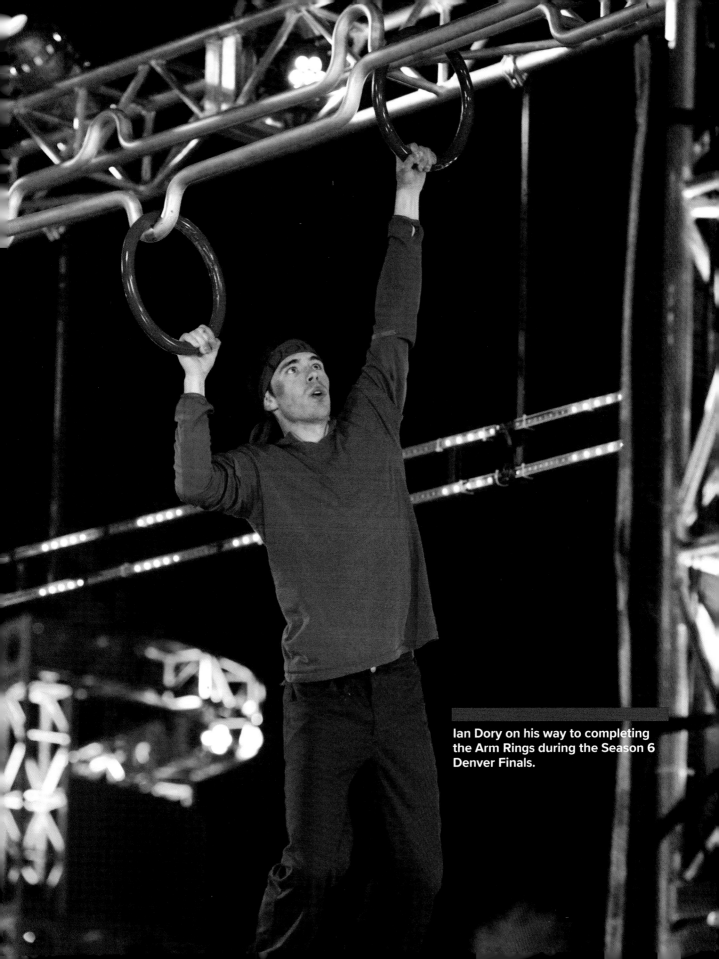

Ian Dory on his way to completing the Arm Rings during the Season 6 Denver Finals.

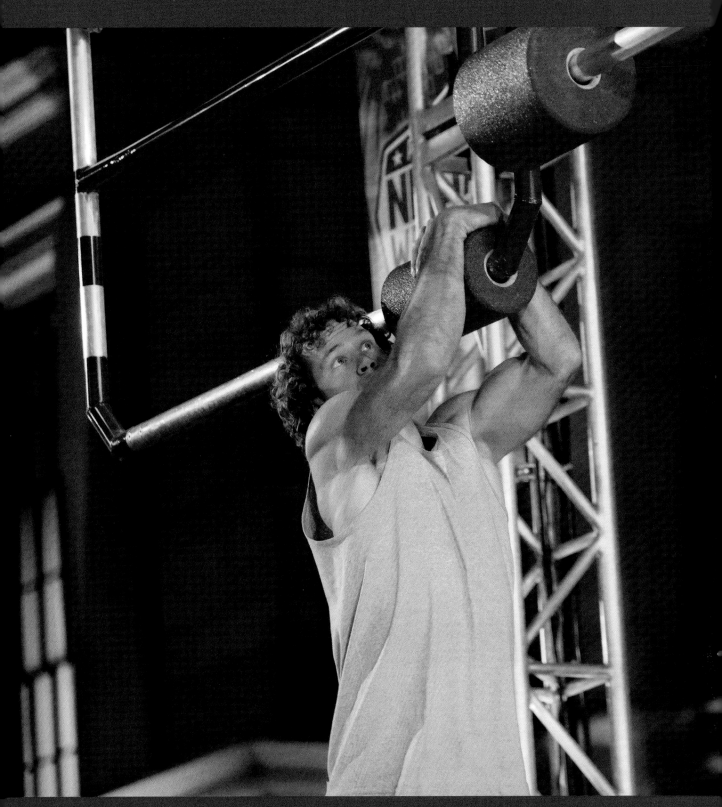

In Season 9, "Island Ninja" Grant McCartney shows the Battering Ram who's boss during the Los Angeles Finals.

a cylindrical barrel while it rolls over a downward-slanted track. As it descends, the athletes have to constantly move their feet in order to keep up with the increasing velocity of the barrel. The obstacle took out some big names in Season 4, but the following year "The Weatherman" Joe Moravsky breezed through the Balance Tank on his way to completing Stage Two as a rookie!

WARRIOR WORDS

KIPPING: The act of thrusting your hips to help generate momentum. Kipping is an essential component to clearing obstacles such as the Salmon Ladder or Crank It Up that require vertical movement.

NINJA KNOW-HOW

"Never look down at the water. Never even *think* you're going to fall in the water. Mentally, you have to know that you can't or you're not going to. It really does help."
—"Island Ninja" Grant McCartney

BAR GLIDER

The Bar Glider appeared only in Stage Three of Season 3, the last season *American Ninja Warrior* traveled to Japan for its Finals round. Similar to the Pipe Slider (see page 101), Bar Glider involves using momentum to push a bar down a track. When competitors get to the end of the first track, they need to build momentum to get to the second half of the track, which they have to traverse in a similar fashion.

BAR HOP

The inspiration for the Bar Hop came from three different places—the Flying Bar from Vegas, the Pipe Slider from Season 4, and a circus trapeze. Course designers meshed them all together for a perfect trifecta of suffering. Bar Hop was the fifth obstacle in the Oklahoma City Qualifying round of Season 8 and also in Season 9's Kansas City. Using their upper body, athletes have to hop a bar across a series of cradles. Not sure ninjas had this in mind when they heard there would be bar hopping on the course.

BATTERING RAM

The Battering Ram took out 10 ninjas when it first appeared in the Los Angeles Qualifiers in Season 9. To complete the Battering Ram, a fan-designed obstacle, competitors have to wrap their arms around a small red foam cylinder—lock in—and kip their way across a steel pipe. Then they have to transition to two other cylinders and traverse those in a similar fashion. When "Island Ninja" Grant McCartney, one of the show's bigger competitors, was dominating the Battering Ram (McCartney would go on to have the fastest time of the night), host Akbar Gbajabiamila exclaimed, "He ain't playing!"

BIG DIPPER

A modified version of the Slider Drop, the Big Dipper made its debut as the second obstacle in the Kansas City Qualifying round of Season 7 and was crushed by Wolfpack Ninjas Brian Arnold and

> " Having a countdown clock in Vegas is the most challenging obstacle for me. Having to do things faster makes it harder not to make little mistakes.
> —Meagan Martin "

Meagan Martin, among others. To complete the obstacle, athletes have to hold on to a metal pipe while it slides down a track and time their release so they can grab a rope ladder and pull themselves onto a landing mat.

BLOCK RUN

Block Run made its debut in the Qualifying round of Atlanta in Season 8 and returned for Season 9 in Los Angeles. Ninjas have to use their balance and agility to run across tilted cubes on a horizontal pole that rotated and slid under their feet. Fans may remember how mother of three Paige Chapman stumbled on the Block Run in Season 9, but made an awesome save, rolling her way onto the landing mat to complete the obstacle.

BOUNCING SPIDER

The Bouncing Spider made its debut in Season 9's Denver Qualifying course, taking out veteran ninjas such as Jon Stewart, Jake Murray, and "Ninjadoc" Noah Kaufman. To complete this obstacle, competitors use their upper and lower body to prop themselves between two pieces of Plexiglas, similar to the Jumping Spider (see page 96), and make a transition to another pair of Plexiglas plates a few inches away. Then they have to jump down to a tramp and bounce up to grab onto one of three suspended pipes before swinging up to a platform.

> There is not necessarily any individual obstacle that is hard, but to be able to maintain composure and strength across the course as a whole, from Point A to Z, is what makes it difficult.
> —Isaac Caldiero

BRIDGE OF BLADES

The Bridge of Blades challenges ninjas' speed, balance, and agility. It first appeared in Season 2 and then returned in Season 3, Season 4 (Midwest and Midsouth), and in St. Louis in Season 6. The obstacle has four ledges that rotate around a central axis. Ninjas usually try to move across the Bridge of Blades quickly to maintain their balance. Fans may remember firefighter Mike Bernardo tried using a slower, unorthodox method to complete the obstacle during the St. Louis Qualifiers in Season 6 but the Bridge of Blades cut his run short.

NINJA KILLER

BODY PROP

The Body Prop appeared as the ninth obstacle at the Baltimore Finals in Season 5 and also the Los Angeles Finals in Season 6. (Fans may also remember a modified version in Season 7's Kansas City Finals.) To complete this obstacle, ninjas have to engage their core and keep their abs tight as they wedge themselves between two wall panels—hands on one panel, feet on the other—and work their way across, all while facing downward. A curved version, Curved Body Prop, appeared on Stage Three of Seasons 8 and 9 and was a massive 30 feet long! "Real Life Ninja" Drew Drechsel was the only athlete to attempt—and complete—this obstacle in Season 8, while "The Weatherman" Joe Moravsky was the only athlete to attempt—and complete—the obstacle in Season 9. Both athletes went on to become the Last Man Standing of their respective seasons.

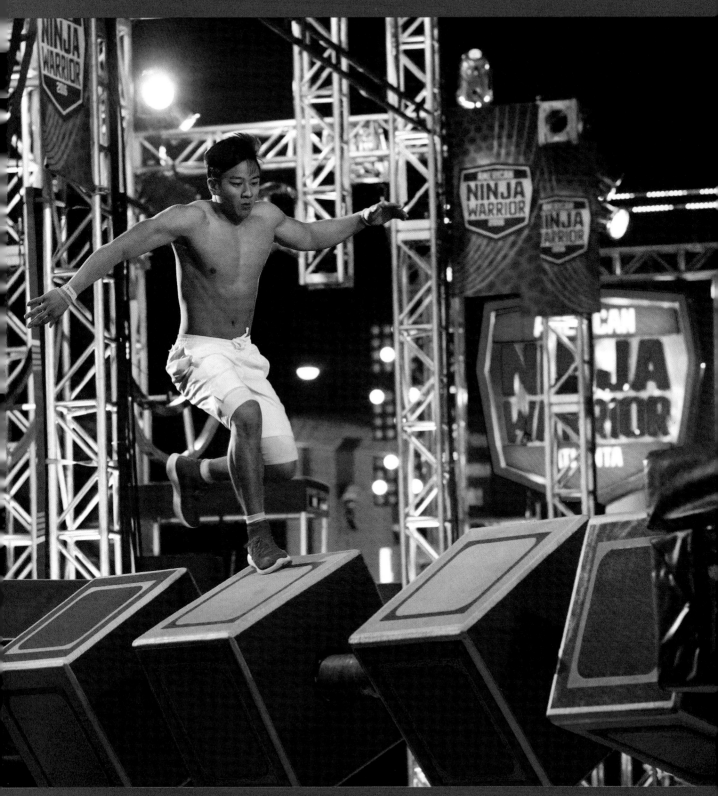

Block Run tests Nikko Galang's agility during the Atlanta Qualifiers of Season 8.

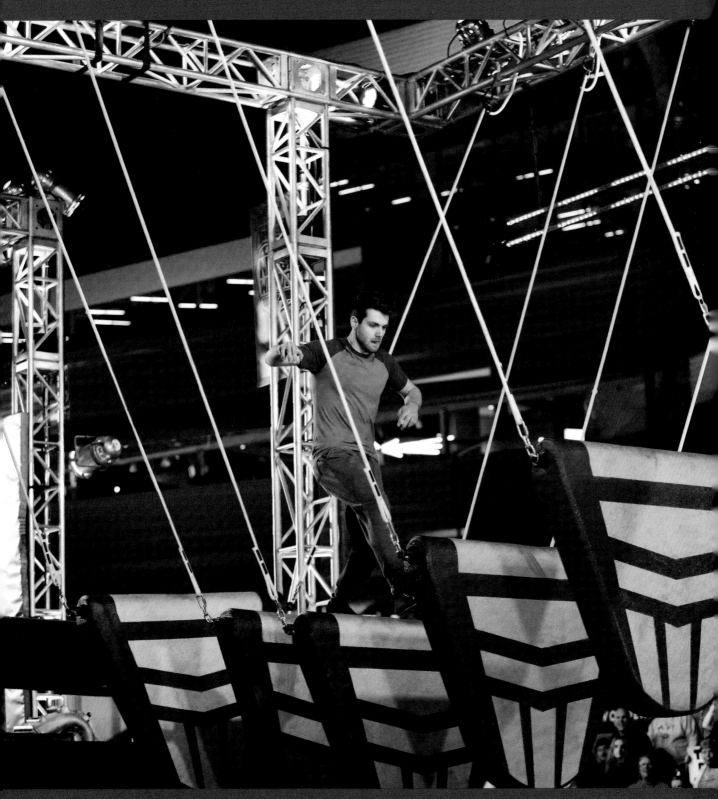
Tyler Gillett crosses the Broken Bridge in Season 9's Daytona Beach Qualifiers.

MEMORABLE MOMENTS

MATT ISEMAN:
"There was one moment we couldn't show, and it was when a guy in a Harry Potter costume ran the course. If you saw *Celebrity Apprentice*, you know there are not many bigger Harry Potter fans than me. So getting to call the run of the Boy Who Lived was magical."

BROKEN BRIDGE

The Broken Bridge premiered in Stage One of Season 8 and returned in Daytona in Season 9. It consists of six unstable triangles hanging at slightly different heights and with gaps between them. Competitors have to use their agility and speed to get across the triangles. Overall, ninjas didn't seem to have too much trouble with the Broken Bridge, which had a high completion rate in both seasons.

BUNGEE BRIDGE

Bungee Bridge appeared only in Season 4, at the Northeast and Southeast regionals. The obstacle is made up of five sections of unstable bungee cords, each of varying size. Competitors have to use those five sections to cross to the other side. Fans may remember that Ryan Stratis had a shocking early exit when he stumbled on the Bungee Bridge in Season 4.

BUNGEE ROAD

Bungee Road, which premiered in the Kansas City Qualifying round of Season 7 (and also appeared in the Oklahoma City Finals of Season 8), consists of a mini-trampoline, four sets of stretching ropes, and an angled suspended log. Competitors jump from the tramp to reach the first set of ropes and use their upper body to traverse each set until they reach the log. Once athletes are on the log, they must slide down to reach a landing mat in order to complete the obstacle. (Using the lower body will result in disqualification.) In Season 7, Meagan Martin became the first woman to complete Bungee Road.

BUNGEE ROPE CLIMB

Bungee Rope Climb appeared in Stage Three of four seasons of *American Ninja Warrior*—Seasons 2 to 5. To complete the obstacle, ninjas must grab onto an elasticized rope and use their momentum to transfer to another rope and so on. The ropes decrease in length as competitors move farther along the obstacle. Veteran ninjas Brent Steffenson and Brian Arnold both completed the Bungee Rope Climb in Seasons 4 and 5 respectively.

NINJA KILLER

BROKEN PIPES

The Broken Pipes, introduced in Kansas City in Season 9, is one of those balance and agility obstacles that look deceivingly simple. It consists of two spinning logs and a small bobblehead between them. The logs, which are not aligned, spin on an axis, and ninjas must run across one and then the other, continuing on to a landing mat in order to complete the obstacle. However, in the Kansas City Qualifiers, the Broken Pipes took out a whopping 33 ninjas (only 12 were televised hitting the water). And in the City Finals, the Broken Pipes took out seven of the night's athletes.

NINJA KILLER

CANNONBALL ALLEY

Cannonball Alley consists of three differently sized balls that increase in size on a slight decline, swinging back and forth from two secured lines. Competitors must swing from one to the other and jump to a platform in order to complete the obstacle. In Season 6, 28-year-old stock trader Kevin Bull, a walk-on, famously crushed this obstacle, which had been stymieing ninjas, by hanging from his legs—rather than his arms—and becoming the first man to survive Cannonball Alley in the Los Angeles Finals.

BUTTERFLY WALL

The Butterfly Wall made its Stage Two debut in Season 6 as the fourth obstacle. Although the wall in earlier *SASUKE* competitions had been rectangular, this rotating padded wall is shaped like butterfly wings with rounded corners and inclined ledges. Ninjas have to jump and grab onto the wall, which spins around a central vertical axis, to reach a platform on the other side. The Butterfly Wall never proved too difficult for ninjas—with only two fails in its history—but it often served as a critical time sapper.

CANNONBALL DROP

Brand new to Season 9, Cannonball Drop held the second position at the Los Angeles Qualifying course. To complete the obstacle, competitors have to grab onto a 9-inch diameter cannonball and ride it down a track that is slightly steeper at the start, making the cannonball accelerate quickly. The track also has two drops that test the grip strength of competitors, but veteran ninjas such as Flip Rodriguez and "Island Ninja" Grant McCartney were able to get through the obstacle without a hitch.

CANNONBALL INCLINE

Cannonball Incline appeared only one time—as the first obstacle in Stage Three of Season 6. Cannonball Incline features three hanging cannonballs that ascend in height—rather than descending, as in Cannonball Alley—with the largest ball in the middle. Both Elet Hall and "The Weatherman" Joe Moravsky, the only competitors to make it to Stage Three that season, got through the obstacle easily.

CARGO CLIMB

Cargo Climb served as the last obstacle of the Semifinals and City Finals in Seasons 1 through 4 of *American Ninja Warrior*, before being replaced with the Spider Climb. Also called the Rope Ladder, this obstacle is one of the more straightforward obstacles derived from *SASUKE*, consisting of a net bridge that athletes must climb to reach a platform.

CARGO CROSSING

Cargo Crossing may be best known as the obstacle that took out "Mighty" Kacy Catanzaro during the Houston Qualifying round of Season 7, a year after Catanzaro's history-making run. The obstacle consists of three parts—a springboard, a seesaw-like suspended cargo net with a horizontal metal bar at each end, and a trapeze bar. Competitors must jump from the springboard to the cargo net, which they must climb under to reach the second metal bar. From there, they swing 6 feet to the trapeze bar, before lacheing to a landing mat. Catanzaro's height, at 5 feet, made it difficult for her to close the gap from the cargo net to the trapeze bar, resulting in her anguishing fall into the water.

CARGO NET

The Cargo Net is a familiar sight on *American Ninja Warrior*, as it often works in tandem with other obstacles. Although in general practice, cargo nets are used to transfer cargo to and from ships, on *American Ninja Warrior* athletes must cross them to complete an obstacle. Usually, ninjas will either swing or jump their way onto the squares of the thick-roped Cargo Net and traverse the net from below to an awaiting platform—all, of course, without getting wet.

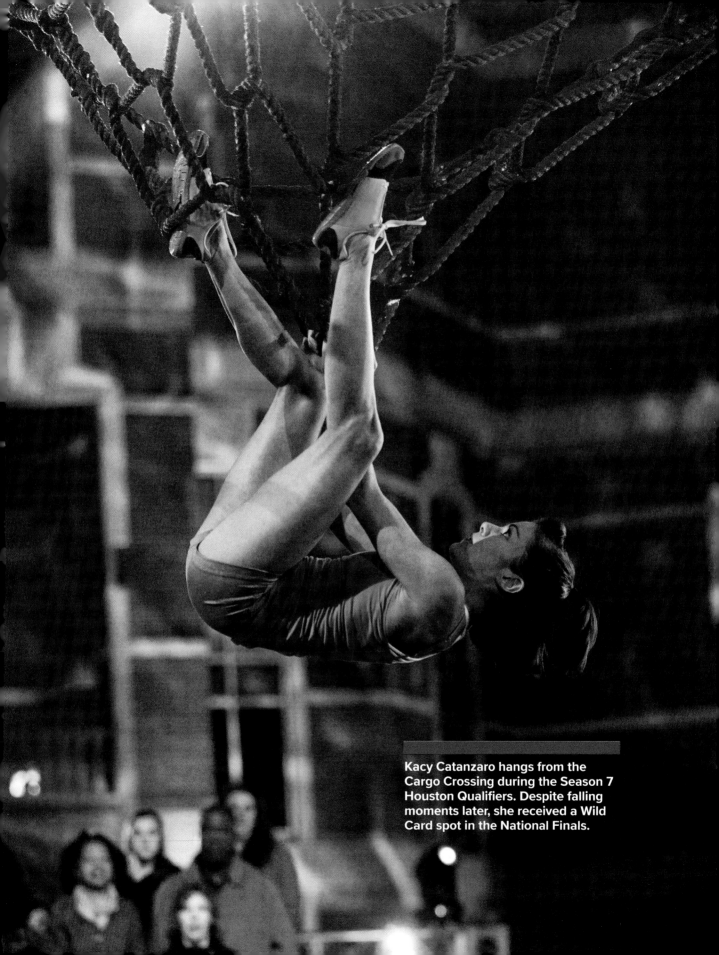

Kacy Catanzaro hangs from the Cargo Crossing during the Season 7 Houston Qualifiers. Despite falling moments later, she received a Wild Card spot in the National Finals.

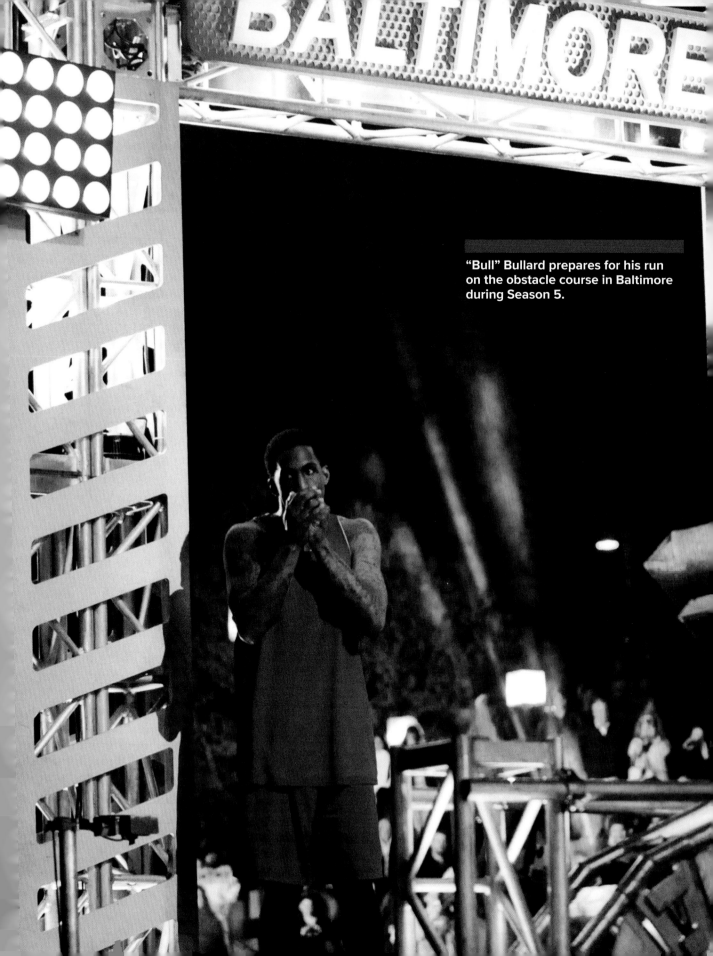

"Bull" Bullard prepares for his run on the obstacle course in Baltimore during Season 5.

> I've never tried the course myself, although every year I say I want to. I think to say that I'd be able to even complete one or two obstacles would take away from the serious training the ninjas go through in order to be successful. I cover professional sports, and 99 percent of the athletes wouldn't be able to do what the ninjas do on the course. It takes serious dedication and training. Maybe one year I'll take up training at one of the ninja gyms and give it a shot myself.
>
> –Cohost Kristine Leahy

CAT GRAB

Surely, ninjas feel like there are big walls trying to keep them from conquering the *American Ninja Warrior* obstacle course, but the Cat Grab obstacle is just that—a series of walls! Cat Grab took the second position in Denver in Season 6, the only season it appeared. To complete the obstacle, ninjas have to jump onto a wall and then onto a second and higher wall. Then, once they crest that second wall, they jump to a landing platform below. The Cat Grab proved relatively trouble-free for most competitors, including veteran ninjas Jon Stewart and Meagan Martin, who made it through the obstacle with ease.

CHAIN SEESAW

Making its only appearance on *American Ninja Warrior* during Stage Three of the Season 3 Finals, the Chain Seesaw requires tremendous balance on the part of ninjas. The obstacle consists of two long chains, each with its own pulley mechanism. If ninjas don't grab the ends of the chains at the same time, then the chain with the most weight will lengthen while the other shortens, likely forcing them into the water.

CIRCLE CROSS

Positioned just before the Warped Wall in Baltimore in Season 5, Circle Cross took out the most competitors in the Qualifying round. The obstacle consists of three rings and two ropes. Ninjas have to jump to the first ring, grasp it with their hands, and from there alternate—rope, ring, rope, ring—before landing safely onto a platform.

CRASHING THE COURSE

Who doesn't love bonus material? NBC's popular digital series *Crashing the Course* offers a behind-the-scenes look at what it takes to conquer an *American Ninja Warrior* obstacle course. Hosted by Alex Weber, *Crashing the Course* features episodes that run between three and seven minutes in length and appear online over the course of a season. Plus, look for your favorite ninjas—as well as producers, course builders, and more!—to stop by and provide insights, info, and even a towel for Weber, who likes to give the obstacles a try.

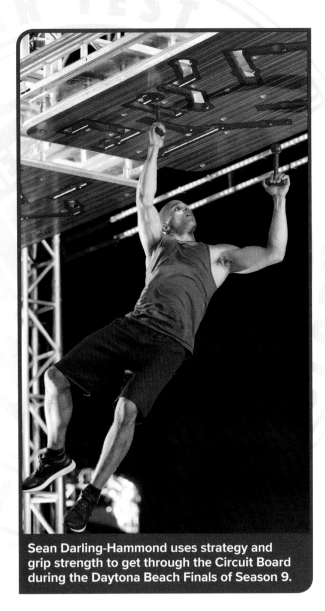

Sean Darling-Hammond uses strategy and grip strength to get through the Circuit Board during the Daytona Beach Finals of Season 9.

CIRCLE SLIDER

Circle Slider was a recurring obstacle on *SASUKE*, but its only *American Ninja Warrior* appearance was in the Season 2 Semifinals. Completion of the obstacle is straightforward: Athletes jump off a springboard in order to latch onto a ring that slides down a sloping path.

CIRCUIT BOARD

Both a physical and mental obstacle, Circuit Board held Position Nine in the Season 8 Indianapolis Finals and also Season 9's Daytona Beach Finals. The obstacle—the idea for which came from a traditional gym pegboard—challenges competitors to use their upper-body strength and core to go across a 25-foot pool while they're hanging 15 feet in the air. All the while, they are traversing the obstacle by inserting handles into four panels of curved paths. It's like doing a puzzle while hanging from your fingertips!

THE CLACKER

The idea for The Clacker came from a wooden ratchet instrument and the piercingly loud clacking sound it makes. This obstacle appeared in the Atlanta Finals of Season 8—taking out three ninjas—and again in the Cleveland Finals of Season 9. The Clacker is 20 feet long and has 10 clackers in total. Using only their upper body, competitors must bring each set of clackers up and over before transitioning to the next set in order to complete the obstacle (the last set of clackers is optional).

CLEAR CLIMB

The Clear Climb, which made its first and only appearance as the ninth obstacle in the Los Angeles Finals of Season 7, consists of a 24-foot-long climbing wall. The wall is tilted back 35 degrees with a final section that is tilted back an additional 10 degrees. Competitors must climb across the wall; they are allowed to use both their hands and feet. Of the six competitors who attempted the Clear Climb, only three were successful—Nicholas Coolridge, Kevin Bull, and "The Godfather" David Campbell.

WARRIOR WORDS

LACHE: A parkour term, this move can be used by ninjas to swing off a bar, usually to another bar or to a dismount. Lacheing requires a lot of core strength. In basic terms, when hanging from a bar, ninjas kick their legs forward—like children do on swing sets—to build momentum. Then they pull their legs up with their core, shoot them out as far as they can get them, and ride that forward extension.

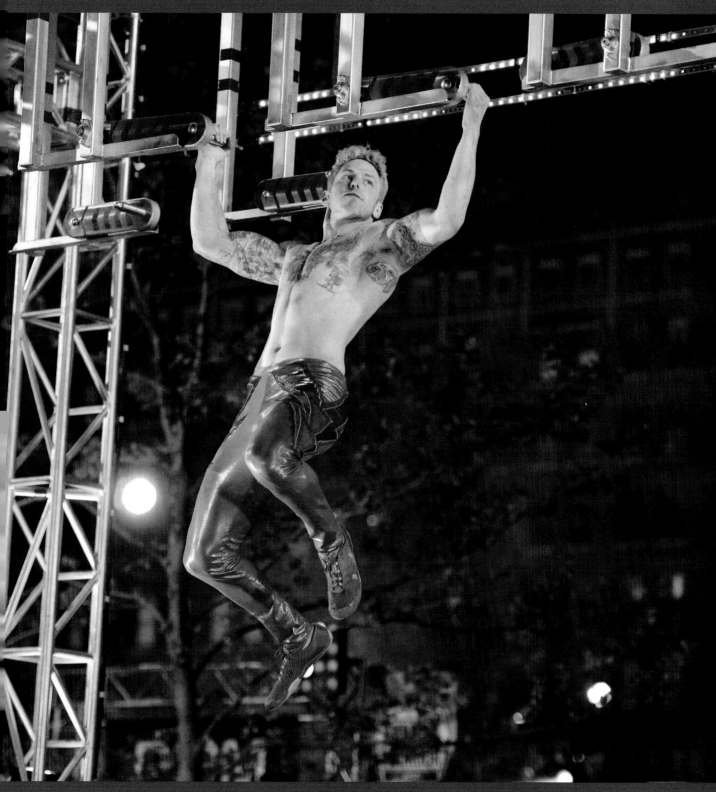

"Captain NBC" Jamie Rahn on his way to defeating The Clacker in the Season 9 Cleveland Finals, marking the fifth consecutive year that he qualified for the Las Vegas National Finals.

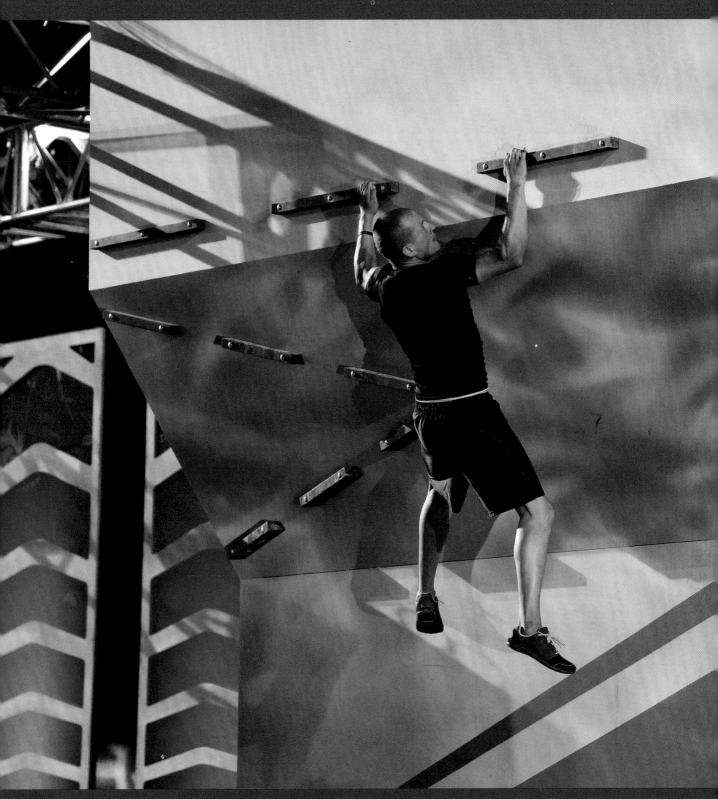

Brent Steffensen hangs on the Ulimate Cliffhanger during the 2016 *American Ninja Warrior All-Star Special: Skills Challenge.*

COIN FLIP

Coin Flip tests balance and agility. It made its only appearance on *American Ninja Warrior* as the seventh obstacle in Stage One of Season 7 and challenges competitors to run across three free-floating discs in order to reach a landing mat. Fans may remember that it was on the Coin Flip that "The Godfather" David Campbell slipped and fell into the water, marking the fourth consecutive year that the ninja veteran ended his run on Stage One. (Campbell would go on to complete Stage One in Season 9.)

CRANK IT UP

A winner of *American Ninja Warrior*'s 2016 Obstacle Design Challenge, show fan Kevin Brekke designed Crank It Up, which made its debut in Kansas City in Season 9. The obstacle taxes competitors' forearms as they use the momentum of their body to crank up a set of handles until the handles move up and forward—a distance of 6 feet! This exhausting motion has to be repeated a total of three times (in the City Finals, there were only two sets of handles with a bigger space between them). Showing grit and stamina, an emotional Maggi Thorne became the first woman to conquer Crank It Up in the Kansas City Finals.

CLIFFHANGER

A direct import from *SASUKE*, the Cliffhanger is one of the most enduring obstacles of *American Ninja Warrior* and has appeared throughout the series in several forms—as the Shin-Cliffhanger from Season 1's Stage Three; as the ninja-killing Ultimate Cliffhanger, which appeared in Stage Three for Seasons 2 to 9 (fans may recall in Season 4 veteran ninja Brent Steffensen became the first American to defeat the Ultimate Cliffhanger); as simply the Cliffhanger in Season 5's Los Angeles Finals, and as the Crazy Cliffhanger in the City Finals of St. Louis in Season 6 and Houston in Season 7. In each version, athletes have to traverse narrow ledges just wide enough to support the fingertips. As ninjas familiar with the various versions of the Cliffhanger know, even minor alterations can cause major headaches on *American Ninja Warrior*.

NINJA KNOW-HOW

When hanging by your fingertips on an obstacle like the Cliffhanger, keeping your arms at 90 degrees—in an L shape—allows you to use the biceps as well as the back muscles.

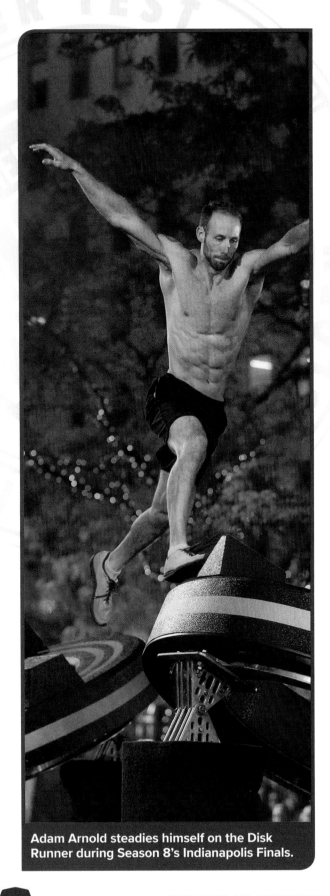

Adam Arnold steadies himself on the Disk Runner during Season 8's Indianapolis Finals.

CURTAIN SLIDER

It was curtains for ninjas when the Curtain Slider appeared in Stage One of *American Ninja Warrior*'s inaugural season. This obstacle, which was also in Season 4's Midwest location and in Miami in Season 6, consists of three curtains (one large, sheetlike curtain and two long, narrow curtains). Competitors must grab the first large curtain and use their momentum to slide the curtain toward the next two. Then they must grab the next two long curtains and traverse those in order to get to a landing platform. In Miami, where athletes such as JJ Woods and Ryan Stratis (with a growl!) conquered the obstacle, the number of long curtains was reduced from two to just one.

CURVED BODY PROP
(SEE BODY PROP)

CYCLE ROAD

Cycle Road—first appearing as the third obstacle of Stage Three in the National Finals of Season 2 and then in Season 4's Northeast and Southeast regionals—proved to be strength-draining rather than difficult for ninjas, who mostly were able to complete it. The obstacle consists of four hanging wheels spaced out unevenly over a distance, and athletes need to throw enough momentum on each wheel to reach the next.

DANCING STONES

Ninjas showed us their moves on the Dancing Stones, which held the fourth position in Season 6's Miami rounds. The obstacle consists of eight small spherical objects attached to the tops of short square poles, and many veteran athletes, including "Real Life Ninja" Drew Drechsel and JJ Woods, moved across them with ease.

DESCENDING LAMP GRASPER
(SEE GLOBE GRASPER)

DEVIL STEPS

Devil Steps—Geoff Britten's favorite obstacle—features a set of ascending and descending stairs.

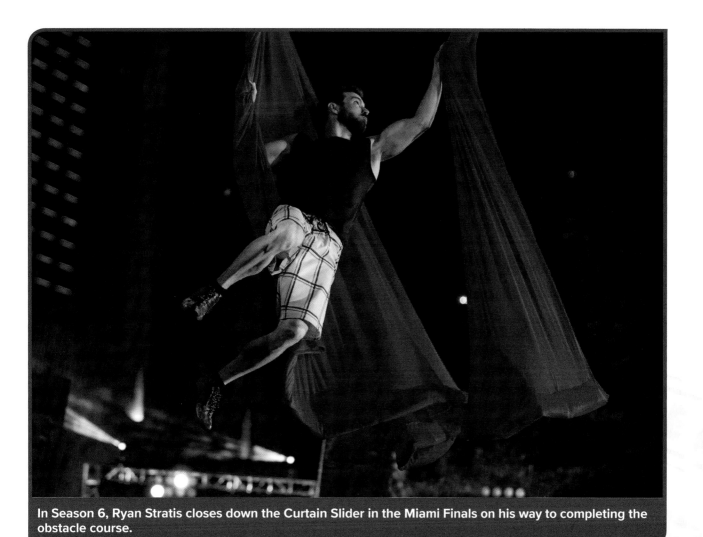

In Season 6, Ryan Stratis closes down the Curtain Slider in the Miami Finals on his way to completing the obstacle course.

There are three intervals of steps, with the first two going upward, and the last one going down. Athletes must climb under the steps to reach the next obstacle. Devil Steps appeared in the very first season of *American Ninja Warrior* in Stage Three, and again in Seasons 4 (Southwest and Northwest), 6 (Denver), and 7 (Pittsburgh).

DISK RUNNER

Inspired by a children's playground in Sweden, Disk Runner was the fourth obstacle in the Indianapolis Qualifying round of Season 8. To complete the obstacle, competitors first have to jump to an off-axis spinning disk (there is a pole at the center that they can use to steady themselves, as no upper-

body is allowed to touch the disks). Next, they jump 5 feet to another off-axis (in the other direction!) spinning disk with three large stumbling blocks, before jumping to a landing platform. Most of the eliminations on Disk Runner were a result of either a foot touching the water, hands touching the wheel, or athletes falling off the side of the course.

DOMINO HILL

Appearing only in Los Angeles in Season 5, Domino Hill resembles seven large dominoes lined up in a row. "Mighty" Kacy Catanzaro and Brent Steffensen were just two of the ninjas who were able to glide successfully across this balance obstacle.

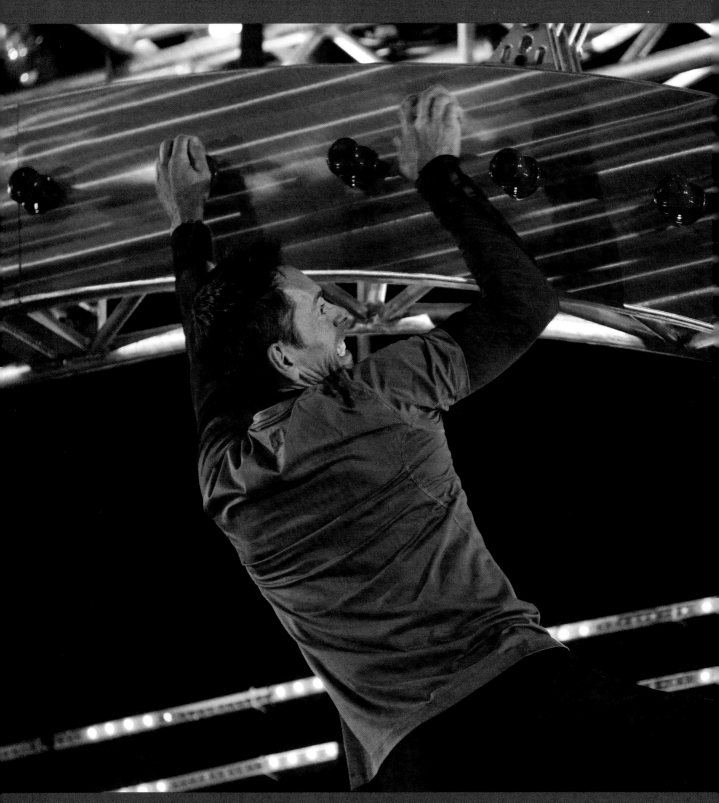

Jon Stewart reaches for the next knob on the Doorknob Arch in the Denver Finals.

DOMINO PIPES

The Domino Pipes premiered in Stage One of the Season 9 National Finals. Competitors have to use their balance and agility to run through five ascending top-heavy spinning pipes to reach a landing platform. Nearly all the ninjas who reached the Domino Pipes completed it, although the obstacle took out personal trainer Karsten Williams, marking the fourth year in a row that the athlete failed Stage One.

DOORKNOB ARCH

The Doorknob Arch first appeared in the Denver Finals of Season 6 and again in the Pittsburgh Finals of Season 7 as the ninth obstacle. It consists of an arch lined with 24 doorknobs (in Denver) and 28 doorknobs (in Pittsburgh). Competitors have to use their hands—and their arm and grip strength—to traverse the obstacle until they are close enough to make a jump for a landing mat. Geoff Britten's massive forearms enabled an aggressive arm-over-arm approach that helped Britten zip through the Doorknob Arch, causing host Matt Iseman to exclaim, "You can see why they call him Popeye!"

DOORKNOB GRASPER

First appearing on *SASUKE*, the Doorknob Grasper was a Stage Three staple on *American Ninja Warrior* from Seasons 4 to 7. It consists of four knobs protruding from a wall (on Seasons 6 and 7, the obstacle was angled with a fifth doorknob added). Ninjas must grab onto that first knob and transition to the next and so on. Although some of the knobs turn, taxing grip strength, most ninjas prevailed on this obstacle. The Doorknob Grasper has a high completion rate—of the 16 athletes ever to attempt it, 15 were able to complete it.

DOUBLE DIPPER

Inspired by a nine-year-old *American Ninja Warrior* fan from California, the Double Dipper made its debut in Season 9 in Stage One. The obstacle is similar to the Big Dipper of Season 7 but doubles down the challenge: Ninjas must slide down a track holding on to a bar and use that momentum—and time their leap!—to lache to another bar on a second track. Eighteen ninjas ended their Stage One run on the Double Dipper.

DOUBLE SALMON LADDER
(SEE SALMON LADDER)

DOUBLE TILT LADDER

The Double Tilt Ladder, which appeared in St. Louis in Season 6 and Orlando in Season 7, consists of two sets of suspended tilting monkey bars. Competitors use their hands to move up the first set of monkey bars until their weight causes the ladder to tilt and they continue on a downslope to the end. Then they must transition—a 6-foot gap—to a second set of bars and navigate it just as the first before swinging to a landing mat. When Michelle Warnky completed the Double Tilt Ladder in Season 6, she became the fourth woman to complete five obstacles.

DOUBLE WEDGE
(SEE WEDGE)

DOWN UP SALMON LADDER
(SEE SALMON LADDER)

> " The most difficult obstacle is the Double Wedge. I think it requires incredible levels of precision. It is a very tough obstacle for athletes to figure out, especially if they are seeing it for the first time.
> –Chris Wilczewski
> "

DOWNHILL JUMP

Originally appearing in Season 1, Downhill Jump returned as the second obstacle in Baltimore during Season 5. Competitors have to slide down a track on an object resembling a snowboard and then jump to a rope on another track that swings toward a landing mat. The obstacle proved no problem for many ninjas in Season 5, including "The Weatherman" Joe Moravsky, who had the right stuff even without the white stuff!

DOWNHILL PIPE DROP

The Downhill Pipe Drop made only one appearance on *American Ninja Warrior* but it was a notorious one, taking out "Real Life Ninja" Drew Drechsel in the Miami City Finals of Season 6. To complete the obstacle, athletes must slide a red pipe down a track and then time their release to grab a rope in order to transition to a landing platform. Drechsel mistimed his rope grab, forcing his stunning early exit from the competition.

ELEVATOR CLIMB

An upper-body beatdown, the Elevator Climb made its debut in Season 9 as the final obstacle in every City Finals course. Ninjas pump their arms to move two levers up a grueling 35 feet. (The Elevator Climb may remind fans of the famed Invisible Ladder, which held that same position in the City Finals in previous seasons.) A select few ninjas, such as "Kingdom Ninja" Daniel Gil, were able to dominate the Elevator Climb, but the brutal obstacle caused many ninjas to gas out, including JJ Woods and Jessie Graff.

ESCALATOR

The Escalator made its only appearance in Los Angeles in Season 8. Competitors have to run up four free-swinging planks and then down two free-swinging planks without using their hands. Although most athletes made it through the Escalator unscathed, "Papal Ninja" Sean Bryan made a shocking exit on the obstacle that season, his rookie year.

FLOATING BOARDS

The Floating Boards obstacle has been a staple of the National Finals' Stage Three since Season 4. It consists of four boards (five boards in *SASUKE*) hanging from a scaffolding. Using their upper body, ninjas must cling onto the first board and transfer

> " I think the Elevator Climb is the toughest obstacle on the course and is often featured in the City Finals. Most of the people who even make it to that round don't get to the Elevator Climb, and if they do, many of them pump out and 'fail.' It's the obstacle that forces ninjas to push past complete exhaustion and somehow find a way to get to the top. Their faces show just how grueling it is to hang up in the air and try to ascend 30 feet after they've already been through nine extremely taxing obstacles.
> —Cohost Kristine Leahy "

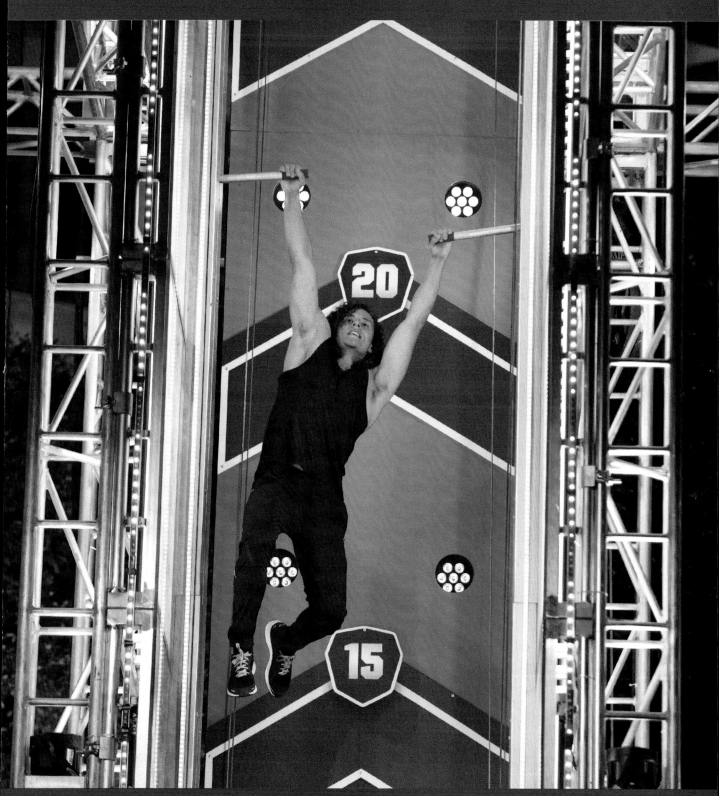

In Season 9, "Kingdom Ninja" Daniel Gil powers through the Elevator Climb during the San Antonio Finals.

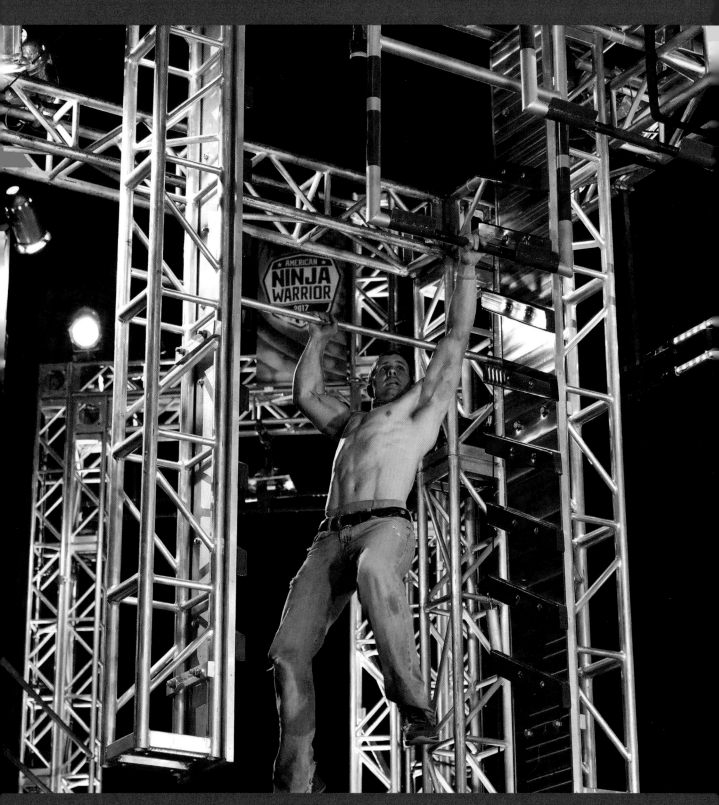

Lance Pekus transitions from the Salmon Ladder to the Floating Monkey Bars in Season 9's Kansas City Finals.

onto the next and so on. Fans may remember that it was the Floating Boards that ended the inspirational run of "The Weatherman" Joe Moravsky in Season 5, his rookie season.

FLOATING CHAINS

Appearing only in Los Angeles in Season 5, the Floating Chains—a modified version of Hang Move, an obstacle that was featured in an early season of *SASUKE*—consists of five hanging chains. The second and fourth chain have a small prism-shaped foothold at the bottom, and ninjas must grab the first chain and swing Tarzan-like to the next and so on in order to complete the obstacle.

FLOATING MONKEY BARS

Positioned right after the Salmon Ladder, the Floating Monkey Bars intensified ninjas' upper-body workout when it appeared in the Pittsburgh Finals of Season 7, the Atlanta Finals of Season 8, and the Kansas City Finals of Season 9. Consisting of two free bars and six suspended trays, the obstacle challenges ninjas to hang from a bar and move forward by placing bars in trays until they are close enough to jump to a landing mat. In Season 8, veterans such as Travis Rosen and "Real Life Ninja" Drew Drechsel were able to conquer the intense Floating Monkey Bars, although the obstacle did trip up some ninjas, including "Cowboy Ninja" Lance Pekus in Season 9.

FLOATING STAIRS

First appearing after the Salmon Ladder in the Denver Finals of Season 5, the Floating Stairs requires intense upper-body strength, grip strength, and core strength. Athletes must traverse three sets of planks that are attached to beams angled up, down, and up again. As taxing as it is on the upper body, it was no match for ninjas such as Brian Arnold and Isaac Caldiero who completed it with ease in Season 5.

FLOATING STEPS

The Floating Steps premiered in Season 8 as the first obstacle of the Qualifying and City Finals courses. Similar to its predecessors, the Quad Steps and the Quintuple Steps, the Floating Steps uses five

> The Floating Steps look so easy. I'm 6 foot 6, I've got long legs—most of my height is legs—and I thought I could just go right through them. I ended up doing what they call the cat grab, where you just—'yeooooooooow'—fly to each step, one by one. It's so intimidating when you see the water below you. It messes with your head. You think, *Oh, I better do what's safe*. It really does say a lot about what type of competitor you are, and I didn't take the risk. Maybe I could do it, but I didn't want to fail, so I went with what was safe. Usually, the saying is, 'it's not how you start, it's how you finish,' but I can tell a lot about a competitor by the Floating Steps.
>
> —Host Akbar Gbajabiamila

> I really enjoy the Flying Bar, not only because of the awkward flying sensation with a bar but also for where it's placed at the end of Stage Three after so many upper-body challenges.
>
> —Isaac Caldiero

> Certain athletes have that 'it' factor, the passion, or heart it takes to go that extra inch when you were done 5 inches ago. When I think about athletes with that 'it' factor, I think about Geoff Britten almost peeling off on the final Flying Bar jump. Geoff needed that heart and determination to make it through that last movement.
>
> —Chris Wilczewski

steps, which get steeper as they ascend in height. Once ninjas reach the fifth and final step, they jump to a hanging rope and swing to a platform to complete the obstacle. While it's true that the Floating Steps have a high completion percentage, ninjas have failed this obstacle when they tried to rush through rather than take their time.

FLOATING TILES

Ninjas got to flaunt their balance and agility as they scooted across the Floating Tiles, which appeared only in Kansas City in Season 7. The Floating Tiles features four suspended tiles that are held by elastic, making them unstable, but the obstacle didn't pose much of a challenge for most ninjas, including Brian Arnold and Lance Pekus who completed it easily.

FLY WHEELS

Ninjas such as "Wolfpup" Ian Dory and "SheWolf" Meagan Martin showed off their grip strength when they defeated the Fly Wheels when it served as the third obstacle in Indianapolis during Season 8. To complete the obstacle, competitors must use their upper body to swing across three hanging wheels (only two wheels in the City Finals) with a mere 1-inch ledge on either side.

FLYING BAR

The Flying Bar has been a regular of Stage Three, appearing in Seasons 2 through 9. The obstacle requires incredible grip and core strength and is sort of a horizontal version of the Salmon Ladder. Athletes must work a free bar across a track by lacheing from one rung to another while holding on to the bar. Fans may remember the excruciating fall into the water by Brian Arnold when he nearly conquered the Flying Bar in Season 5, only feet away from completing Stage Three.

WARRIOR WORDS

BACK HALF: The obstacles in the City Finals courses that appear after the Warped Wall.

BECOME AN AMERICAN NINJA WARRIOR: THE ULTIMATE INSIDER'S GUIDE

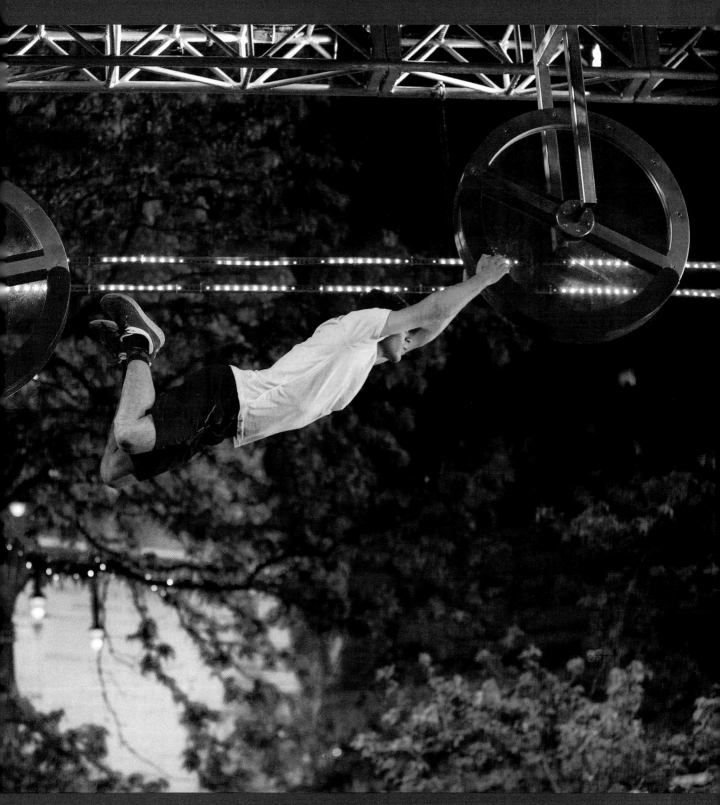

"Wolfpup" Ian Dory grabs hold of a wheel in the Fly Wheels obstacle at the Indianapolis Qualifiers in Season 8.

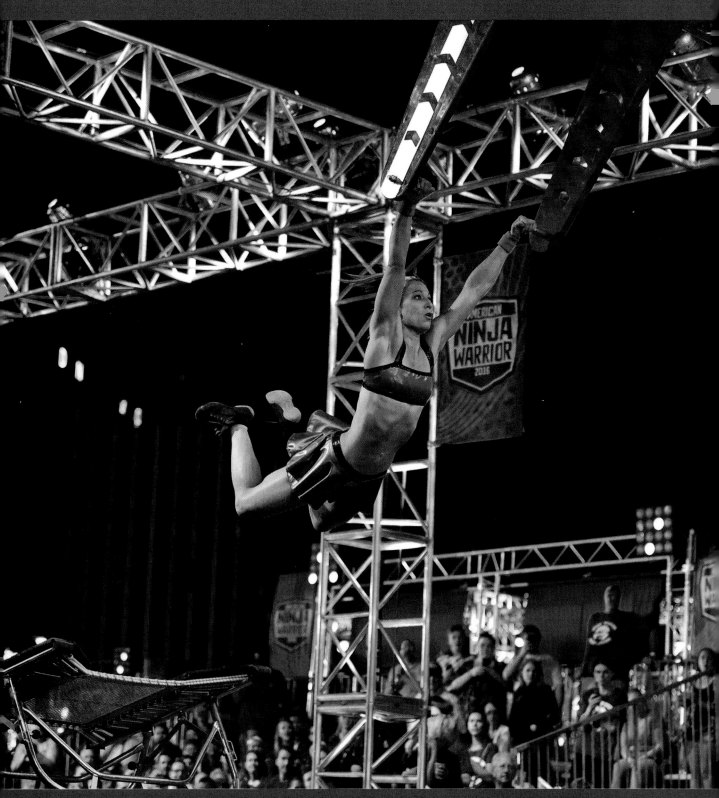

In the Season 8 National Finals, Jessie Graff swings on the Flying Squirrel just before she becomes the first woman ever to complete Stage One in *American Ninja Warrior* history.

FLYING NUNCHUCKS

The Flying Nunchucks appeared as the fifth obstacle in Los Angeles in Season 5. To complete the obstacle, ninjas have to leap off a mini-tramp and grab onto a pair of side-by-side nunchucks that hang from a swing. From there, they must swing to a second set of nunchucks before dismounting onto a platform. "Mighty" Kacy Catanzaro couldn't hold on to the first set of nunchucks when she tackled this obstacle in the Qualifiers, but as fans know Catanzaro would go on to make *American Ninja Warrior* history the following season.

NINJA KNOW-HOW

SWITCH GRIP

Using a switch grip—also called a cross or alternating grip—can help ninjas gain more stability on obstacles that require them to move a free bar, such as the Salmon Ladder. Ninjas employ a switch grip by grasping the bar with one palm facing away from them and one facing toward them. This grip can also keep the bar from spinning or rolling out of their fingertips.

FLYING SQUIRREL

The Flying Squirrel may go down in *American Ninja Warrior* history as the obstacle that prevented Jessie Graff from completing Stage One in Season 9! The Flying Squirrel, which first appeared in Season 8, challenges competitors to jump 11 feet from a mini-tramp to two separate handles that swing independently of each other, similar to The Clacker. Athletes must then lache to another set of handles, which are also 11 feet away, before lacheing 10 feet to a Cargo Net, which they must climb to clear Stage One.

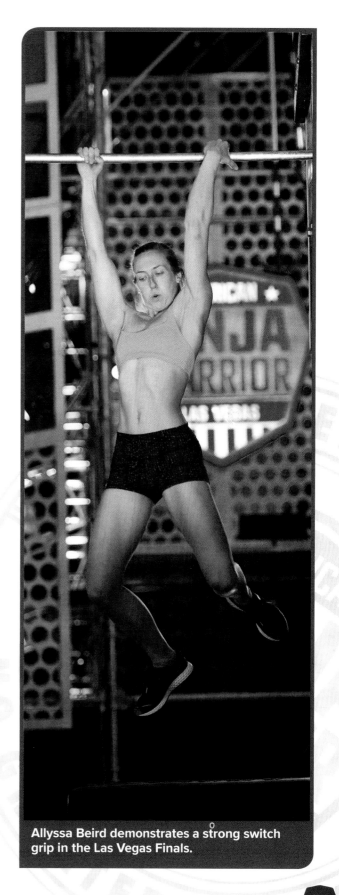

Allyssa Beird demonstrates a strong switch grip in the Las Vegas Finals.

FLYING SHELF GRAB

The Flying Shelf Grab first appeared as the eighth obstacle in the Kansas City Finals of Season 7—knocking out veteran ninja Jon Stewart—and held the same position in Season 8 in Philadelphia. The Flying Shelf Grab challenges competitors' upper-body and grip strength and consists of two suspended shelves with narrow 3-inch ledges. Ninjas must swing to the first shelf and then the second, which is 8 feet away, before lacheing to a landing mat.

FRAME SLIDER

Appearing in Los Angeles during Season 5, the Frame Slider challenges ninjas to wedge themselves inside a hanging frame and then slide down a track with both a drop and a sudden stop at the end. Most ninjas, including Jessie Graff, who that season became the first woman to advance past a Qualifying round, didn't get hung up on the Frame Slider and completed it with ease.

G-ROPE

Making its first and only appearance on Season 1 as the second half of Stage Four, G-Rope was a grand finale 10-meter rope climb, at the end of which was the final buzzer and Total Victory.

GIANT CYCLE

The Giant Cycle, a hybrid of the Giant Swing and Cycle Road, made its debut in Stage One during

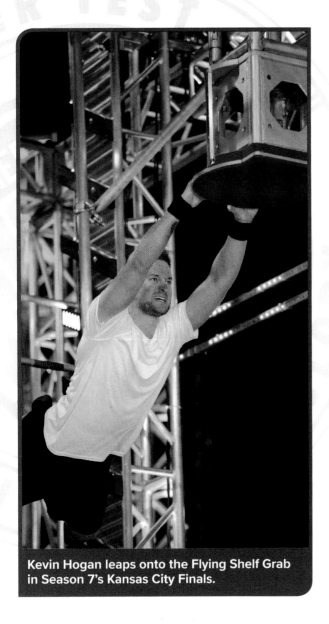

Kevin Hogan leaps onto the Flying Shelf Grab in Season 7's Kansas City Finals.

NINJA KILLER

GIANT CUBES

The Giant Cubes hung up quite a few ninjas when it made its debut in Season 9 during the Daytona Beach Finals. (Host Akbar Gbajabiamila said that the Cubes were "more like Rubik's Cubes," because ninjas were having trouble figuring them out!) This obstacle requires some rock climbing and a bit of parkour leaping—and, in the case of Jessie Graff, a little gymnastic ingenuity. Ninjas traverse down a slanted pole coming directly from the Salmon Ladder and transition onto the first of two Giant Cubes with three Cliffhanger-esque ledges. Athletes have to traverse the cube and then position themselves to leap to a second cube, which they also have to traverse before leaping to safety on a landing mat.

Season 5. The Giant Cycle requires ninjas to jump off a trampoline and use their upper body to grab onto a large wheel, which spins. Athletes then use the momentum from their swing to dismount to a landing pad. (In Season 6, it was renamed the Giant Ring, but still had the same function.) The obstacle didn't pose much of a problem for ninjas such as "The Weatherman" Joe Moravsky and "The Godfather" David Campbell, although a bit of showboating almost cost Campbell completion of the obstacle.

GIANT LOG GRIP
(SEE LOG GRIP)

GIANT RING
(SEE GIANT CYCLE)

GIANT SWING
The Giant Swing appeared in Stage One of Seasons 2 through 4. The concept is simple: Competitors had to jump from a springboard to a giant bar that swings to a net, much like a trapeze. The obstacle posed little trouble for ninjas such as "Real Life Ninja" Drew Drechsel who sailed through it easily.

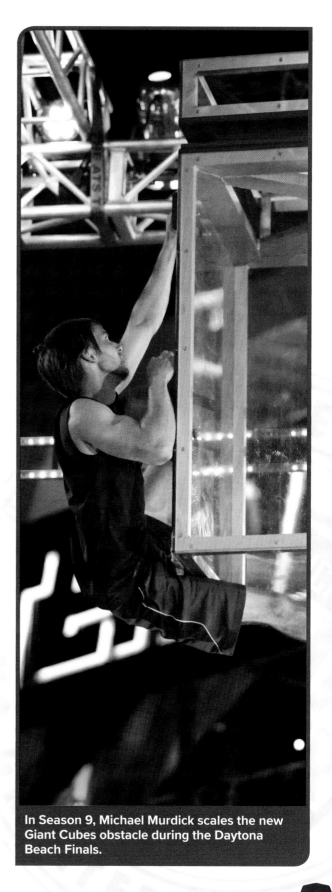

In Season 9, Michael Murdick scales the new Giant Cubes obstacle during the Daytona Beach Finals.

GIANT RING SWING
(SEE RING SWING)

GLIDING RING

The completion rules for the Gliding Ring—which appeared only once, as the final obstacle of Stage Three in Season 1—are pretty straightforward, as with many of the earlier *American Ninja Warrior* obstacles. Competitors are tasked with using their upper body to push a ring down a track to the end position and then swinging off onto a finishing platform.

GLOBE GRASPER

Ninjas had the whole world in their hands when they took on the Globe Grasper, also referred to as the Lamp Grasper, which is a grip-strength gauntlet. The obstacle popped up in several seasons of *American Ninja Warrior*, including Seasons 4 and 7. To successfully complete the Globe Grasper, competitors have to grab onto a series of small spheres attached to scaffolding/poles and work their way across until they can dismount. (A version of this obstacle, Descending Lamp Grasper, appeared in Season 1's Stage Three.)

GRIP HANG

The Grip Hang taxed not only ninjas' grip strength but core strength when it made its only appearance on *American Ninja Warrior* in Denver during Season 5. The obstacle challenges competitors to use their upper body to traverse a series of hanging curved mechanisms and also to transition between them. Although the Grip Hang's wide width makes hanging on a challenge, the obstacle proved to be no match for athletes such as Brian Arnold and Isaac Caldiero, who made it through with no problem.

HALF-PIPE ATTACK

A staple of the Stage One Finals from Seasons 1 to 6, Half-Pipe Attack challenges competitors to run across a vertical half-pipe and then make a leap onto a rope that swings them onto a narrow landing pad. *American Ninja Warrior* fans may remember

WARRIOR WORDS

LAST MAN STANDING: A competitor who has made it farther than any other competitor on a season of *American Ninja Warrior* when no one has achieved Total Victory.

that "Real Life Ninja" Drew Drechsel injured his knee on the Half-Pipe Attack in Season 3. The following year, the obstacle took out JJ Woods, who grasped the rope too low, causing his feet to graze the water and ending his run.

HANG CLIMB

Hang Climb is perhaps best known as the obstacle that took down "Real Life Ninja" Drew Drechsel in Stage Three in back-to-back seasons (Seasons 7 and 8) of *American Ninja Warrior*. (In 2017, Drechsel did go on to conquer the obstacle in *American Ninja Warrior: USA vs. The World*.) Hang Climb consists of an angled wall with only small handholds to grab onto. It is one of the few Stage Three obstacles that allows ninjas to use their lower body.

HANG GLIDER

Hang Glider premiered in Kansas City during *American Ninja Warrior*'s Season 9. There are two components to this obstacle: First, competitors have to grab onto two hanging handles connected to a ring that slides down a track with two drops. At the bottom of the track, athletes need to swing their legs to latch onto a suspended pipe, which they have to grab hold of before swinging to a platform. The Hang Glider took out a solid 13 ninjas in the Qualifiers, about 10 percent of all competitors.

HAZARD SWING

The Hazard Swing made its only appearance on *American Ninja Warrior* in the second position of Stage One during Season 2. It requires competitors to stand on a swing, on which they have to use their body momentum to swing onto a high platform.

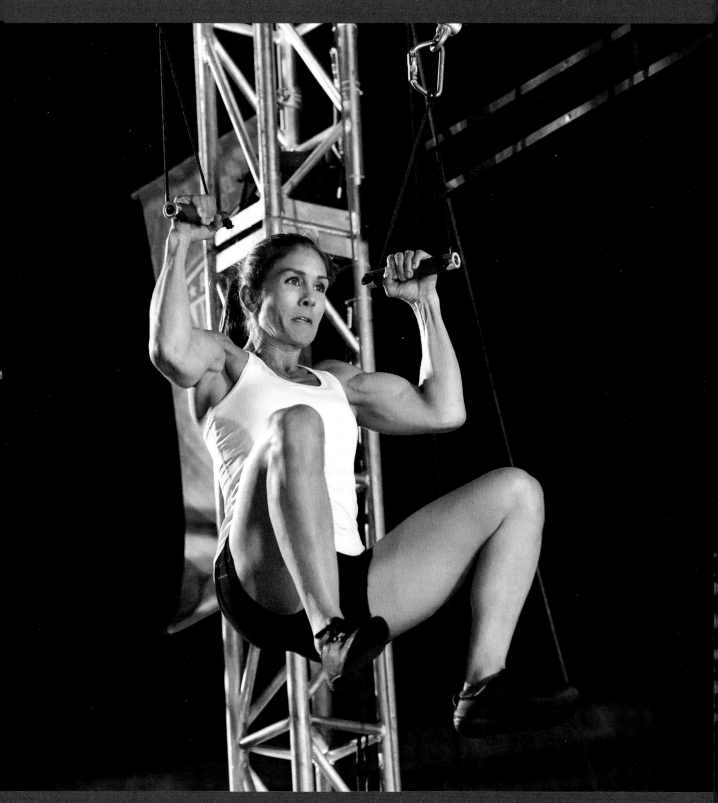

Abby Paul takes on the first challenge of the Hang Glider obstacle during the Season 9 Kansas City Finals.

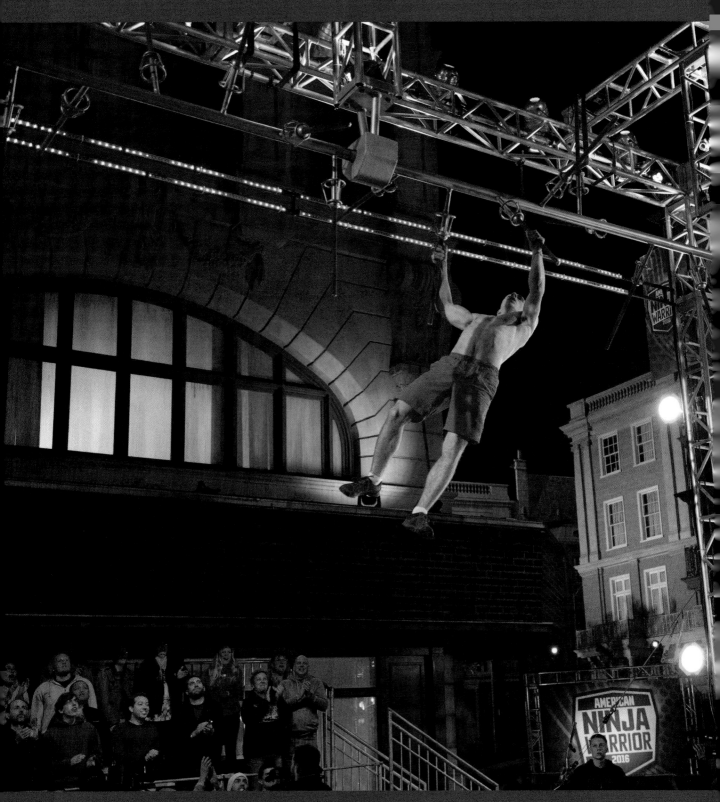

Josh Levin holds on tight to the Helix Hang during the Los Angeles Finals in Season 8.

Once there, they can use a bar to pull themselves up to a landing mat.

HEAVENLY LADDER

The Heavenly Ladder made its only appearance on *American Ninja Warrior* in Stage Four of Season 1. The obstacle consists of a 13-meter rope ladder that forms the first half of that Final Stage; the second half is the G-Rope. The following season, the Heavenly Ladder and G-Rope would merge into the Rope Climb, which would become the final obstacle for the rest of the series.

HELIX HANG

The Helix Hang made its debut in the Orlando Finals of Season 7. The obstacle consists of two center axes, one after the other, each with rods sticking out of them forming two helices. Competitors must traverse the first helix's rods with their hands, causing it to turn counterclockwise. Then they must transfer to the second helix and traverse its rods, causing it to turn clockwise, until they are close enough to jump to a landing mat. During the Orlando Finals, seven competitors attempted the Double Helix Hang and five completed it, including "Real Life Ninja" Drew Drechsel, James "The Beast" McGrath, and Flip Rodriguez.

I-BEAM CROSS

Josh Levin showed some smooth moves on the I-Beam Cross when he completed the obstacle—feet first—in the Los Angeles Finals during Season 8. I-Beam Cross, which first appeared in San Pedro in Season 7, consists of an angled beam, similar to the Spider Flip. Competitors have to traverse the beam from underneath, using their arms and legs, but their grip strength is critical because the beam's ledges vary in width—in Season 8, a small part of the beam had no ledges at all! The beam also gets a little tricky near the middle where it shifts 90 degrees, going vertical and challenging ninjas to adjust their body position in order to fight gravity.

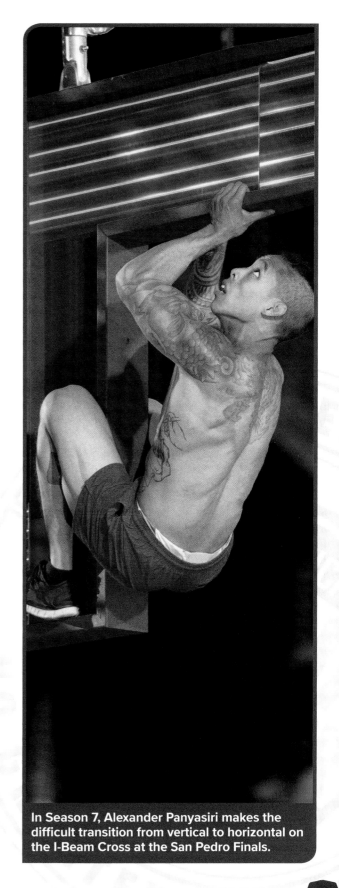

In Season 7, Alexander Panyasiri makes the difficult transition from vertical to horizontal on the I-Beam Cross at the San Pedro Finals.

NINJA KILLER

HOURGLASS DROP

One of "SheWolf" Meagan Martin's favorite obstacles, the Hourglass Drop had a pretty impressive knockout rate when it first appeared in Season 7's Los Angeles Qualifying course, making it one of the biggest ninja killers in *American Ninja Warrior* history. The obstacle features two consecutive hanging planks that wobble. Using their hands, competitors have to traverse the first plank, drop onto a mini-tramp, grab onto the second, and traverse that one just like the first. Many competitors not only found it hard to get bounce from the mini-tramp but were even disqualified for getting to the landing without grabbing the second plank. (The Hourglass Drop appeared again in Seasons 8 and 9 with slight modifications.) The Hourglass Drop took out Jessie Graff in the Qualifying round, but Graff came back strong in the City Finals, exhibiting perfect technique to beat the obstacle the second time around.

There are some obstacles that are uniquely challenging. I think of the Hourglass Drop with the supertramp. That may have been the most unforgiving obstacle we've ever had.

–Host Matt Iseman

The Hourglass Drop is my favorite. It requires a great amount of precision, aerial control, and strength, and it is just very exciting.

–Kevin Bull

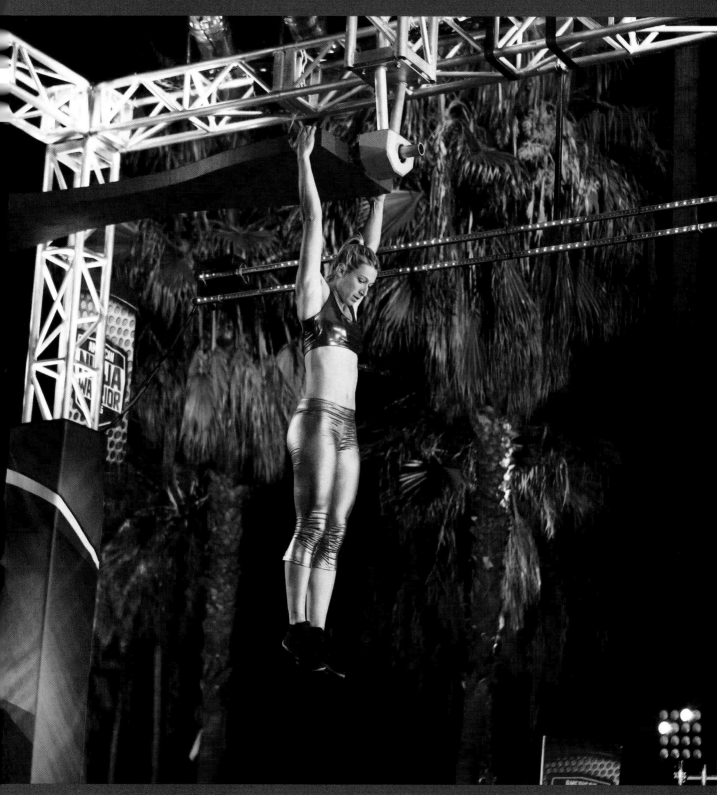

Jessie Graff prepares her fall onto the mini-tramp as part of the Hourglass Drop in Los Angeles during Season 7.

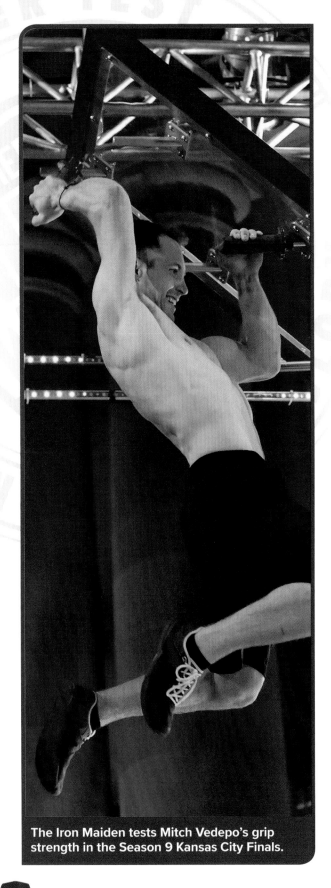

The Iron Maiden tests Mitch Vedepo's grip strength in the Season 9 Kansas City Finals.

I-BEAM GAP

As if the I-Beam Cross weren't difficult enough, an upgraded version called the I-Beam Gap premiered in the Cleveland Qualifying round of Season 9. As with the I-Beam Cross, ninjas have to traverse a horizontal—and then vertical—beam using their arms and legs. However, next they have to perform a 180-degree jump onto another beam, which they have to climb down and across in order to dismount. Fifteen competitors were able to complete this obstacle during the Cleveland Qualifiers, including Jesse Labreck and Allyssa Beird.

INVISIBLE LADDER

The Invisible Ladder did some visible damage to ninjas when it appeared in Seasons 7 and 8 as the final obstacle in every City Finals course, replacing the Spider Climb from the previous two seasons. The obstacle features two hanging rings in a 30-foot chute. Ninjas have to hold one ring in each hand and pump their arms upward, as if climbing an invisible ladder, all the way up the chute—a brutal challenge, especially coming off the upper-body-intensive Back Half. In Season 7, the Invisible Ladder took out veterans such as Ryan Stratis, "Real Life Ninja" Drew Drechsel, Kevin Bull, "The Godfather" David Campbell, and Flip Rodriguez, who managed to get one of his feet onto the finishing platform before his arms gave out in an anguishing fall.

IRON MAIDEN

Making its debut at Position Nine at the Kansas City Finals in Season 9, the Iron Maiden became one of the newest ninja torture devices. Consisting of three inclined reverse pegboards, the Iron Maiden was designed by longtime *American Ninja Warrior* competitor and one of the Obstacle Design Challenge winners Brett Sims. It requires ninjas to make their way down the first, then up the second, and back down the third pegboard before dismounting onto a platform. What makes this obstacle unique is that instead of inserting pegs, ninjas have to pull out hollow sleeves that have to be accurately replaced on peg-shaped spikes as they make their way

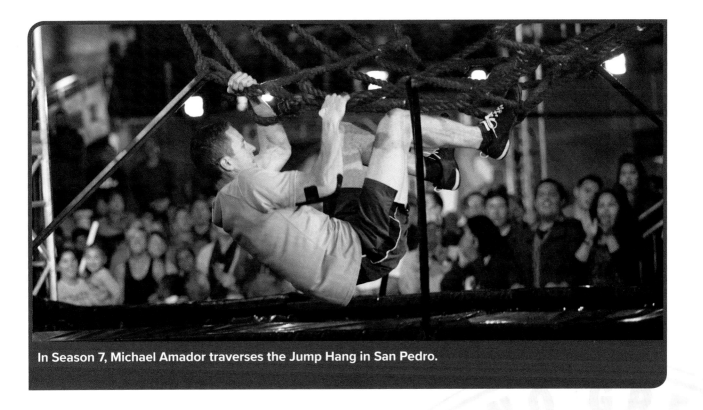

In Season 7, Michael Amador traverses the Jump Hang in San Pedro.

down the first and third panels. Precision is crucial. Show executives were really getting medieval on ninjas with this one!

JUMP HANG

The Jump Hang has hung around quite a bit on *American Ninja Warrior* over the years. It appeared as the fourth obstacle in Season 3, in every regional Qualifying round of Season 4, in Season 6's Miami rounds, and also as the second obstacle in San Pedro during Season 7. To complete this obstacle, ninjas have to leap off a tramp in order to grasp the underside of a cargo net, which they have to traverse to get to a landing platform. Fans may remember that in Miami Flip Rodriguez failed the obstacle when his body grazed the water while he maneuvered across the cargo net. However, the setback would only set the stage for Rodriguez's triumphant comeback in seasons to follow.

JUMP HANG KAI

A lot of obstacles on *American Ninja Warrior* feature cargo nets. This one is nothing but net.

Appearing in Denver during Season 5, Jump Hang Kai features two cargo nets—one on the left, one on the right, with a space between them. To complete the obstacle, ninjas have to climb through the two nets, which aren't taut; therefore, speed and a straightforward direction are paramount to success.

JUMPING BARS

This obstacle may bring back memories of childhood playground days! To complete the Jumping Bars, ninjas simply have to swing, or lache, from one bar to another. Seems simple enough, but as with so many other obstacles, the show ingeniously makes it a little more challenging season by season-- because ninjas are smart, and when one sees how to conquer an obstacle, many other ninjas soon can do it, too. When this obstacle appeared in Seasons 1, 2, 3, and 4, there was a trampoline at the starting platform. When it made a return in Los Angeles during Season 6, the obstacle was combined with the Cargo Net to create a hybrid called the Jumping Bars into Cargo Net—ninjas had the added challenge of traversing a cargo net to reach a landing platform.

JUMPING RINGS

The Jumping Rings, a *SASUKE* obstacle, appeared only in Stage Three of Season 3. Competitors have to jump across two rings and then use their feet to help grab a ladder to assist in getting to the next obstacle. The obstacle had a 100 percent completion rate.

KEY LOCK HANG

Who knew picking a lock would come in handy on the course? Key Lock Hang, which appeared in Stage Three in Seasons 8 and 9, challenges ninjas to traverse a series of panels by inserting "keys" into locks. Ninjas often employ what's called the "Vulcan" here—putting the handles between their middle and ring fingers, which helps them secure grip strength. Fans may remember that Najee Richardson fell from his dismount on this obstacle in Season 9, but was able to recover by grabbing onto the landing mat and pulling himself to safety.

LAMP GRASPER
(SEE GLOBE GRASPER)

LEDGE JUMP

The Ledge Jump made only one appearance on *American Ninja Warrior*, in Season 5's Miami Finals. The obstacle, positioned just after the Salmon Ladder, consists of three hanging boards, each with a bottom ledge that gets smaller—from 3 inches to

WARRIOR WORDS

SUPERTRAMP: The hyper-responsive, oversized trampoline that stretches the width of an obstacle, such as the Hourglass Drop, to launch athletes up when necessary to traverse an obstacle.

1 inch—as ninjas transition from board to board. Ninjas have to traverse each board consecutively before jumping to a landing platform. Ninjas such as Ryan Stratis and Travis Rosen were able to complete the obstacle with relative ease.

LOG GRIP

For the Log Grip, which made its debut in the Qualifiers in Season 3, athletes cling onto a large vertical log with their arms and legs for 25 feet as it slides down a track. The log contains small indentations to provide some grip assistance (in later seasons, it was modified with handles instead of holes). An intimidating Giant Log Grip appeared in Stage One of Season 8 and gave ninjas a wild ride, banging its way down a 52-foot-long track and requiring a precision dismount onto a small landing pad floating in the water. Competitors have to time their landing correctly to keep from getting wet.

NINJA KILLER

JUMPING SPIDER

"SheWolf" Meagan Martin made *American Ninja Warrior* history in Season 6 when she became the first woman ever to complete the brutal Jumping Spider, one of the direct imports from *SASUKE* and a mainstay of *American Ninja Warrior*, appearing consistently in Stage One of the National Finals. To complete this obstacle, ninjas, after a running start, jump from a mini-tramp straight up between two parallel walls. Once they find a grip on this Spider Walk portion of the obstacle, they travel forward until they reach the end of the obstacle and drop down onto a landing mat (a modified version, the Bouncing Spider, appeared in Season 9). Fans may remember it was the Jumping Spider that took out "Mighty" Kacy Catanzaro in the Season 6 National Finals, ending her inspiring run.

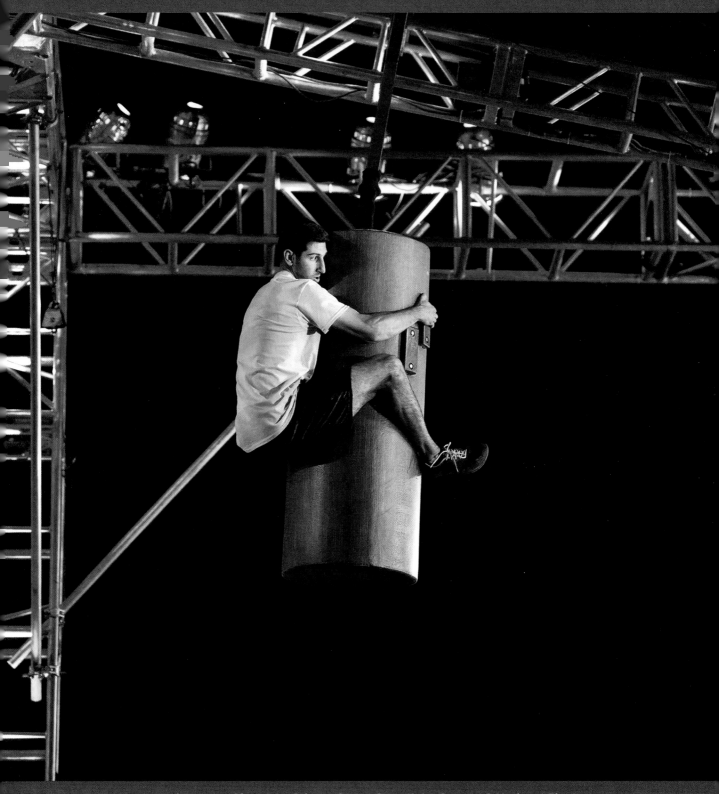

Anthony DeFranco locks in on the Giant Log Grip on Stage One of the Season 8 National Finals.

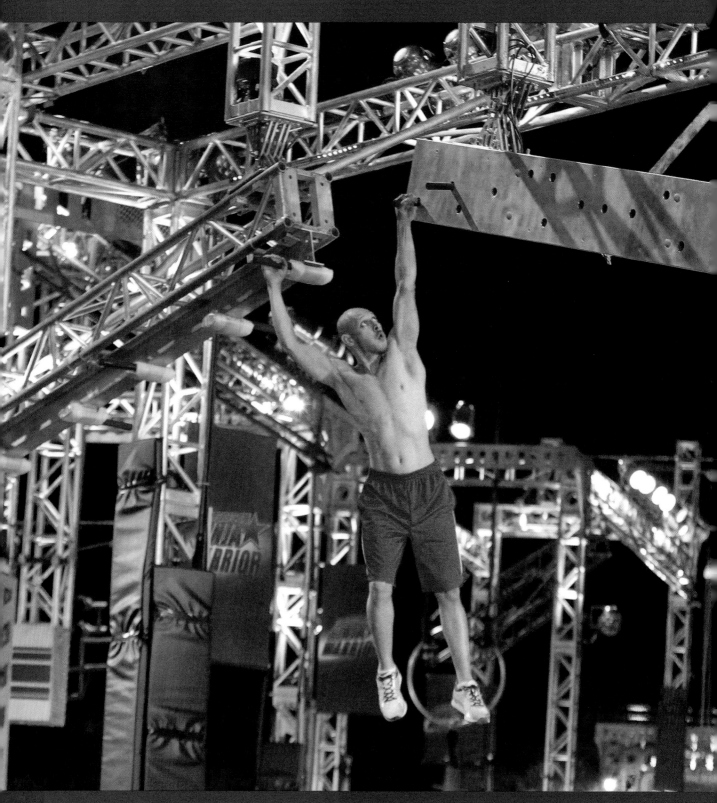

Edgardo Osorio takes on the Monkey Peg in Miami during Season 5.

180 ROTATION: Facing one direction and then, when transitioning on an obstacle, flipping your body with a spinning, 180-degree jump. This technique is often employed for obstacles such as the Giant Cubes or the Ledge Jump.

LOG RUNNER

The Log Runner first appeared in the San Pedro Qualifying round of Season 7. It consists of four free-spinning logs—four feet from one another—that competitors have to run across, using their agility and balance. In Season 8, the obstacle came back with a vengeance in the Oklahoma City Qualifiers, featuring five logs instead of four. This time around, there was also a consistent difference in elevation among the logs; however, the fourth log was level with the third, which tripped up some of the ninjas. It was on that fourth log that "Cowboy Ninja" Lance Pekus lost his balance, causing him to crash into the final log and then fall into the water.

METAL SPIN

Resembling both a chandelier and a jellyfish, Metal Spin features an array of chains that dangle from a horizontal wheel that spins. To complete the obstacle, ninjas must jump to grasp one of the chains, spinning the wheel so they can dismount on the other side. This obstacle was used in Stage Two on the first six seasons of *American Ninja Warrior*. Fans may remember "The Weatherman" Joe Moravsky breezing through this obstacle on his way to completing Stage Two in Season 5, his rookie year! Fans may also recall Sean McColl's miraculous diving dismount on the Metal Spin during his first run on a ninja course in *USA vs. The World*.

MINEFIELD

The Minefield was the eighth obstacle in the Miami Finals of Season 6. Ninjas have to hang from any of 12 dangling shape-grips—eight cannonballs, two nunchucks, and two cones—to swing across to a landing pad. It's important that they stay in control of their swing. JJ Woods got a little hung up at the end of the obstacle and had trouble sticking his landing but was able to complete it.

MINI SILK SLIDER
(SEE SILK SLIDER)

MONKEY PEG

The Monkey Peg first appeared in Miami in Season 5 and returned for the Los Angeles rounds of Season 6. It consists of two sections: the first features pegs on an upwardly slanted wall that ninjas must swing across like monkey bars, and

NINJA KILLER

NAIL CLIPPER

The Nail Clipper cut off a whopping 20 ninjas before they could finish the course when it made its debut at the Cleveland Finals in Season 9 (it returned for Stage Three). Designed by Calvin Boyce, a 16-year-old fan from Provo, Utah, the Nail Clipper challenges athletes to get across four horizontal cylinders with rows of short ledges, a feat that requires tremendous grip strength. And because the Nail Clipper took the grueling eighth position, right after the Salmon Ladder, it proved to be too much for most of the Finals' ninjas, whose runs were clipped short. Only two—"The Weatherman" Joe Moravsky and "Captain NBC" Jamie Rahn—were able to complete this daunting obstacle.

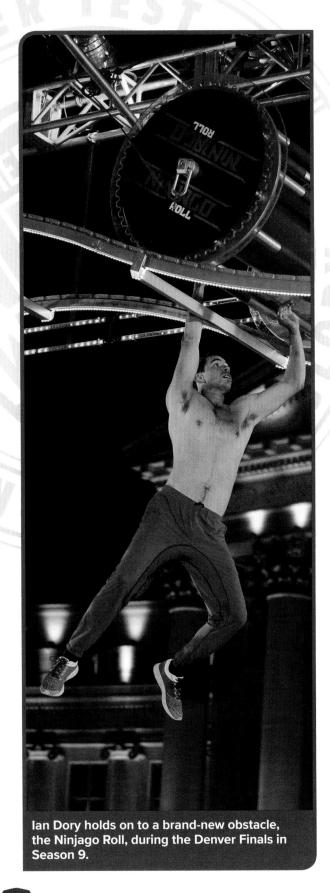

Ian Dory holds on to a brand-new obstacle, the Ninjago Roll, during the Denver Finals in Season 9.

the second section has a pegboard on a downward slant that they traverse toward a landing mat. "Real Life Ninja" Drew Drechsel blew through the Monkey Peg in the Season 5 Miami Qualifiers on his way to annihilating the course.

MONKEY PEGS

What a difference one little letter makes! A modified version of the Monkey Peg, called the Monkey Pegs, appeared in the San Pedro Qualifying round of Season 7. It consists of an arched board with two sections like its predecessor, but instead of the pegs in the first section extending from both sides of the wall, they are all on one side.

NINJAGO ROLL

American Ninja Warrior partnered with Warner Bros. and *The Lego Ninjago Movie* for the Ninjago Roll obstacle, which took the ninth position in the Denver Finals in Season 9. Ninjas have to hang from a giant 150-pound cylinder and use their hands to roll it up and down a track. This obstacle idea came from the 2016 Obstacle Design Challenge and was inspired by 11-year-old fan Josephine Starr Stevenson.

PADDLE BOARDS

Some ninjas are board to run! The Paddle Boards obstacle made its debut in the Orlando Qualifying round of Season 7 and returned in Season 8's Philly and Season 9's Denver courses. It consists of six (eight in Denver) paddles that are supported by a center axis. Competitors have to maintain their balance while running across the paddles, without touching the center axis. Fans may recall in Season 9's Denver Finals that veteran ninja Sam Sann was disqualified on the Paddle Boards when he stepped on the center beam.

PARKOUR RUN

This obstacle made its debut in Stage One of the Season 9 National Finals. Parkour Run is similar to Season 8's Sonic Curve in that athletes run along a series of angled tiles—here there are five—arranged in a semicircle before jumping to a rope and swinging to a landing platform. However, in Parkour Run the fourth tile is flipped, switching competitors' momentum. Fans may remember Jesse "Flex" Labreck got a bit hung up on this obstacle, which ate up a lot of her time, forcing her to rush through the rest of the course and resulting in her eventual fall on the Flying Squirrel.

PEG CLOUD

Peg Cloud was anything but heavenly when it appeared on Stage Three in Season 9. The new obstacle challenges ninjas to traverse a series of downward beams using footholds and removable pegs that athletes need to take along with them as they maneuver through the obstacle. "The Weatherman" Joe Moravsky was the only ninja to take on the Peg Cloud, and while it gave him some trouble, he emerged victorious. Peg Cloud would be the last obstacle Moravsky completed before he became Last Man Standing in Season 9.

PIPE FITTER

Pipe Fitter, introduced in Season 8, was inspired by the historic Carrie Furnace, a former blast furnace located in the Pittsburgh-area industrial town of Swissvale, Pennsylvania—the town that served as the backdrop for Season 7's Pittsburgh rounds. Pipe Fitter consists of several pipes: Ninjas have to shinny up the first pipe to transition to two smaller hanging pipes, one after the other. The key is to wrap both of their arms—not just their hands— around the pipes. They then have to grab hold of another pipe to dismount. Ninjas weren't allowed to use their lower body on the two hanging pipes—nor for Season 9, on the final pipe.

PIPE SLIDER

A longtime *SASUKE* obstacle, the Pipe Slider appeared in the very first season of *American Ninja Warrior* and also in the Northwest Qualifier of Season 4. To complete this obstacle, ninjas have to hang from a metal bar, sliding it across a track with several drops. Although Pipe Slider didn't appear again after Season 4, its influence can be seen in many of the show's track-oriented obstacles.

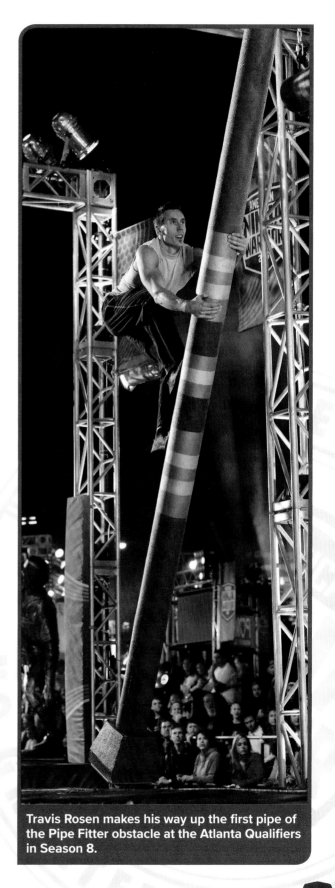

Travis Rosen makes his way up the first pipe of the Pipe Fitter obstacle at the Atlanta Qualifiers in Season 8.

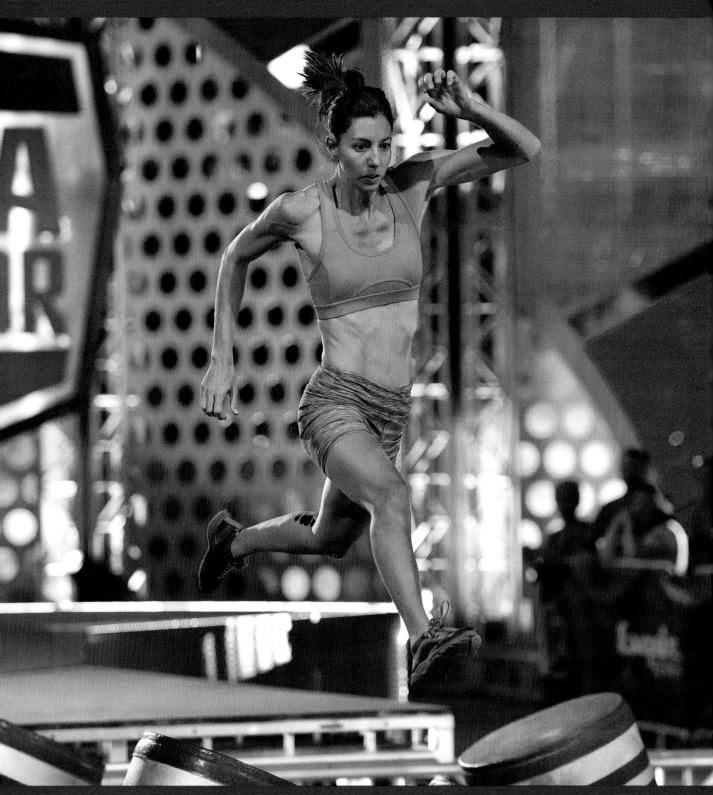

Marybeth Wang shows her agility on Piston Road during Stage One of the Season 7 National Finals.

PISTON ROAD

Appearing as the first obstacle of Stage One in Season 6 and returning in Season 7, Piston Road consists of six tilted cylinders. Ninjas must jump from one piston to the other to clear the obstacle. Piston Road had a high completion rate and was replaced by Snake Run in Season 8.

POLE GRASPER

Fans got their first look at Pole Grasper in the Denver Finals in Season 5 and then again in the Dallas Finals in Season 6. To complete this obstacle, ninjas have to traverse five suspended poles using their hands and feet. Pole Grasper became the first obstacle from a city course to be used in Vegas when it appeared as the fifth obstacle in Stage Three of the National Finals in Season 7. But there was one change . . . one of the poles was suspended from a bungee cord!

PRISM TILT

First seen in *American Ninja Warrior* during the Baltimore Qualifiers of Season 5, the Prism Tilt is made up of a triangular prism that's on an axis, allowing it to spin. Athletes have to jump onto the prism and then scramble to the other side before it tips over. Ninjas such as "Captain NBC" Jamie Rahn used their own body weight to counter-balance the prism, allowing them to successfully complete the obstacle.

PROPELLER BAR

A variation of *SASUKE*'s Propeller Untei, Propeller Bar first appeared on Season 6 and consists of one wooden propeller that spins freely. Ninjas have to jump off a mini-tramp, grab the propeller, spin around, and then grab a rope before transitioning to the Hang Climb. The obstacle returned in Seasons 7, 8, and 9 as the second obstacle of Stage One, with ninjas having the added challenge of landing on a sloped platform that they must climb to complete the obstacle. The Propeller Bar has taken out a lot of top competitors, including Allyssa Beird in Season 8. Fans may remember that "SheWolf" Meagan Martin got hung up on the Propeller Bar in

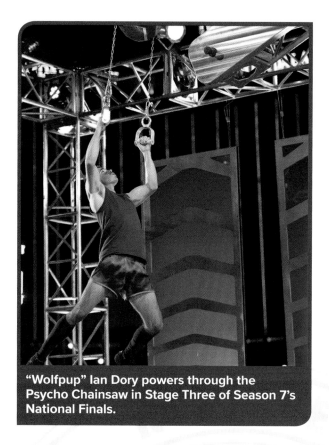

"Wolfpup" Ian Dory powers through the Psycho Chainsaw in Stage Three of Season 7's National Finals.

Season 9, and although she managed to complete the obstacle, it sapped a lot of her time, and she eventually timed out.

PSYCHO CHAINSAW

The Psycho Chainsaw was the first obstacle in Season 7's Stage Three of the National Finals. Competitors have to grab two chains and pump their arms up and down, resembling the motion of a chainsaw, in order to move a large disk looming over them down a track. Despite its horror-movie name, Psycho Chainsaw had a 100 percent completion rate—all eight athletes who attempted it were able to clear it.

QUAD STEPS

A classic *American Ninja Warrior* obstacle, the Quad Steps served as the gateway to the obstacle course in Seasons 2, 3, and 4. Consisting of four angled steps, the Quad Steps was retired for Season 5, replaced by the Quintuple Steps (see page 104).

QUINTUPLE STEPS

The Quintuple Steps appeared as the first obstacle in the Qualifying round of Season 1 and then again as the first obstacle in Seasons 5, 6, and 7. The Quintuple Steps consists of angled steps like its predecessor, the Quad Steps (see page 103), only with farther spacing, an extra step, and a slightly different design. While ninjas often cleared both the Quad Steps and Quintuple Steps with ease, these obstacles were easy to underestimate, which could lead to sloppy mistakes that landed competitors in the water. In Season 6's Denver Qualifiers, "Ninjadoc" Noah Kaufman had a tiny slip on the last Quintuple Step that turned into a near fall into the water on the final sloped landing platform, but he was able to recover.

RAZOR'S EDGE

Razor's Edge made its first appearance in Cleveland during Season 9. To complete the obstacle, competitors have to sprint across the tops of three unstable vertical boards—that can tilt left or right, depending on the ninjas' footwork and weight distribution—until they reach the landing platform. The Razor's Edge cut out 19 ninjas in the Qualifiers and three in the City Finals.

RING JUMP

The Ring Jump made its *American Ninja Warrior* debut in Season 8's Los Angeles rounds (it appeared again in Cleveland during Season 9). Using their upper body, competitors have to move rings across two slanted beams—the first beam slants up, while the second slants down—that feature pegs of various heights. Fans may remember Natalie Duran's left foot was just inches away from touching the water during her dismount from the Ring Jump in Season 8, but Duran completed the obstacle successfully.

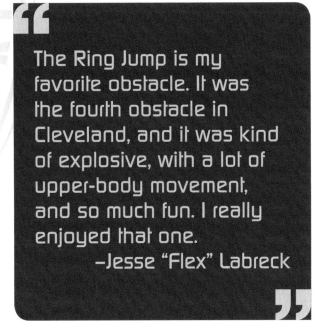

The Ring Jump is my favorite obstacle. It was the fourth obstacle in Cleveland, and it was kind of explosive, with a lot of upper-body movement, and so much fun. I really enjoyed that one.

—Jesse "Flex" Labreck

NINJA KILLER

RAIL RUNNER

One of the newest and deadliest obstacles on *American Ninja Warrior*, the Rail Runner made its debut in Season 9 as the fifth obstacle of the Denver Qualifiers. To complete the obstacle, athletes have to slide a pair of handles, resembling an upside-down bicycle handlebar, across an 11-foot track and then make a 3-foot transition to grab onto a pair of perpendicular handles, which they have to slide along a second 11-foot track. A total of 24 competitors, including "SheWolf" Meagan Martin, Sam Sann, and Brian Arnold (who broke his nose making the transition to the second set of handles), failed to complete this obstacle. This set records for the second lowest number of finishers in an *American Ninja Warrior* Qualifying course as well as the second lowest number of finishers in a Qualifying obstacle, behind the Hourglass Drop in Season 7.

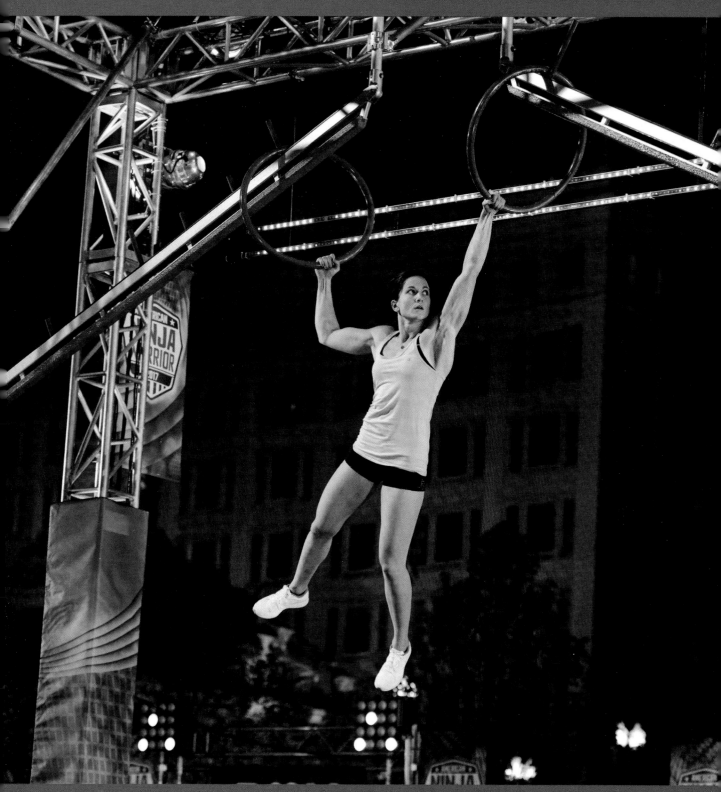

Jesse "Flex" Labreck demonstrates her powerful upper body on the Ring Jump in the Season 9 Cleveland Qualifiers.

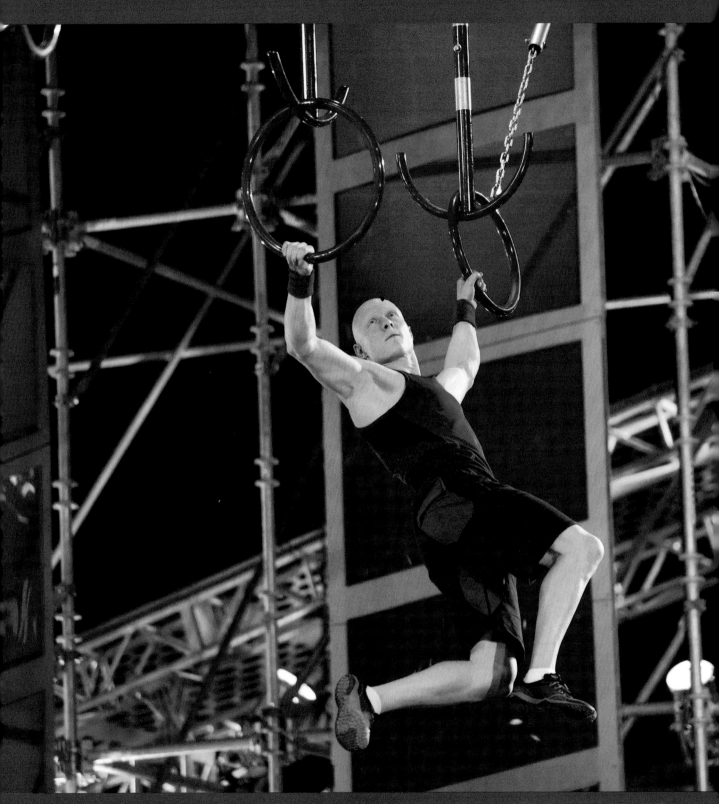

Kevin Bull takes on a super-sized Ring Swing—called the Giant Ring Swing—in Stage Two of the Season 9 National Finals.

RING SWING

The Ring Swing first appeared in Season 8's Oklahoma City Qualifiers. To complete the obstacle, athletes have to grab a ring, swing it to a post, and lock it on. Then they have to transition to a second ring, hop it over a post, and swing to a landing platform. Fans may remember Old Man Brent Steffensen getting a little hung up on the Ring Swing during the Qualifiers before completeing the obstacle on his way to finishing the course. The Ring Swing returned bigger and better as a Giant Ring Swing in Stage Two of the National Finals in Seasons 8 and 9.

RING TOSS

The Ring Toss premiered in the Dallas Qualifiers in Season 6 and consists of three sections of pegs and two rings. To complete the obstacle, ninjas have to use the rings to traverse the pegs. It was right after "Mighty" Kacy Catanzaro completed the Ring Toss in her history-making Dallas Finals run that host Akbar Gbajabiamila exclaimed, "Somebody call security, because this girl is going to need a bodyguard. She is a superstar!"

ROLLING ESCARGOT

The Rolling Escargot appeared early on in *American Ninja Warrior*, in Stage One of Seasons 2 and 3. To complete this obstacle, athletes have to latch on to a giant disc—that they must face—by holding on to handles and jamming their feet into toe clips. They have to hang on tight while the disk starts rolling down a track—turning them into a human wheel!

ROLLING LOG

Fans may remember quick-moving Lorin Ball made a shocking exit when he fell off the Rolling Log during the Indianapolis Finals in Season 8. The Rolling Log has appeared in six seasons of *American Ninja Warrior* and challenges athletes to wrap themselves around a horizontal log and hang on as it spins down a track, building speed and torque. The key to surviving this daunting obstacle is for ninjas to lock in with their body—using their hands and ankles, if they can—and then simply to hold on tight!

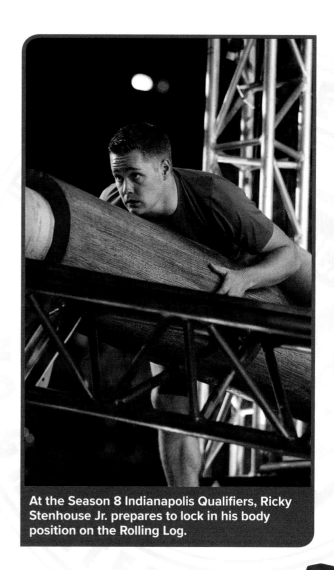

At the Season 8 Indianapolis Qualifiers, Ricky Stenhouse Jr. prepares to lock in his body position on the Rolling Log.

ROLLING PIN

Ninjas have to lock in their grip to complete the Rolling Pin, which first appeared on Season 9 in Daytona. Two red cylinders circle a bar (kind of like toilet paper) on a swing-like contraption, and ninjas have to use their upper body to hold on as it travels down two uneven tracks with sudden jolts.

ROLLING STEEL

Rolling Steel made its only appearance in Season 5's Miami Finals and looked like a cross between a pull-up bar and the Arm Bike. To complete the obstacle, athletes have to hold on to two handles and pedal across a track. Only two competitors failed this obstacle, while ninjas such as Travis Rosen and "Real Life Ninja" Drew Drechsel were able to complete it easily.

ROPE CLIMB

If there were a final frontier to *American Ninja Warrior*, it would be the Rope Climb, the last obstacle of Mount Midoriyama in Seasons 2 to 9. The Rope Climb is just that—a 75-foot rope climb that ninjas must complete in under 30 seconds. To date, every athlete has been chewed up and spit out

> Rolling Thunder from the Season 8 Philly Qualifiers was an incredibly hard obstacle. It was 30 moves, with just your arms. It also clattered all about and had drops that took out some great ninjas.
>
> —Geoff Britten

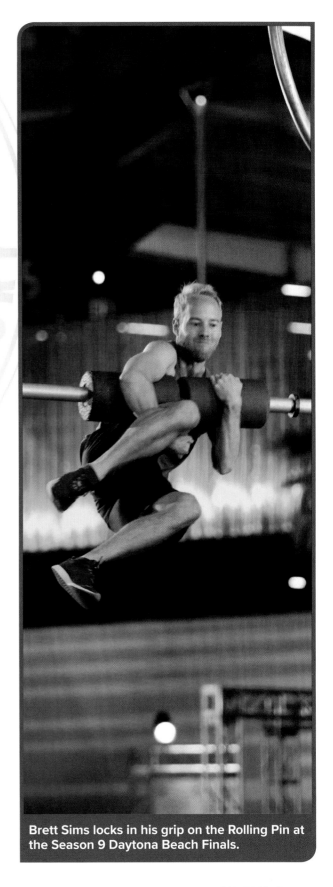

Brett Sims locks in his grip on the Rolling Pin at the Season 9 Daytona Beach Finals.

BECOME AN AMERICAN NINJA WARRIOR: THE ULTIMATE INSIDER'S GUIDE

NINJA KILLER

ROLLING THUNDER

In Season 8, when Rolling Thunder made its *American Ninja Warrior* debut at the Philadelphia Qualifying course, it had the second lowest completion percentage of any Qualifying obstacle (only Season 7's Hourglass Drop was lower). To complete this ninja killer, athletes have to hang from a giant wheel weighing 100 pounds and, using their upper body, roll it down a 25-foot track with two drops. After wreaking havoc in the Qualifiers, Rolling Thunder went on to take out eight ninjas, including Michelle Warnky, Allyssa Beird, and Chris DiGangi, in the Philly Finals.

by Mount Midoriyama except two—Geoff Britten and Isaac Caldiero, who have been the only ninjas to reach Stage Four's Rope Climb thus far. In Season 7, both successfully cleared the Rope Climb, Caldiero with the faster time.

> Rolling Thunder takes so many moves to complete, and you try to be in a lock off, but as soon as you lose that lock off and go to a straight arm, it gets really hard. The moves are super small. It really taxes your arms.
>
> —Jesse "Flex" Labreck

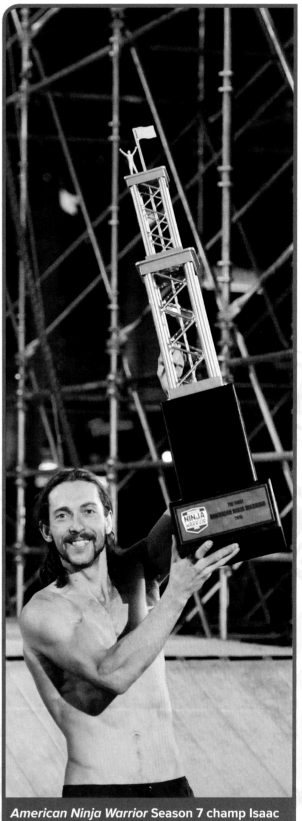

American Ninja Warrior Season 7 champ Isaac Caldiero holds up his trophy.

ROPE GLIDER

The Rope Glider made its only appearance on *American Ninja Warrior* during Stage One of the Vegas National Finals in Season 5. Fashioned like a zip line, the Rope Glider has competitors grab onto a rope and slide down a track, timing their dismount so that they land on a long mat floating in the water.

ROPE LADDER
(SEE CARGO CLIMB)

ROPE JUNCTION

Rock climbers tend to do well on Rope Junction, which first appeared on Season 4's Midsouth Qualifiers. The upper-body obstacle consists of six ropes, and ninjas have to traverse all six—Tarzan-style—in order to get to a landing mount to complete the obstacle.

ROPE JUNGLE

Like Rope Junction (above), Rope Jungle—which first appeared in Stage Two of Season 6—requires ninjas to traverse a series of ropes. What makes this obstacle challenging is that some of ropes are elasticized and some slide on tracks. Figuring out how best to maneuver through them can turn into a massive time waster and strength drainer, if ninjas aren't careful. Brian Arnold discovered just as much when he used a lot of time and upper-body strength to complete this obstacle in Season 6.

ROPE MAZE

The Rope Maze made its first and only appearance at the Los Angeles Finals of Season 5 (a round that, fans may remember, saw a chicken-outfitted Jessie Graff become the first j171
 ever to take on a City Final). Rope Maze challenges ninjas to hang from a rope and use their upper body to navigate it through a grid of piping track.

ROPE SWING

The Rope Swing that was featured during the Qualifiers of the first two seasons of *American Ninja Warrior* almost looks like child's play when compared to the other rope obstacles that would appear in later seasons. To complete this obstacle, competitors have to simply grab a rope and jump, like Tarzan, off a platform and land on the other side of the obstacle. In Season 6's St. Louis Qualifiers, the Rope Swing was modified into Rope Swing into Cargo Net. This version had ninjas jump from a tramp and then swing from two consecutive ropes into a cargo net.

ROTATING BRIDGE

No obstacle had taken out more athletes in Denver in Season 5 than the Rotating Bridge. That season, this balance obstacle—featuring three spinning rectangular cutouts along an axis—made its only appearance on *American Ninja Warrior*. Ninjas need both speed and balance to have success on the obstacle, as evidenced by Isaac Caldiero and Brian Arnold, who completed it with ease.

> "
> The challenge an obstacle poses always depends on the athlete facing it. What might be tough for a shorter gymnast could prove easy for a taller rock climber, and vice versa. The reality is, we never know how difficult an obstacle is until we see it in competition. But if there's one thing we've learned, it's that the ninjas will find a way.
> —Host Matt Iseman
> "

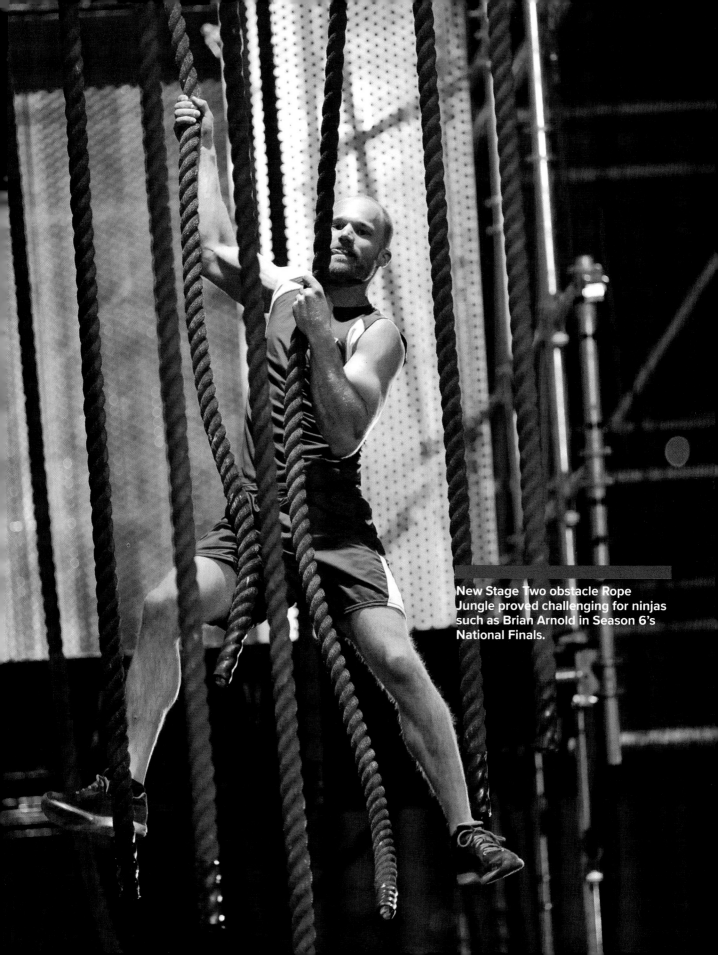

New Stage Two obstacle Rope Jungle proved challenging for ninjas such as Brian Arnold in Season 6's National Finals.

ROULETTE CYLINDER

The Roulette Cylinder was featured in Seasons 2, 4, and 5 as the first obstacle of Stage Three. It challenges competitors to negotiate a pronged cylinder (that resembles a large spool) down a pipe track using only their upper body. "The Weatherman" Joe Moravsky showed solid technique—arms at 90 degrees, eyes focused—when he completed the obstacle in Season 5.

ROULETTE ROW

Host Matt Iseman called Roulette Row the "make or break" obstacle when it appeared in Stage Two of Season 7 because ninjas only had one shot to complete it. After a running start to launch off a tramp, athletes have to use their arms and body momentum to quickly transition between two large Spin Cycles. Of the 20 competitors who attempted the obstacle, only eight completed it, including Geoff Britten and Isaac Caldiero, both of whom would go on to become American Ninja Warriors that season.

NINJA KNOW-HOW

When you pull up with your arms on the Salmon Ladder, drive up with your legs too. This engages your whole body in the movement. Use your abs to pull up your lower body and then your arms to pull up whatever is left.

RUMBLING DICE

In various versions, the Rumbling Dice obstacle has appeared in three City Finals courses on *American Ninja Warrior*—Season 5 in Baltimore, Season 6 in St. Louis, and Season 7 in Los Angeles. To complete the obstacle, ninjas have to hang from a rectangular metal box and "roll" it along a track. Fans may remember that, in St. Louis, "The Weatherman" Joe Moravsky pulled one side of the dice off the track. (He was able to complete the obstacle with an early dismount.)

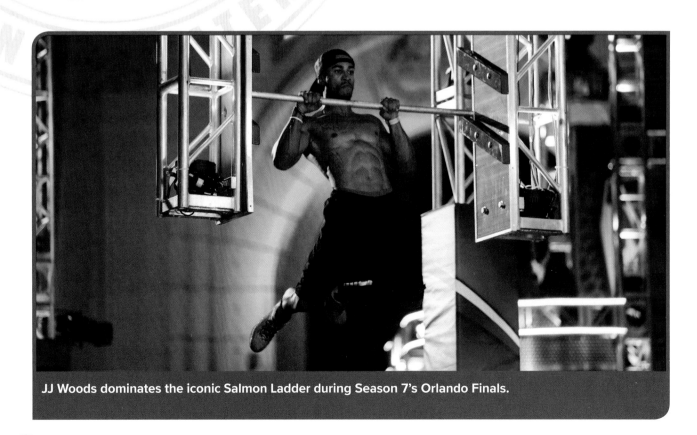

JJ Woods dominates the iconic Salmon Ladder during Season 7's Orlando Finals.

BECOME AN AMERICAN NINJA WARRIOR: THE ULTIMATE INSIDER'S GUIDE

SALMON LADDER

One of the iconic *SASUKE* obstacles, the Salmon Ladder first appeared in Season 2 of *American Ninja Warrior*, giving ninjas the chance to defy gravity. The obstacle gets its name from a traditional fish ladder, which is designed to enable fish to swim past a dam or other barrier by jumping up a series of steps. To complete the obstacle, competitors have to grab a free bar, the bottom rung of the Salmon Ladder, and using mainly upper-body strength, propel their bodies up, moving the bar vertically up the ladder. Variations of the Salmon Ladder include the Double Salmon Ladder, the Down Up Salmon Ladder, and the Criss Cross Salmon Ladder.

SHIN-CLIFFHANGER (SEE CLIFFHANGER)

SILK SLIDER

The Silk Slider eliminated some top competitors—including James McGrath, Kevin Bull, and "The Godfather" David Campbell—when it first appeared on *American Ninja Warrior* in Stage One during Season 6. To complete the obstacle, athletes have to grab two connected curtains and slide them down a track, making sure they correctly time their landing onto a floating platform. (A modified version of this obstacle, the Mini Silk Slider, appeared in Los Angeles in Season 7.)

SKY HOOKS

Making its debut in San Antonio in Season 9, the Sky Hooks challenges ninjas to maneuver three separate rings across a series of hooks in order to complete the obstacle. Designed by a seven-year-old fan, Sky Hooks requires tremendous grip strength and body control. The key is to maintain momentum and keep from "orbiting," or wobbling, in the air—something "Mighty" Kacy Catanzaro struggled with when she took on the Sky Hooks that season. Although she managed to reclaim her momentum, a misstep on the Sky Hooks brought her down; however, she still qualified for the City Finals.

SLACK LADDER

Just before Kevin Bull tackled the Slack Ladder in the Los Angeles Finals during Season 6, host Matt Iseman said that Bull claimed having alopecia—a condition that rendered him hairless since he was 21 years old—made him more aerodynamic. That was certainly the case as the then-rookie used his lower body to sail across the sensitive 18-foot nylon ladder with little trouble.

SLIDER DROP

Used as the first obstacle in Stage Two on Seasons 2, 3, and 4, Slider Drop is all about upper-body control. Ninjas have to grab onto a pole, slide it down a track—surviving the jolt of a drop—and then dismount onto a landing mat. The key to success for this obstacle is keeping the bar relatively straight to prevent it from sliding off the track. In Season 4, the Slider Drop did considerable damage, eliminating ninja heavyweights James "The Beast" McGrath and Chris Wilczewski.

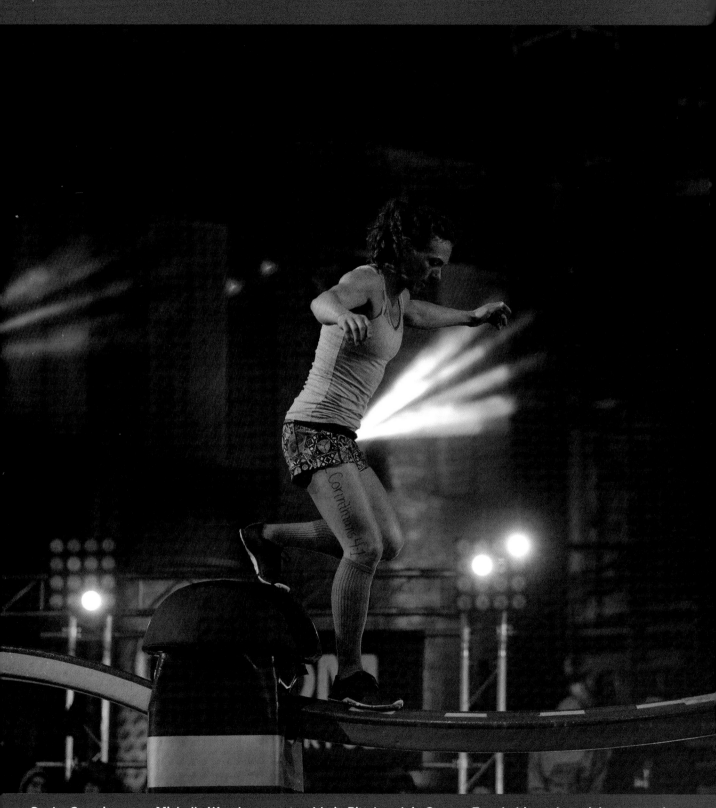

Snake Crossing gave Michelle Warnky some trouble in Pittsburgh in Season 7 and ultimately took her out at the City Finals.

SLIDER JUMP

Slider Jump set the bar—literally!—for many of the bar/track obstacles that would become part of the *American Ninja Warrior* obstacle family, such as the Double Dipper. First appearing in Stage One of Season 1 and later in Miami for Season 5, Slider Jump challenges athletes to hang from a bar as they slide down a track, with drops, and then to launch onto a net that they must traverse to complete the obstacle.

SNAKE CROSSING

Snake Crossing looked deceptively simple when it made its first and only appearance in Pittsburgh during Season 7, but it rattled quite a few ninjas! The obstacle consists of two S-shaped, tilting balance beams that separate three Dancing Stones. Without using their hands, athletes have to get across, using their balance and agility. Fans may remember Michelle Warnky had a little difficulty taming this obstacle in the Qualifiers, but was able to pull through. However, she was unable to complete Snake Crossing in the City Finals—due to what host Matt Iseman described as a "mental lapse."

SNAKE RUN

Inspired by Sonic Curve, Snake Run appeared as the first obstacle of Stage One in Season 8—taking out veteran ninja Geoff Britten!—and also in Season 9. Athletes have to cross a series of angled disks, resembling stepping-stones, that formed the letter S. Competitors are allowed to skip some of the disks in this obstacle, but at their own peril! Brian Wilczewski got bitten by the Snake Run in Season 9 when he skipped the first disk and slipped right off the second into the water.

SONIC CURVE

Sonic Curve was looking to test ninjas' agility when it appeared on *American Ninja Warrior* in Stage One of Seasons 7 and 8. To complete the obstacle, athletes have to run full speed along a series of six arced and angled tiles—that increase in height—in order to jump to a rope. In Season 7, Isaac Caldiero looked like he was going down after that last tile but was saved by the rope from falling into the water. As fans know, Caldiero would go on to win *American Ninja Warrior* that season.

WARRIOR WORDS

PERFECT SEASON: Completing all six courses and hitting all six buzzers. To date, only one ninja—cameraman Geoff Britten in Season 7—has done it on *American Ninja Warrior*.

SPIDER CLIMB

Taking on the Spider Climb is like taking an elevator to the third floor of a building when there is no elevator! Representing the final obstacle of all the City Finals in Seasons 5 and 6, the Spider Climb has ninjas using both their upper and lower body—hands and feet pressed against the walls—to go straight up a chute. Perhaps it would be easier if ninjas had eight legs? Not for "Mighty" Kacy Catanzaro, who stunned hosts Matt Iseman and Akbar Gbajabiamila by dominating the obstacle and, as Iseman said, going on to "elevate the standards for female competitors."

SPIDER FLIP

A fixture in *American Ninja Warrior*'s Stage Three at the National Finals—it appeared in the seventh position in Seasons 1, 4, 5, and 6—Spider Flip is a grip-strength gauntlet. Ninjas have to hang on to a small lip on a ledge, much like an I-beam girder, which they have to traverse horizontally and then vertically. Then they have to do a 180-rotation to grab onto a second ledge to traverse. In Season 5, Brian Arnold became the first American to complete the Spider Flip.

SPIKES INTO CARGO NET

Just as Brian Arnold was completing Spikes into Cargo Net in the Denver Qualifying round of Season 6, host Matt Iseman revealed that Arnold had told him that he was "nervous as hell" right before go time. Yet Arnold was not only able to dominate this obstacle—which requires ninjas to hang from a pair of suspended cones and then transition to another cone before swinging to a cargo net—but he also completed the Denver Qualifying course with ease.

SPIN CYCLE

What's a Spin Cycle? It looks like a hanging, tilted, upside-down wastepaper basket. And the Spin Cycle obstacle, which first appeared in the Los Angeles Qualifiers of Season 7, features three of them. To complete the obstacle, athletes have to use their upper body to transition from Spin Cycle to Spin Cycle, swinging like Tarzan and using their body weight in unison with each Spin Cycle's rotation.

SPINBALL WIZARD

Spinning handlebars. Off-axis body movement. Multiple laches. The Spinball Wizard has them all! Making its debut in Season 9 at the San Antonio Finals, the Spinball Wizard consists of five free-moving sets of inverted handlebars with spherical grips. Competitors have to grab hold of the first set of grips and lache 4 feet to another set. They repeat the process until they can make the last swing to a platform. It's easier said than done, as personal trainer Karsten Williams learned—he was the first to encounter and fall on Spinball Wizard.

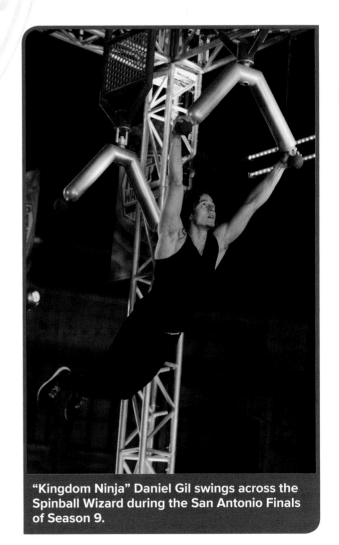

"Kingdom Ninja" Daniel Gil swings across the Spinball Wizard during the San Antonio Finals of Season 9.

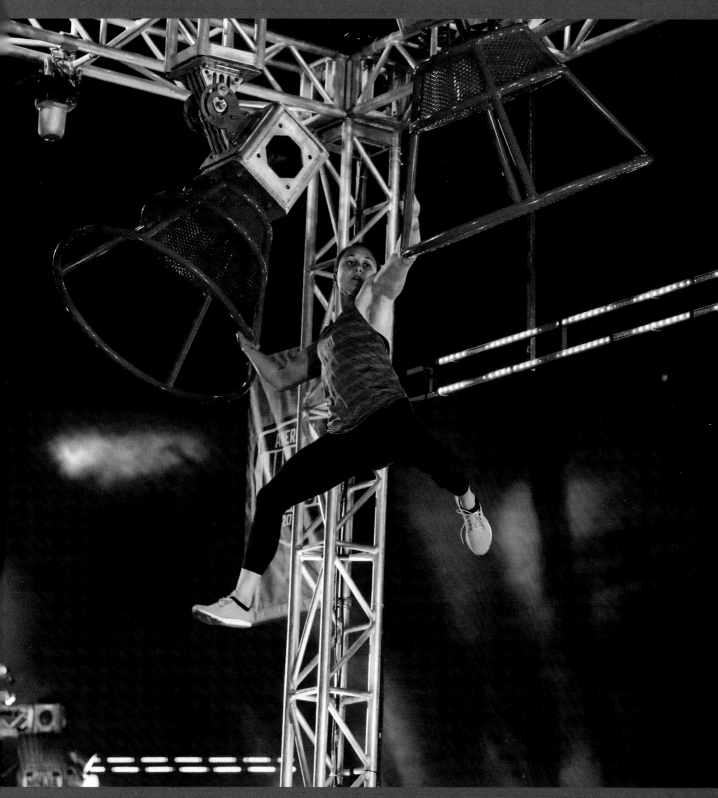

Erica Cook times her transition on the Spin Cycle in Season 8's Atlanta Qualifier.

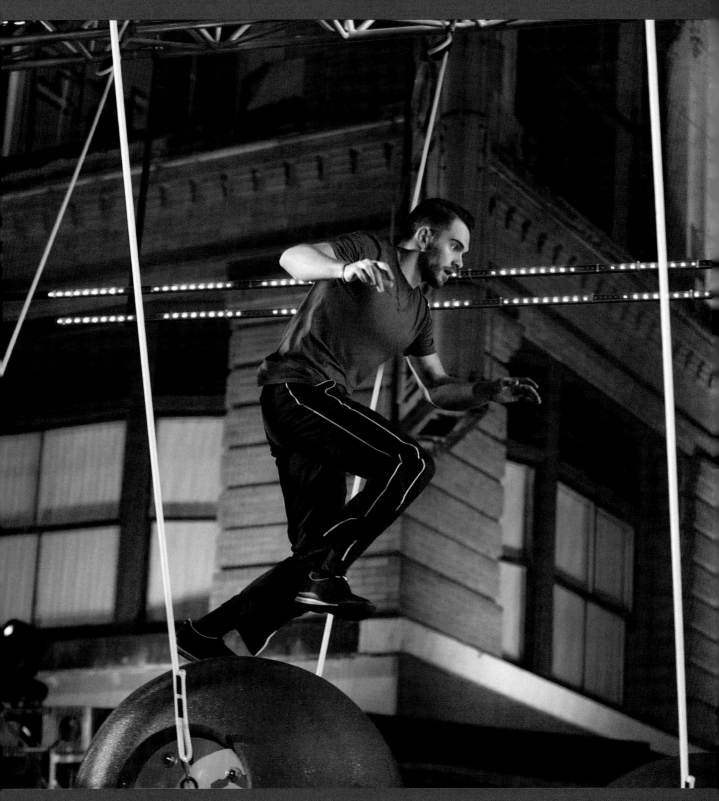

Brian Burkhardt attempts to make it across the Spinning Bridge in the San Antonio Finals, Season 9.

SPINNING BRIDGE

Fans may remember the Spinning Bridge in Season 4 as the obstacle that took out "The Godfather" David Campbell, whose misstep resulted in a shocking fall. The Spinning Bridge held the seventh position in Stage One during Seasons 4 to 6, and it also returned in Season 9 as the third obstacle in San Antonio. Like many of the other bridge obstacles on *American Ninja Warrior*, the Spinning Bridge tests balance and agility. Competitors have to run across four large suspended spheres, which spin, in order to complete the obstacle.

SPINNING LOG

The Spinning Log, originally called the Rolling Barrel, appeared in several seasons of *American Ninja Warrior* and challenges ninjas to cross a balance-beam-like Spinning Log, which, not surprisingly, spins on its axis. In Season 4, competitors could use their hands to complete the obstacle—fans may remember Ryoga Vee, in his red-and-black ninja outfit, doing what host Matt Iseman dubbed the "ninja crawl." However, in Seasons 6 and 7, upper body use was not allowed, and, in Season 7, a barrier was placed in the middle of the log to add to the challenge.

SPINNING WHEEL

The Spinning Wheel made its only appearance on *American Ninja Warrior* in Los Angeles in Season 6.

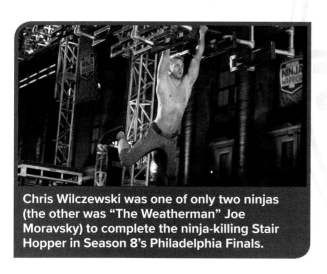

Chris Wilczewski was one of only two ninjas (the other was "The Weatherman" Joe Moravsky) to complete the ninja-killing Stair Hopper in Season 8's Philadelphia Finals.

Similar to the Rolling Escargot, the obstacle features a giant disk that ninjas have to hang on to as it rolls down a track. Brian Orosco was one of the ninjas who succumbed to the Spinning Wheel.

STAIR HOPPER

Bar placement is crucial to completing the Stair Hopper, which made its debut at the Philadelphia Finals of Season 8 and appeared again at the Los Angeles Finals of Season 9. A mash-up of the Pipe Slider and the Bar Hop, the Stair Hopper challenges ninjas to hang from a four-foot bar and then "hop" down and up a series of levels. In Season 8, among the ten competitors who reached the Stair Hopper, only two could complete it—"The Weatherman" Joe Moravsky and Chris Wilczewski. One of the Stair Hopper's most notable casualties that season was Geoff Britten, who, until that fall, had hit a buzzer seven times in a row.

STEP SLIDER

The Step Slider appeared early on in *American Ninja Warrior*—in Stage One of Seasons 2, 3, and 4—and seemed to be an early version of the Floating Steps, which premiered in Season 8. To complete the obstacle, competitors have to hop across four slanted steps and then jump to a rope in order to swing to a landing platform.

STICK SLIDER

Stick Slider was a Stage Two obstacle from *SASUKE* 18 to 23, appearing only in Season 1's Stage Two Finals of *American Ninja Warrior*. Immediately following the Salmon Ladder, Stick Slider challenges ninjas to navigate a free bar along two descending tracks that come together in a V shape. Athletes have to keep the bar on the tracks and let go at the right time to reach a landing mat.

SWING CIRCLE

Imagine four large hoop earrings hanging from scaffolding. That's what makes up Swing Circle, which appeared early on in *American Ninja Warrior*'s history—in Season 2's Stage Three Finals and Season 4's Southeast regionals. Ninjas have to swing from one ring to the next, using only their upper body and make it to a platform on the other side.

SWING JUMP

After injuring his ankle on the preceding obstacle, Sam Sann used an unconventional method to complete the Swing Jump in the Season 6 Dallas Qualifiers. The Swing Jump—which also appeared in Baltimore in Season 5—challenges ninjas to use a large swing to build momentum to reach a cargo net. While most athletes stood on the swing, Sann instead swung while hanging on to one of the support chains in order to keep from putting pressure on his ankle and was able to complete the obstacle.

SWING SURFER

Ninjas test their leaping skills on the Swing Surfer, which is reminiscent of the Tic Toc obstacle. Making its first appearance in Stage Two of Season 9, Swing Surfer challenges ninjas to jump to a pendulum and then carefully time their next jump to a rope—a jump that hit hard on impact. "Wolfpup" Ian Dory was the first ninja to succumb to this new obstacle after a small miscalculation in direction.

SWINGING FRAMES

When Sam Sann got hung up on the Swinging Frames during the Season 6 Dallas Finals (he ultimately fell), host Akbar Gbajabiamila exclaimed, "Believe me, it is taxing him more than the United States government!" Indeed, the Swinging Frames is an upper-body-intensive obstacle that appeared in the City Finals of Dallas in Season 6 and San Pedro in Season 7, both times in the intimidating eighth position after the Salmon Ladder. Ninjas have to hang from frames that swing and tilt with every move of their body weight while they try to transition from frame to frame to complete the obstacle.

SWINGING PEGBOARD

The Swinging Pegboard premiered on a special edition of *American Ninja Warrior* titled *Celebrity Ninja Warrior: Red Nose Day* (see page 40) but made its official debut in the Los Angeles Finals of Season 9. The obstacle is made up of two swinging panels with holes, and ninjas have to use pegs to traverse each panel, transferring between them. Six ninjas were taken out by the Swinging Pegboard, including Rebekah Bonilla and "The Godfather" David Campbell.

SWINGING SPIKES

The Swinging Spikes, which appeared in Houston in Season 7 and returned in Indianapolis in Season 8, consists of eight suspended nunchuck-like spikes that ninjas have to traverse to reach a landing mat. The spikes are unpredictable—some move side to side, forward, and backward, and others are attached to a bungee. Fans may remember, during the Season 7 Houston Finals, that Brent Steffensen gave a quick shout-out to then-girlfriend Kacy Catanzaro, who was in the host tower with Matt Iseman and Akbar Gbajabiamila, just before he tackled the Swinging Spikes during his run.

WARRIOR WORDS

KNOCKOUT RATE: The percentage of ninjas who fail to complete an obstacle. For example, if 20 athletes attempt an obstacle and only 5 are able to clear it, the knockout rate is 75 percent.

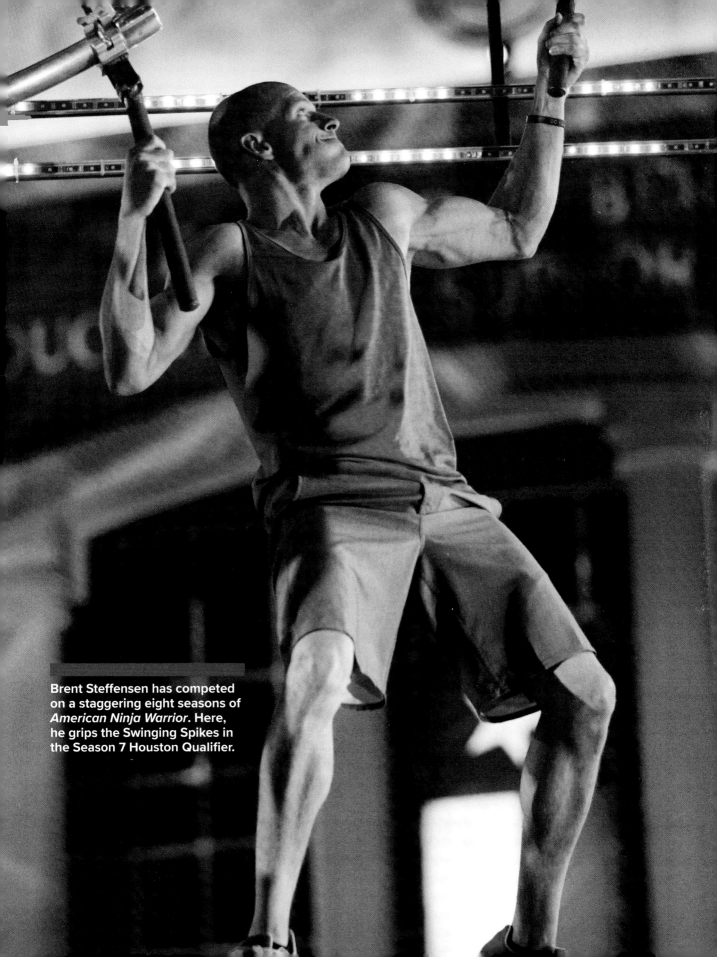

Brent Steffensen has competed on a staggering eight seasons of *American Ninja Warrior*. Here, he grips the Swinging Spikes in the Season 7 Houston Qualifier.

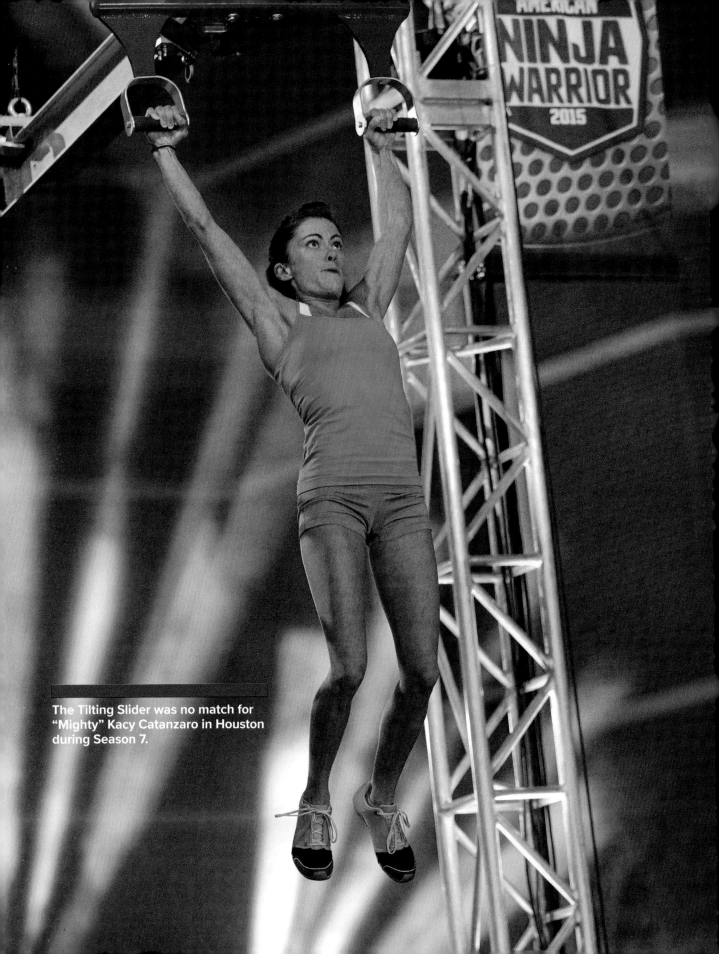

The Tilting Slider was no match for "Mighty" Kacy Catanzaro in Houston during Season 7.

TARZAN ROPE

The Tarzan Rope is an obstacle that has been around for a long time—appearing very early on in *SASUKE* and in Stage One of *American Ninja Warrior* Seasons 1 to 6. To complete the Tarzan Rope, competitors simply have to grab onto a rope and swing—a la Tarzan—to the next obstacle.

TARZAN SWING

A predecessor of Rope Jungle, the Tarzan Swing appeared in the Semifinal round of *American Ninja Warrior*'s Season 1. Unlike the Tarzan Rope, which consists of a single rope, this obstacle features several ropes, and competitors have to transition from rope to rope in order to complete the obstacle.

TIC TOC

The idea for Tic Toc, introduced during Season 8's Los Angeles Qualifiers, came from a punching bag. The actual obstacle has three parts: First, ninjas have to swing with their hands on a trapeze swing. Next, they have to transition to a large pendulum with a very narrow ledge at the bottom. Once on the pendulum, athletes have to shinny around and use the momentum of the pendulum to jump to a cargo net attached to a landing platform.

TILTING SLIDER

This obstacle made its first and only appearance in *American Ninja Warrior*'s Season 7 in Houston. It features a seesaw-like suspended track that has two handles. Ninjas have to grab those handles—which can be a long reach for some of the shorter competitors, such as Kacy Catanzaro—and work their way up the angled track until it pivots from their weight, allowing them to slide the rest of the way. At the end of the track, athletes have to swing to a pole before transitioning to a landing mat.

TILTING TABLE

Also known as the Balance Bridge in *SASUKE*, the Tilting Table made an appearance in Season 6 in Dallas as well as Season 7 in Los Angeles. Ninjas have to be careful not to underestimate this agility and balance obstacle. As it tilts, ninjas have to run

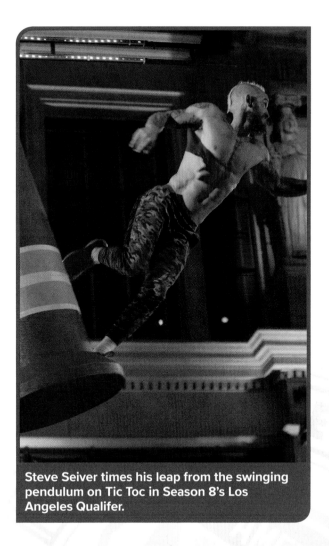

Steve Seiver times his leap from the swinging pendulum on Tic Toc in Season 8's Los Angeles Qualifer.

over barriers—resembling the skirt or apron of a table—that can surprise them and trip them up if they aren't ready.

TIMBERS
(SEE TWELVE TIMBERS)

TIME BOMB

A grip-strength gauntlet, the Time Bomb is an explosive new obstacle that made its debut in Stage Three of Season 9. Athletes have to traverse a series of hooks by hanging on to spheres, or Globe Grasps, attached to rings dangling from hooks. Fans may recall that it was the Time Bomb that finally brought down "The Weatherman" Joe Moravsky, who was Last Man Standing in Season 9.

Season 9's Last Man Standing, "The Weather-man" Joe Moravsky, gassed out on the new Time Bomb obstacle, ending an inspiring run.

TIRE SWING

The Tire Swing premiered in Orlando in Season 7 (it returned in Oklahoma in Season 8) and features three suspended tires that ninjas have to get across using their upper body. Fans may remember that when Flip Rodriguez returned to *American Ninja Warrior* in Season 7, he was coming off a disappointing season during which a tiny mistake on a cargo net eliminated him from the competition. However, in Season 7, Rodriguez was newly focused, and as he was dominating the Tire Swing host Akbar Gbajabiamila remarked, "You can measure height, you can measure weight, but the one thing you can't measure is heart, and this kid has a lot of heart."

TRAPEZE SWING

When the Trapeze Swing appeared in Los Angeles in Season 5, it didn't seem to give ninjas any trouble—all who attempted it completed it. This may be why the Trapeze Swing—which challenges ninjas to transition between two consecutive swings—would appear in only one season of *American Ninja Warrior*.

TRIPLE SWING

The Triple Swing had a single appearance on *American Ninja Warrior*—as the eighth and final obstacle of Stage One in the National Finals of Season 7. However, that was enough to give it its notorious reputation. The Triple Swing—which consists of an angled platform, hanging bars, and a cargo net—knocked out veteran ninja Paul Kasemir, ending his attempt at a sixth straight Stage One completion.

TWELVE TIMBERS

Twelve Timbers appeared as the first obstacle of Stage One in *American Ninja Warrior*'s inaugural season. Ninjas have to jump across a set of 11 slanted planks to get to a landing platform, which is the twelfth timber. The logs are angled slightly differently, which increases the difficulty. This obstacle also appeared in Season 5's Stage One of the National Finals with only eight logs to clear and was called simply Timbers.

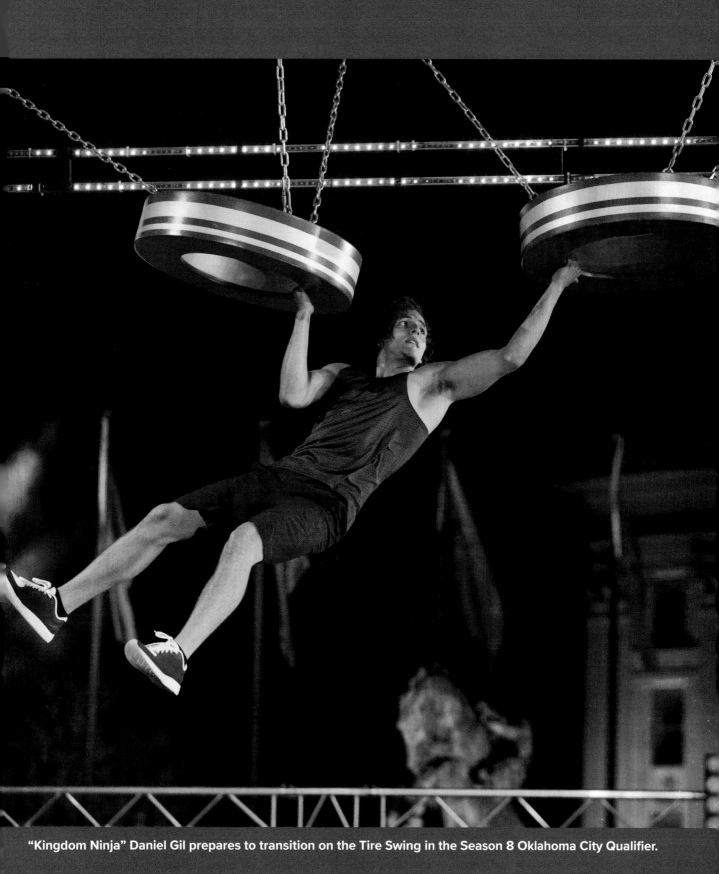

"Kingdom Ninja" Daniel Gil prepares to transition on the Tire Swing in the Season 8 Oklahoma City Qualifier.

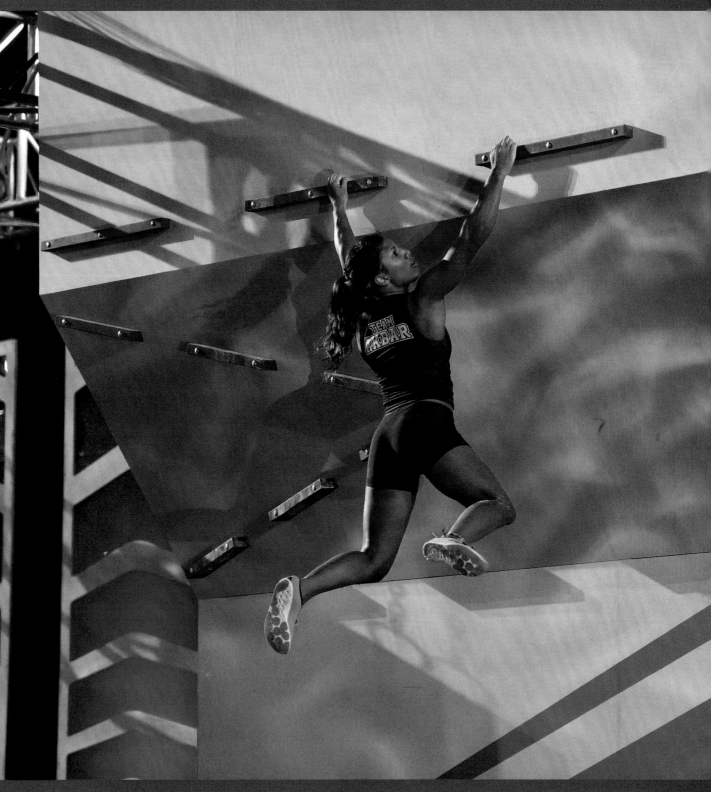

Meagan Martin takes on the Ultimate Cliffhanger in the first-ever *American Ninja Warrior All-Star Special: Skills Challenge* as a member of Team Akbar.

ULTIMATE CLIFFHANGER
(SEE CLIFFHANGER)

UTILITY POLE SLIDER

The Utility Pole Slider appeared for the first and only time in Miami during Season 5 in the second position. To complete this obstacle, ninjas have to grab hold of a utility-type pole, either by wrapping their legs around it or hanging on to bars at its top (or they can do both, like "Real Life Ninja" Drew Drechsel), and then ride it down a track.

WALKING BAR

The Walking Bar made its debut during the Season 7 Houston Finals. Similar to the Flying Bar, the Walking Bar challenges ninjas to move a bar using their upper body. However, this time they have to move the bar *one side at a time* into staggered cradles before transitioning to a rope. Fans may remember that Brent Steffensen clinched a spot in the National Finals once he grabbed onto the Walking Bar in Season 7, but he wound up getting wet right after making his first move.

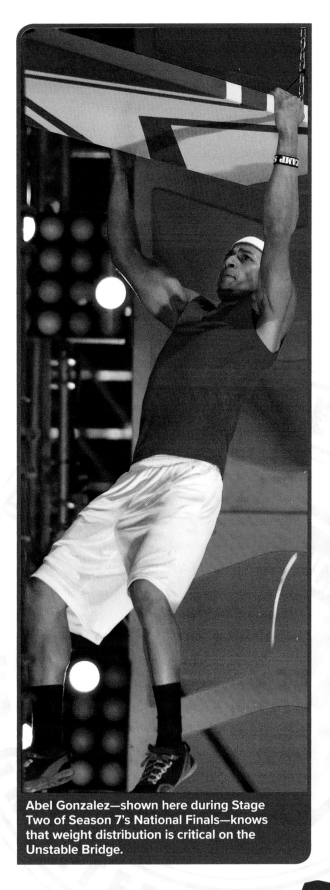

Abel Gonzalez—shown here during Stage Two of Season 7's National Finals—knows that weight distribution is critical on the Unstable Bridge.

NINJA KILLER

UNSTABLE BRIDGE

During its tenure, the Unstable Bridge, a Stage Two obstacle that appeared in the first seven seasons of *American Ninja Warrior* and also in the Semifinal round of Season 3, has knocked out some heavyweight ninjas, including Lorin Ball, Brian Arnold, "Ninjadoc" Noah Kaufmann, and "Real Life Ninja" Drew Drechsel. The obstacle, which was replaced by the Wave Runner in Season 8, features two suspended wooden planks that ninjas have to traverse—one after the other—using their upper body. Weight distribution is key to the completion of this obstacle, since the planks can easily tilt.

An obstacle like the Ultimate Cliffhanger is such a grip-strength gauntlet. It's going to be a brutal challenge for anyone who hasn't spent years developing their upper body and forearm strength.
—Host Matt Iseman

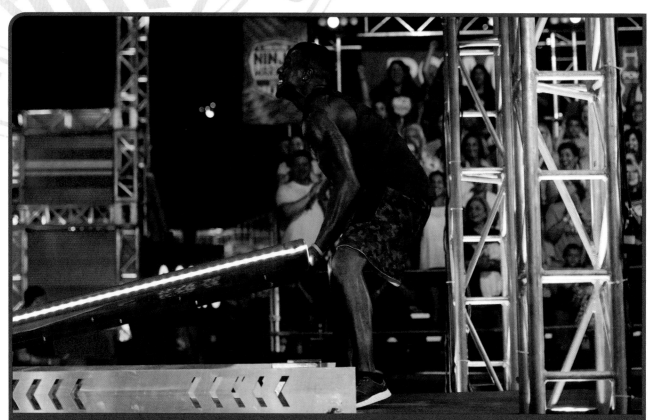

"Philly Phoenix" Najee Richardson was one of three ninjas to dominate the Wall Flip on Stage Two of the Season 9 National Finals.

BECOME AN AMERICAN NINJA WARRIOR: THE ULTIMATE INSIDER'S GUIDE

WALL DROP

The Wall Drop, which made its only appearance in Philadelphia during Season 8, challenges ninjas' entire body—the upper body on a series of hanging objects, a cannonball and a pair of nunchucks; core to balance on an unstable wall; legs on a trampoline; and then upper body again on a pair of hanging pendulums. However, even though the Wall Drop threw everything it had at ninjas, veterans such as Geoff Britten and "The Weatherman" Joe Moravsky were able to prevail.

WALL FLIP

There's something climactic about seeing ninjas take on the Wall Flip. Positioned as the final obstacle of Stage Two in Seasons 8 and 9, the Wall Flip challenges ninjas to lift and flip over three walls—weighing approximately 95, 115, and 135 pounds—before hitting that stage-ending buzzer. The three competitors who made it to the Wall Flip in Season 9 all completed it—Najee Richardson, Sean Bryan, and Joe Moravsky—pushing down those walls with satisfaction.

WALL LIFT

It's hard not to think of Hercules while watching ninjas take on the Wall Lift, which was the final obstacle of Stage Two in *American Ninja Warrior*'s first seven seasons. (A modified version of the Wall Lift also made an appearance in the Season 4 Northeast and Southeast regional courses.) Ninjas have to dig deep and lift three walls of increasing weights—approximately 70, 90, and 110 pounds, respectively—and then pass underneath to transition through the obstacle. Nearly every competitor who has reached this obstacle has been able to complete it.

WARPED WALL

Perhaps the most recognizable of all the obstacles, the Warped Wall is the centerpiece of the *American Ninja Warrior* course and one of the oldest obstacles in *SASUKE* history, appearing in all seasons except for the first four. It consists of a short runway and a steeply curving wall that extends up $14^1/_2$ feet. (The Wall originally was 14 feet, but was extended 6 inches, beginning in Season 8.) The Warped

> Everything after the Warped Wall—the Back Half—is the toughest. There's just no break. It's so intense. I don't know what you have to do to be able to block out the pain that is associated with the Back Half. I mean, you get fatigued, and I always challenge people: Think about a time where you've been working out and you're, like, I have no more left. That's what some of them feel when they get on the seventh and eighth obstacle, and there's still number 9 and number 10 they have to complete. I just don't know how they do it.
>
> —Chris Wilczewski

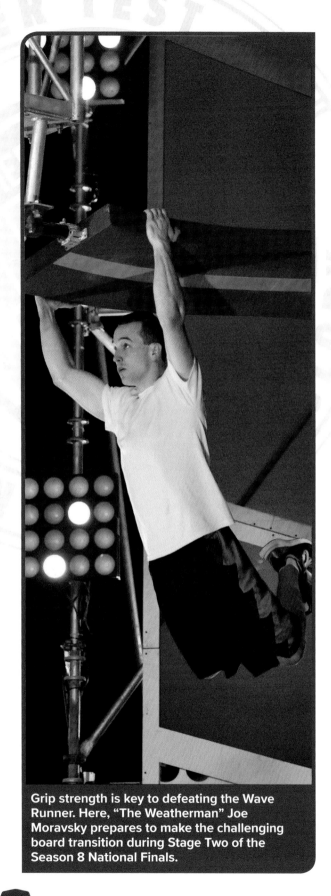

Grip strength is key to defeating the Wave Runner. Here, "The Weatherman" Joe Moravsky prepares to make the challenging board transition during Stage Two of the Season 8 National Finals.

Wall is the finale of the Qualifying course and the entranceway to the Back Half of the City Finals. It has become a *Ninja Warrior* tradition to chant "Beat that wall!" as athletes build up speed that they convert to vertical momentum, launching up to grip the Wall's ledge and hurling themselves over the top. In the Qualifying and City Finals rounds, ninjas get three chances to make it up the Warped Wall; in the National Finals, they run the risk of getting timed out.

> When I get to the Warped Wall in a Qualifying round, I know that I'm almost done, because there's the buzzer at the top, and I know that I've got it. At my height, I'm not going to struggle getting up.
>
> —"Island Ninja" Grant McCartney

WAVE RUNNER

Premiering in Stage Two of Season 8, Wave Runner consists of two boards—the first is an uneven S-board, the second an uneven pyramid board. Ninjas have to hang from both boards, transitioning from one to the other. The transition from board to board proved challenging for some competitors. Fans may remember, in Season 8, that Flip Rodriguez bypassed the second board, resulting in disqualification, and "Real Life Ninja" Drew Drechsel came dangerously close to disqualification but was able to grab hold of the second board before a quick dismount to complete the obstacle.

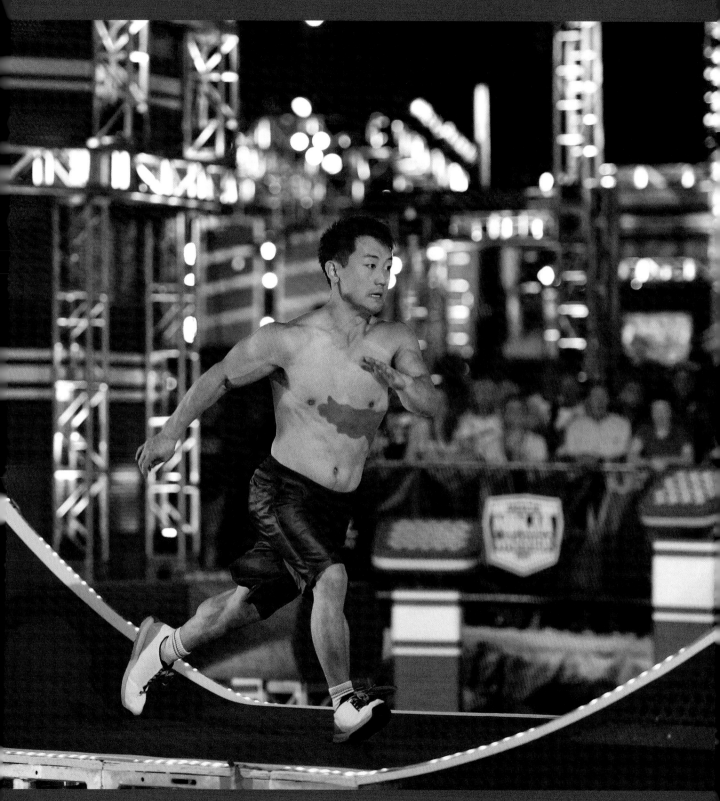

Tyler Yamauchi tries to work up a good speed to make it over the iconic Warped Wall during the Season 8 National Finals in Las Vegas.

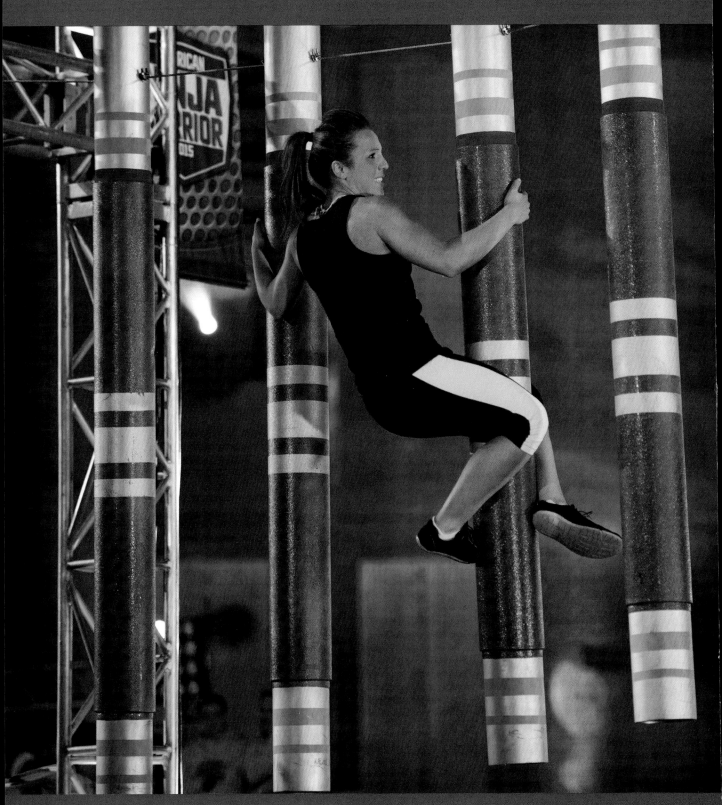

Amber Holbrook uses her upper- and lower-body to traverse the Wind Chimes in Pittsburgh in Season 7.

NINJA KILLER

THE WEDGE

Sixteen competitors were taken out by the Wedge when it made its debut at the Los Angeles Finals in Season 8. The idea for this obstacle came from the Flying Bar (see page 82) and the Wedge, a surfing spot in Newport Beach, California, known for its large wedge-shaped waves.

To complete it, ninjas need core body control as they jump a bar between two angled walls. Once they reach the end, they have to lache a whopping 8 feet in order to dismount to a landing platform.

WIND CHIMES

Premiering in Pittsburgh during Season 7, the Wind Chimes—a series of large suspended poles—challenges ninjas to use both their upper and lower body to complete the obstacle. Fans may recall that Michelle Warnky used a powerful move to navigate a large gap between two chimes, planting both her hands and feet between the chimes in order to transition between them. "It looked like the Spider Climb right there!" exclaimed host Akbar Gbajabiamila.

WINDOW HANG

The Window Hang is the ultimate test of ninjas' grip-strength. It made its first and only appearance as the ninth obstacle in Season 8's Oklahoma City Finals. Competitors have to move across five panels that vary in distance and height and have extremely narrow ledges—decreasing from $2^1/_2$ inches to $1^1/_2$ inches. Although ninjas are allowed to use their legs to complete the obstacle, some, such as "Kingdom Ninja" Daniel Gil, preferred to go all upper body, relying solely on their grip strength.

WINGNUTS

The Wingnuts, designed by *American Ninja Warrior* fan and competitor Kevin Carbone, made its debut in Season 9 in Daytona Beach. It features three "wingnuts"—large, nutlike levers with one projecting ledge on each side. To complete this

obstacle, competitors have to swing sideways, like the pendulum of a clock, from wingnut to wingnut. Carbone was able to dominate his own creation in competition, but not all ninjas were so lucky. John Loobey, who became the oldest competitor to finish an obstacle at age 65 on *American Ninja Warrior* that season, was able to complete two obstacles but then succumbed to the Wingnuts, losing his dentures in the process!

NINJA KILLER

WINGNUT ALLEY

Wingnut Alley showed no mercy when it premiered in Stage Two of Season 9. A next-level version of the Wingnuts, this obstacle forces ninjas to step up their swing game. Here, competitors don't have a straight swing from wingnut to wingnut as they did in the regionals. Instead, they have to shift their body momentum to deal with angle changes while lacheing across longer gaps. Wingnut Alley took out a whopping 23 ninjas—more than half of the 41 athletes who made it to Stage Two!

NINJA SPOTLIGHT:

KEVIN CARBONE

Next-gen ninja Kevin Carbone, known as "The Maker," is a tennis instructor from Alpharetta, Georgia. Not only does he have the distinction of being one of the winners of *American Ninja Warrior*'s first Obstacle Design Challenge, but he is also the only ninja in the show's history to defeat an obstacle of his own creation in competition. Plus, he went on to hit the buzzer of the Qualifying course in his rookie debut! A fan of the original *SASUKE* (he used to stay up late while his parents were asleep so he could watch), Carbone first appeared on Season 9 of *American Ninja Warrior* as a walk-on.

What do you love about *American Ninja Warrior*?
The exciting athletic challenges are unlike any American sport. I just love the thrill and the do-or-die mentality. *Ninja* presents a challenge to my day-to-day routine, and I love to have something to continually work at and to give me a sense of purpose.

Why did you enter the Obstacle Design Challenge in 2016?
Plain and simple, I'm an inventor. I've always created things, beginning with LEGOs as a kid, and worked my way up to disassembling all kinds of gadgets with motors and moving parts and remaking them into more useful devices. I was inspired to design an obstacle ever since I saw a commercial for the Obstacle Design Challenge.

How did you come up with the design for Wingnuts?
I tend to dream up ideas in the shower and this one started there as well. The Wingnuts design came from my memory of a rope swing that I put up in my backyard, which I built to swing in many directions. I loved the freedom of all the movement without hitting anything and thought I could design an obstacle that moved laterally instead of the typical front to back swinging.

How did you come up with the name for it?
I showed my dad the design—he is also very handy and knows tools and hardware. He thought it looked like a wingnut, and as soon as I said the name aloud a few times, I knew that was the one!

What was it like competing on your own obstacle? And beating it?!
I was never more focused at any point on the course than I was on the Wingnuts. I could hear nothing but my mental instructions and swung to each with a controlled swing. I did not want to fall because I would never hear the end of it from my friends and family, so that may have helped motivate me to hang on for dear life! I'm so glad I made it through and it was more fun than I even imagined.

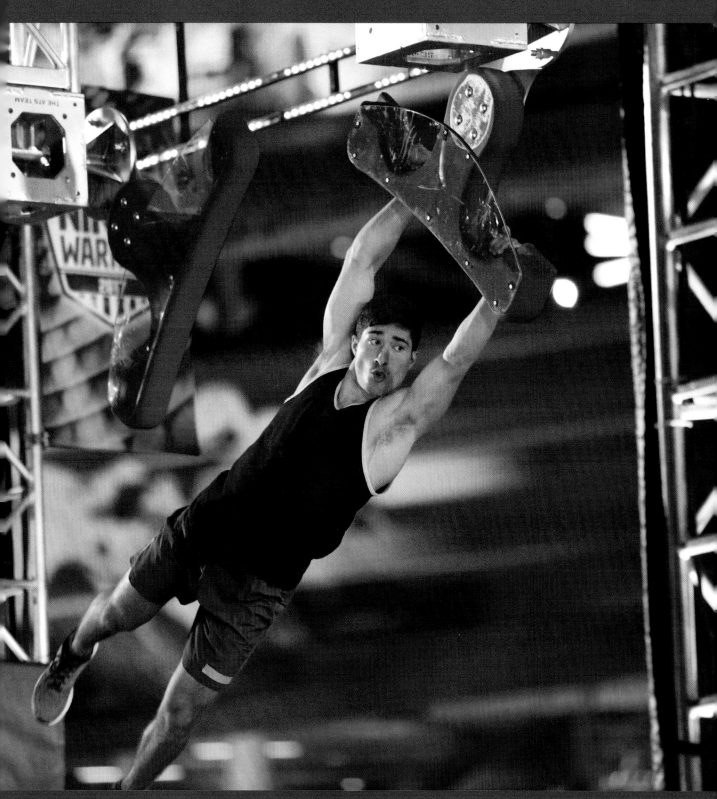

"The Maker" Kevin Carbone first tackled his own obstacle, the Wingnuts, in the Daytona Beach Qualifier in Season 9. To date, he is the only ninja to ever defeat his own obstacle.

Qualifying Obstacles

Season 1	Quintuple Steps	Rope Swing	Rolling Barrel	Jumping Spider	Pipe Slider	Warped Wall	
Season 2	Quad Steps	Rope Swing	Bridge of Blades	Jumping Spider	Jumping Bars	Warped Wall	
Season 3	Quad Steps	Log Grip	Bridge of Blades	Jump Hang	Jumping Bars	Warped Wall	
Season 4/Southwest	Quad Steps	Log Grip	Spinning Log	Jump Hang	Devil Steps	Warped Wall	
Season 4/Midwest	Quad Steps	Log Grip	Bridge of Blades	Jump Hang	Curtain Slider	Warped Wall	
Season 4/Northeast	Quad Steps	Log Grip	Bungee Bridge	Jump Hang	Jumping Bars	Wall Lift	Warped Wall
Season 4/Northwest	Quad Steps	Log Grip	Spinning Log	Jump Hang	Pipe Slider /Devil Steps	Warped Wall	
Season 4/Mid-South	Quad Steps	Log Grip	Bridge of Blades	Jump Hang	Rope Junction	Warped Wall	
Season 4/Southeast	Quad Steps	Log Grip	Bungee Bridge	Jump Hang	Swing Circle	Wall Lift	Warped Wall
Season 5/Venice	Quintuple Steps	Frame Slider	Domino Hill	Floating Chains	Flying Nunchucks /Trapeze Swing	Warped Wall	
Season 5/Baltimore	Quintuple Steps	Downhill Jump	Prism Tilt	Swing Jump	Circle Cross	Warped Wall	
Season 5/Miami	Quintuple Steps	Utility Pole Slider	Balance Bridge	Slider Jump	Monkey Peg	Warped Wall	
Season 5/Denver	Quintuple Steps	Rolling Log	Rotating Bridge	Jump Hang Kai	Grip Hang	Warped Wall	
Season 6/Venice	Quintuple Steps	Spinning Wheel	Slack Ladder	Jumping Bars into Cargo Net	Monkey Peg	Warped Wall	
Season 6/Dallas	Quintuple Steps	Log Grip	Tilting Table	Swing Jump	Ring Toss	Warped Wall	
Season 6/St. Louis	Quintuple Steps	Rolling Log	Bridge of Blades	Rope Swing into Cargo Net	Double Tilt Ladder	Warped Wall	
Season 6/Miami	Quintuple Steps	Downhill Pipe Drop	Dancing Stones	Jump Hang	Curtain Slider	Warped Wall	
Season 6/Denver	Quintuple Steps	Cat Grab	Spinning Log	Spikes into Cargo Net	Devil Steps	Warped Wall	
Season 7/Venice	Quintuple Steps	Mini Silk Slider	Tilting Table	Spin Cycle	Hourglass Drop	Warped Wall	
Season 7/Kansas City	Quintuple Steps	Big Dipper	Floating Tiles	(Modified) Ring Toss	Bungee Road	Warped Wall	
Season 7/Houston	Quintuple Steps	Tilting Slider	Spinning Log	Cargo Crossing	Swinging Spikes	Warped Wall	
Season 7/Orlando	Quintuple Steps	Rolling Log	Paddle Boards	Tire Swing	Double Tilt Ladder	Warped Wall	
Season 7/Pittsburgh	Quintuple Steps	Log Grip	Snake Crossing	Wind Chimes	Devil Steps	Warped Wall	
Season 7/San Pedro	Quintuple Steps	Jump Hang	Log Runner	Monkey Pegs	I-Beam Cross	Warped Wall	
Season 8/Los Angeles	Floating Steps	Tic Toc	Escalator	Ring Jump	I-Beam Cross	Warped Wall	
Season 8/Atlanta	Floating Steps	Big Dipper	Block Run	Spin Cycle	Pipe Fitter	Warped Wall	
Season 8/Indianapolis	Floating Steps	Rolling Log	Fly Wheels	Disk Runner	Swinging Spikes	Warped Wall	
Season 8/Oklahoma	Floating Steps	Ring Swing	Log Runner	Tire Swing	Bar Hop	Warped Wall	
Season 8/Philadelphia	Floating Steps	Log Grip	Paddle Boards	Wall Drop	Rolling Thunder	Warped Wall	
Season 9/Los Angeles	Floating Steps	Cannonball Drop	Fly Wheels	Block Run	Battering Ram	Warped Wall	
Season 9/San Antonio	Floating Steps	Tic Toc	Spinning Bridge	Sky Hooks	Pipe Fitter	Warped Wall	
Season 9/Daytona	Floating Steps	Rolling Pin	Wingnuts	Broken Bridge	Rolling Thunder	Warped Wall	
Season 9/Kansas City	Floating Steps	Hang Glider	Broken Pipes	Crank It Up	Bar Hop	Warped Wall	
Season 9/Cleveland	Floating Steps	Rolling Log	Razor's Edge	Ring Jump	I-Beam Gap	Warped Wall	
Season 9/Denver	Floating Steps	Ring Swing	Bouncing Spider	Paddle Boards	Rail Runner	Warped Wall	

City Finals Obstacles

Season 1	Tarzan Swing	Jumping Bars	Cargo Climb	
Season 2	Salmon Ladder	Circle Slider	Cargo Climb	
Season 3	Salmon Ladder	Unstable Bridge	Cargo Climb	
Season 4/Southwest	Salmon Ladder	Arm Rings	Cargo Climb	
Season 4/Midwest	Salmon Ladder	Lamp Grasper	Cargo Climb	
Season 4/Northeast	Salmon Ladder	Cycle Road	Cargo Climb	
Season 4/Northwest	Salmon Ladder	Arm Rings	Cargo Climb	
Season 4/Mid-South	Salmon Ladder	Lamp Grasper	Cargo Climb	
Season 4/Southeast	Salmon Ladder	Cycle Road	Cargo Climb	
Season 5/Venice	Salmon Ladder	Rope Maze	Cliffhanger	Spider Climb
Season 5/Baltimore	Salmon Ladder	Rumbling Dice	Body Prop	Spider Climb
Season 5/Miami	Salmon Ladder	Ledge Jump	Rolling Steel	Spider Climb
Season 5/Denver	Salmon Ladder	Floating Stairs	Pole Grasper	Spider Climb
Season 6/Venice	Salmon Ladder	Cannonball Alley	Body Prop	Spider Climb
Season 6/Dallas	Salmon Ladder	Swinging Frames	Pole Grasper	Spider Climb
Season 6/St. Louis	Salmon Ladder	Rumbling Dice	Crazy Cliffhanger	Spider Climb
Season 6/Miami	Salmon Ladder	Minefield	Floating Stairs	Spider Climb
Season 6/Denver	Salmon Ladder	Arm Rings	Doorknob Arch	Spider Climb
Season 7/Venice	Salmon Ladder	Rumbling Dice	Clear Climb	Invisible Ladder
Season 7/Kansas City	Salmon Ladder	Flying Shelf Grab	Body Prop	Invisible Ladder
Season 7/Houston	Salmon Ladder	Walking Bar	Crazy Cliffhanger	Invisible Ladder
Season 7/Orlando	Salmon Ladder	Cannonball Alley	Helix Hang	Invisible Ladder
Season 7/Pittsburgh	Salmon Ladder	Floating Monkey Bars	Doorknob Arch	Invisible Ladder
Season 7/San Pedro	Salmon Ladder	Swinging Frames	Globe Grasper	Invisible Ladder
Season 8/Los Angeles	Salmon Ladder	The Wedge	Helix Hang	Invisible Ladder
Season 8/Atlanta	Salmon Ladder	Floating Monkey Bars	The Clacker	Invisible Ladder
Season 8/Indianapolis	Salmon Ladder	Hourglass Drop	Circuit Board	Invisible Ladder
Season 8/Oklahoma	Salmon Ladder	Bungee Road	Window Hang	Invisible Ladder
Season 8/Philadelphia	Salmon Ladder	Flying Shelf Grab	Stair Hopper	Invisible Ladder
Season 9/Los Angeles	Salmon Ladder	Swinging Pegboard	Stair Hopper	Elevator Climb
Season 9/San Antonio	Salmon Ladder	Hourglass Drop	Spinball Wizard	Elevator Climb
Season 9/Daytona	Salmon Ladder	Giant Cubes	Circuit Board	Elevator Climb
Season 9/Kansas City	Salmon Ladder	Floating Monkey Bars	Iron Maiden	Elevator Climb
Season 9/Cleveland	Salmon Ladder	Nail Clipper	The Clacker	Elevator Climb
Season 9/Denver	Salmon Ladder	The Wedge	Ninjago Roll	Elevator Climb

Stage 1 Finals

Season 1	Twelve Timbers	Curtain Slider	Log Grip	Jumping Spider	Half-Pipe Attack	Warped Wall	Slider Jump	Tarzan Rope
Season 2	Step Slider	Hazard Swing	Rolling Escargot	Jumping Spider	Half-Pipe Attack	Warped Wall	Giant Swing	Tarzan Rope
Season 3	Step Slider	Rolling Escargot	Giant Swing	Jumping Spider	Half-Pipe Attack	Warped Wall	Spinning Bridge	Tarzan Rope
Season 4	Step Slider	Rolling Log	Giant Swing	Jumping Spider	Half-Pipe Attack	Warped Wall	Spinning Bridge	Tarzan Rope
Season 5	Timbers	Giant Cycle	Rope Glider	Jumping Spider	Half-Pipe Attack	Warped Wall	Spinning Bridge	Tarzan Rope
Season 6	Piston Road	Giant Ring	Silk Slider	Jumping Spider	Half-Pipe Attack	Warped Wall	Spinning Bridge	Tarzan Rope
Season 7	Piston Road	Propeller Bar	Silk Slider	Jumping Spider	Sonic Curve	Warped Wall	Coin Flip	Triple Swing
Season 8	Snake Run	Propeller Bar	Giant Log Grip	Jumping Spider	Sonic Curve	Warped Wall	Broken Bridge	Flying Squirrel
Season 9	Snake Run	Propeller Bar	Double Dipper	Jumping Spider	Parkour Run	Warped Wall	Domino Pipes	Flying Squirrel

Stage 2 Finals

Season 1	Downhill Jump	Salmon Ladder	Stick Slider	Unstable Bridge	Metal Spin	Wall Lift
Season 2	Slider Drop	Double Salmon Ladder	Unstable Bridge	Balance Tank	Metal Spin	Wall Lift
Season 3	Slider Drop	Double Salmon Ladder	Unstable Bridge	Balance Tank	Metal Spin	Wall Lift
Season 4	Slider Drop	Double Salmon Ladder	Unstable Bridge	Balance Tank	Metal Spin	Wall Lift
Season 5	Hang Slider	Double Salmon Ladder	Unstable Bridge	Balance Tank	Metal Spin	Wall Lift
Season 6	Rope Jungle	Double Salmon Ladder	Unstable Bridge	Butterfly Wall	Metal Spin	Wall Lift
Season 7	Rope Jungle	Double Salmon Ladder	Unstable Bridge	Butterfly Wall	Roulette Row	Wall Lift
Season 8	Giant Ring Swing	Down Up Salmon Ladder	Wave Runner	Butterfly Wall	Double Wedge	Wall Flip
Season 9	Giant Ring Swing	Criss Cross Salmon Ladder	Wave Runner	Swing Surfer	Wingnut Alley	Wall Flip

Stage 3 Finals

Season 1	Arm Rings	Descending Lamp Grasper	Devil Steps	Shin-Cliffhanger	Jumping Bars	Hang Climb	Spider Flip	Gliding Ring
Season 2	Roulette Cylinder	Doorknob Grasper	Cycle Road	Ultimate Cliffhanger	Swing Circle	Bungee Rope Climb	Flying Bar	
Season 3	Arm Bike	Flying Bar	Ultimate Cliffhanger	Jumping Rings	Chain Seesaw	Bungee Rope Climb	Bar Glider	
Season 4	Roulette Cylinder	Doorknob Grasper	Floating Boards	Ultimate Cliffhanger	Bungee Rope Climb	Hang Climb	Spider Flip	Flying Bar
Season 5	Roulette Cylinder	Doorknob Grasper	Floating Boards	Ultimate Cliffhanger	Bungee Rope Climb	Hang Climb	Spider Flip	Flying Bar
Season 6	Cannonball Incline	Doorknob Grasper	Floating Boards	Ultimate Cliffhanger	Propeller Bar	Hang Climb	Spider Flip	Flying Bar
Season 7	Psycho Chainsaw	Doorknob Grasper	Floating Boards	Ultimate Cliffhanger	Pole Grasper	Hang Climb	Area 51	Flying Bar
Season 8	Keylock Hang	Floating Boards	Ultimate Cliffhanger	Curved Body Prop	Hang Climb	Walking Bar	Flying Bar	
Season 9	Floating Boards	Keylock Hang	Nail Clipper	Ultimate Cliffhanger	Curved Body Prop	Peg Cloud	Time Bomb	Flying Bar

Stage 4 Finals

DID YOU KNOW?

Geoff Britten, who is the only ninja to have a perfect season to date, used to be very skinny! He was a slim **125 lbs.** into his mid-twenties and still only weighs **150 lbs.**

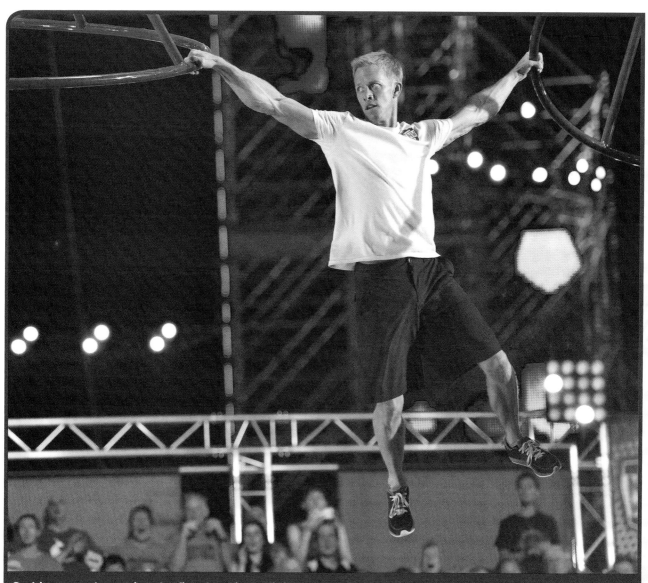

On his way to becoming the first American Ninja Warrior, Geoff Britten swings across Stage Two's Roulette Row during the National Finals of Season 7.

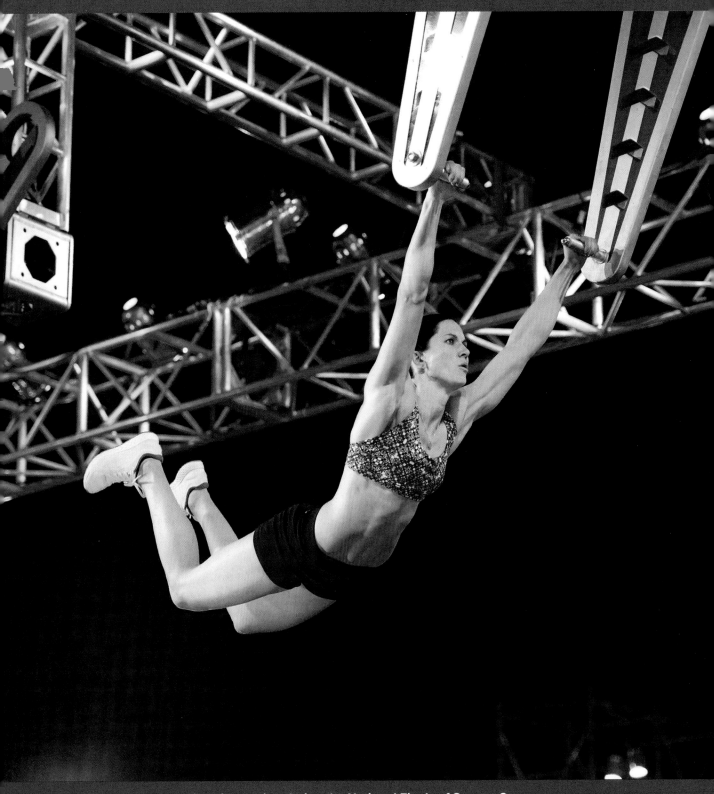

Jesse "Flex" Labreck swings into action during the National Finals of Season 9.

CHAPTER 3

THE NINJAS

Athletes who compete on *American Ninja Warrior* come from virtually every corner of the country. From "Eskimo Ninja" Nick Hanson, who lives in a small town in Alaska—with a population of fewer than 1,000—to "Island Ninja" Grant McCartney who lives in Honolulu, Hawaii, to Jesse "Flex" Labreck, an Oakland, Maine, native who took the course by storm in her rookie year in Season 8, the show's ninjas are as diverse as they are talented.

ELIGIBILITY REQUIREMENTS

Who is eligible to apply to become a competitor on *American Ninja Warrior*? These are the eligibility requirements:

1. You must be a legal resident of the United States.

2. You must be at least 19 years of age. (Prior to Season 10, competitors had to be at least 21 years old to compete.) There is no upper-age limit.

3. You must be in good health and capable of participating in strenuous athletic activities.

4. You must be available to participate in your regional Qualifying round, which will take place sometime in March, April, or May. Additionally, if you qualify or are selected to be a National Finalist, you must be available to participate in the National Finals in Las Vegas later in the year.

5. You must submit a clear digital photo of yourself and a video, approximately 2 to 3 minutes in length, along with your application.

6. To start an application or for more information, visit ANWTryouts.com.

HOW ARE COMPETITORS CHOSEN?

American Ninja Warrior doesn't hold traditional casting calls. Instead, prospective ninjas submit an online application, including a short video of themselves, in order to appear on the show. While in the first few seasons there were only a few hundred submissions, by Season 9 the show was receiving more than 70,000 from all over the country!

"Initially, it was rare to view a submission from someone living in Alaska exercising outside in the snow or from Guam showing their upper-body strength by climbing a large tree outdoors," says Angelou Deign, who serves as casting director for *American Ninja Warrior.* "Nowadays, we see competitors getting visually creative in everyday settings, like an office."

CROSS-SECTION OF AMERICA

"*American Ninja Warrior* is an ensemble," says executive producer Arthur Smith. "During the course of the season, you really want to feel like you have the full spectrum of America represented. You want to have different types, different looks, different personalities, different backgrounds, and that's what the show is."

Executives start the process of selecting ninjas after the new year, in early January, once the deadline for

TECH TALK

The submission video is an important consideration for whether potential ninjas are chosen to compete on the show. According to casting director Angelou Deign, over the years the required length has decreased—from 7 to 8 minutes down to 2 to 3 minutes—while the quality of the videos she has received has increased, mostly due to improvements in high-definition video gadgetry. Still, Deign has two tech tips for would-be ninjas:

- Avoid backlighting: Standing in front of a light while filming yourself will cause the video to appear too dark.
- Always check your volume or audio before sending video.

applications has expired. The casting team watches each competitor's video submission and reads the accompanying application. The team creates a brief bio and notes on the competitors, all of which is then given to casting director Angelou Deign. "The first thing that catches my eye is the competitor's level of energy—vocally and visually," she says. "We hope to find someone with a spark in their eyes, someone who is not over the top, but genuine. We want to mirror America, so we're equally interested in a veterinarian as we are a New York City cab driver. Each season, we hope to share unique stories from everyday people. Even if a story seems sad, those who ultimately become ninjas have a way of sharing that lifts us up and gives us hope that if they can overcome their situation, then we too can conquer our real-life obstacles!"

TEAM EFFORT

Once casting director Angelou Deign narrows down the applications from the tens of thousands to the hundreds, the casting team prepares the remaining applications, with Deign's notes, for the executives from the network and production company. Deign says that the submissions that the executives feel unanimously or most positive about become the selected competitors.

Although athleticism is certainly a key deciding factor for being selected to appear on *American Ninja Warrior*, show executives each have slightly different criteria for choosing ninjas. "Applicants with lots of positive energy tend to stand out," says executive producer Anthony Storm. "Interesting jobs, backgrounds, families, or stories also grab our attention. And anyone that's impressive on ninja obstacles gets serious consideration. We love seeing success on the course!"

"Do they sound genuinely excited and present a great case for why you should select them? And then do they have the athletic ability to at least get through a few obstacles?" notes executive producer Brian Richardson. "You don't expect everyone to finish the course, but you don't want someone to get hurt because they haven't trained properly. And then you look at what that person's story is: whether it's their job, or their family, or a hobby, or even where they're from. Is it unique? Is it relatable? Is this someone Americans will root for? Sometimes it just comes down to numbers. There are a lot of good choices, and there just aren't enough spots for everyone."

"Narrowing it down is one of the toughest things we have to do," adds executive producer Kent Weed. "It's a monster, not because it's a choice between individuals who are good and those who are not good. It's a choice between two goods. Plus, you have to have a certain mix of everything. You have to think about skills and stories, adversity, and gender when you put the story together."

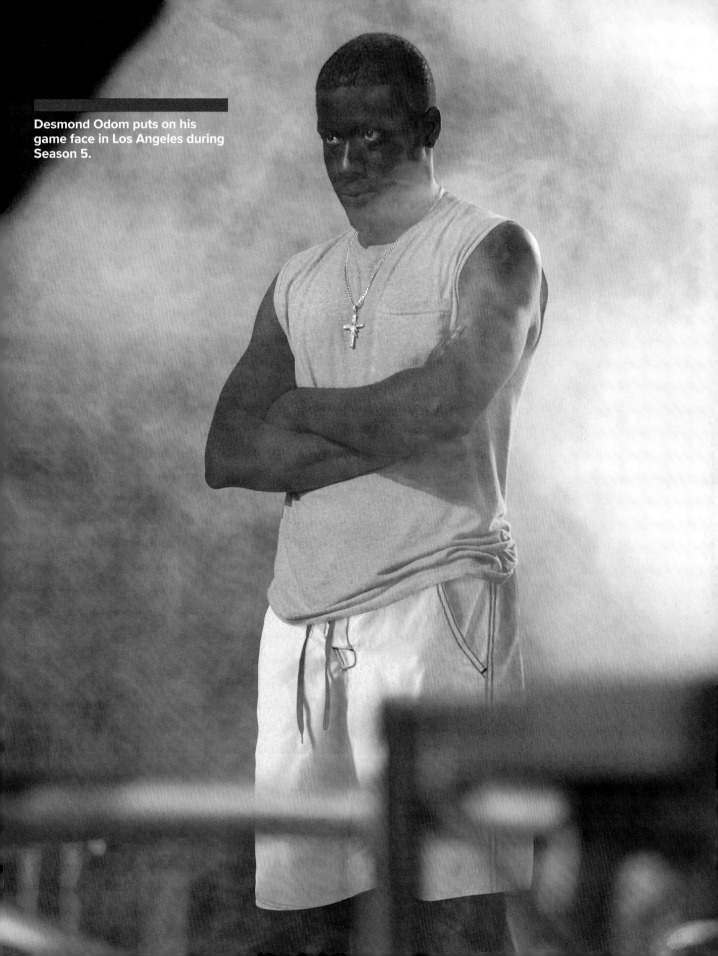

Desmond Odom puts on his game face in Los Angeles during Season 5.

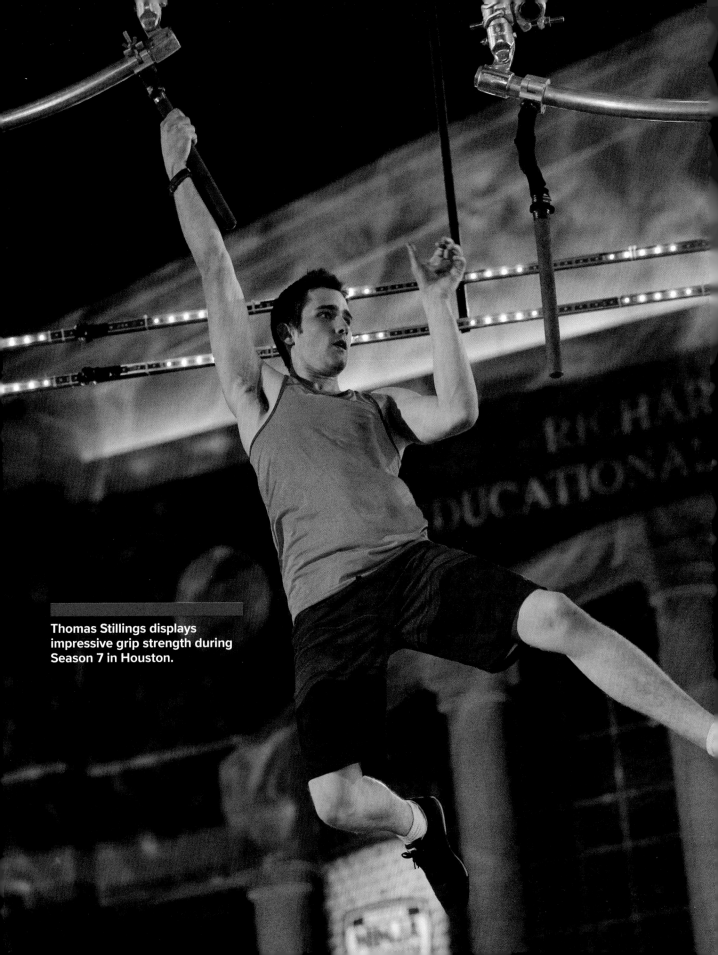

Thomas Stillings displays
impressive grip strength during
Season 7 in Houston.

> The hosts get a big binder with about 100 ninja one-sheets (single documents that provide information and stats on each ninja) a few days before we head to each city to shoot. I go through each one-sheet while I watch the ninja's submission video, and then I make notes on things that stand out or questions I want to make sure to ask. I do about 10 at a time and then take a break... usually while eating M&M's. Then I feel guilty for eating the M&M's as I watch extremely fit and athletic people in videos.
>
> —Cohost Kristine Leahy

EVEN VETERANS NEED TO REAPPLY

Veteran ninjas follow the same application procedures as new competitors, as there is no guarantee that any ninja will be back for another season, even if he or she did well the previous year. Executive producer Brian Richardson says *American Ninja Warrior* executives try to keep roughly a 60/40 mix of new people and ninja veterans. "We want to bring back those who have done well or are fan favorites but also allow new athletes a chance to break in and have a chance at the course," he says.

That means submission videos are just as important for veterans as they are for rookies. "It's very competitive for those slots," Richardson says, "and we want the people who really want to be there. If a veteran sends in a tape that just doesn't show much enthusiasm or seems like they're just going through the motions, then they may not get invited that season."

'NINJA FIT'

Casting director Angelou Deign says that she and the other show executives are looking for whether

an applicant is "ninja fit," meaning that their skill set includes agility, stamina, strength, grip-strength, balance and flexibility. "The only way we'll know if someone can handle the obstacle course is by them showing themselves in their videos," Deign says, "conquering ninja-style obstacles in a continual pattern, as they would be required to do on the show."

STRENGTH-TO-WEIGHT RATIO

Many times in American sports, size and strength are the most important competitive characteristics, but that's not necessarily so on *American Ninja Warrior*. Strength-to-weight ratio—strength, or the amount of weight ninjas can lift, divided by their body weight—plays more of a key role in course success. In other words, the less weight you have to carry on the course, the better your strength—or you can carry a lot of weight as long as you are able to lift that much more.

Size, by itself, is indeterminate as a measure of success. "Mighty" Kacy Catanzaro, at only five feet in height, triumphed over the Qualifying and City Finals courses in Dallas in Season 6. On the other side of

> Isaac Caldiero and Geoff Britten climbing Stage Four in Season 7 was a big moment. It's the only time anyone's made it that far on the course, and the only time someone has won the million dollars. But probably the biggest thing to affect the growth of the show was Kacy Catanzaro in Season 6. During that year, Kacy became the first woman to get up the Warped Wall and then became the first woman to finish a City Finals course. Both were huge accomplishments, but what was extraordinary was that Kacy was 5 feet tall and weighed 100 pounds. She opened the eyes of so many people, both women and men. If she could do it, they could do it. The next year, our submissions increased tenfold, from around 5,000 a year to about 50,000. A huge majority of them cited Kacy as the reason they were trying out. She was also the first to get large-scale media attention, doing commercials, making appearances on the *Today* show, etc., things that had not happened with our athletes before. Since then, another woman, Jessie Graff, has become a huge media star. In the past few years, she has had several history-making, boundary-breaking runs that have garnered a ton of attention and made her one of the most recognized female athletes in the country.
>
> –Executive Producer Brian Richardson

the spectrum, Texan Jody Avila, at 6 feet, 6 inches and 215 pounds, seemed an unlikely ninja victor at the San Antonio Qualifiers in Season 9. However, the HVAC technician had the strength to carry his weight, and he went on to complete all obstacles in his run, earning the nickname of "Big Dawg Ninja" from host Akbar Gbajabiamila.

"Athletes with good strength-to-weight ratios normally do well on the course, regardless of their trained athletic fields," says Deign. "On any given day, it could be anyone's day to succeed. No one can predict the obstacles and how the course will play."

VARYING SKILL SETS

Every ninja brings something different to the course. "When we look at our top competitors, from the physical point of view, we see a history of pretty high-level activity," says host Matt Iseman. "Most Finals of the top ninjas grew up active—gymnastics or rock climbing. Parkour has also been an important skill set for the ninjas. But the thing I really learned is, more than any particular physical skills or experience, the

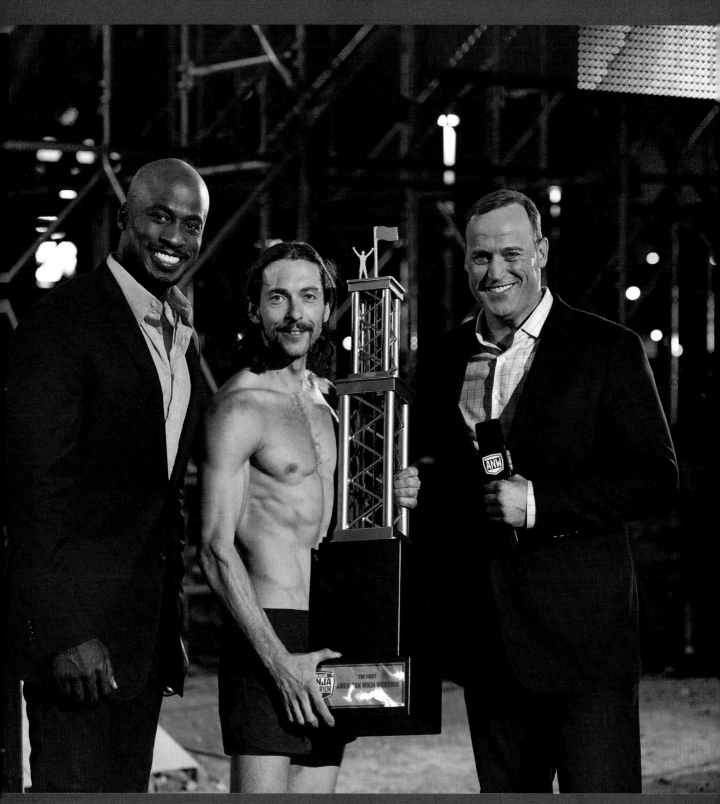

In Season 7, busboy Isaac Caldiero thrilled audiences when he barely beat Geoff Britten's time, completing Stage Four of the National Finals and becoming the first and only winner of *American Ninja Warrior* to date! Holding his well-earned trophy, Caldiero is flanked here by hosts Akbar Gbajabiamila (left) and Matt Iseman.

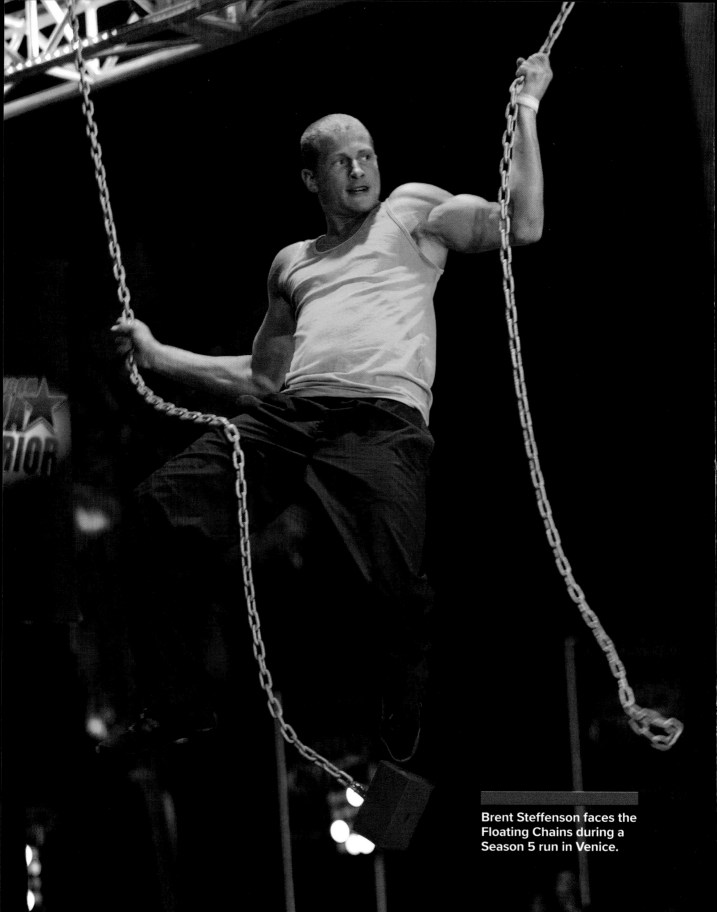

Brent Steffenson faces the
Floating Chains during a
Season 5 run in Venice.

biggest predictor for success is determination. The athletes that do well on *American Ninja Warrior* are the athletes who were willing to work the hardest."

Upper-body strength, core stability, speed—these are integral aspects of ninja success. According to host Akbar Gbajabiamila, parkour practitioners often come alive and go far in the competition, which usually features agility obstacles mixed with upper-body strength obstacles. "Also, climbers are used to operating under stress when their lives are on the line, especially the free climbers. Those guys are nuts," Gbajabiamila says. "When they're in situations where they're starting to feel the burn, they can dig deep in an area where some of the other competitors and ninjas can't. They can't go that far because they've never been there. It's like muscle memory. The climbers know, 'I'm starting to get pumped out, I'm starting to get gassed out, but I know where to go and how to tap into my reserves.'"

> " The ones who have been successful have been the ones who have been in this type of form before where they've been competitive for a long time. Meagan Martin, college athlete. Kacy Catanzaro, college athlete. Kevin Bull has that pedigree. Jessie Graff, college athlete.
> —Host Akbar Gbajabiamila "

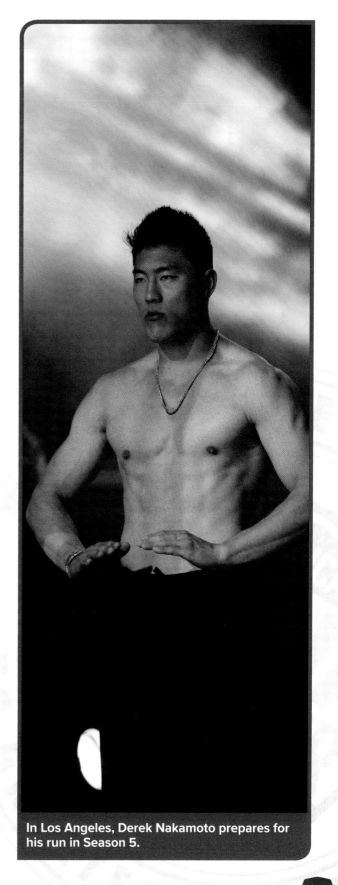

In Los Angeles, Derek Nakamoto prepares for his run in Season 5.

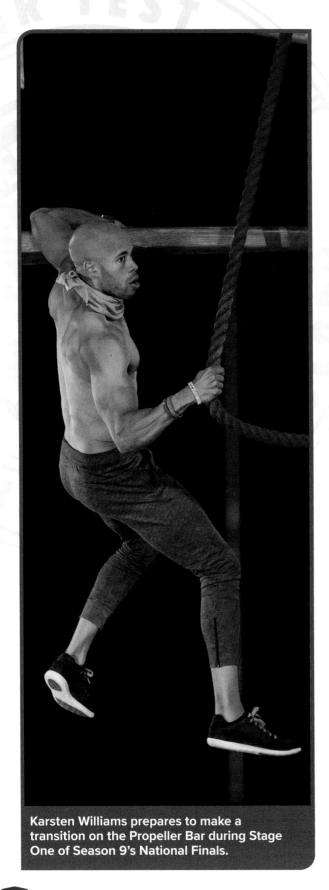

Karsten Williams prepares to make a transition on the Propeller Bar during Stage One of Season 9's National Finals.

> It's not always about going the farthest or winning the money. Sometimes it's just about showing up. When I look at an athlete like Steven Moul who has severe autism but came out of his shell training for *American Ninja Warrior*, he fell on just the second obstacle, but he came out of the water like he won the Super Bowl! That moment really showed me how athletes can truly achieve victory in so many different ways.
>
> –Host Matt Iseman

STORYTELLERS

One of the most popular aspects of *American Ninja Warrior* is the "competitor profiles," the background packages shown just before ninjas run the course that offer an inside look into their lives. As athletes step up to the starting line, viewers discover what led them to the course—a personal or family tragedy, a deep-rooted conviction. They have become tiny movie—and moving—moments within the show.

"The story packages help connect the audience with the athletes," says executive producer Anthony

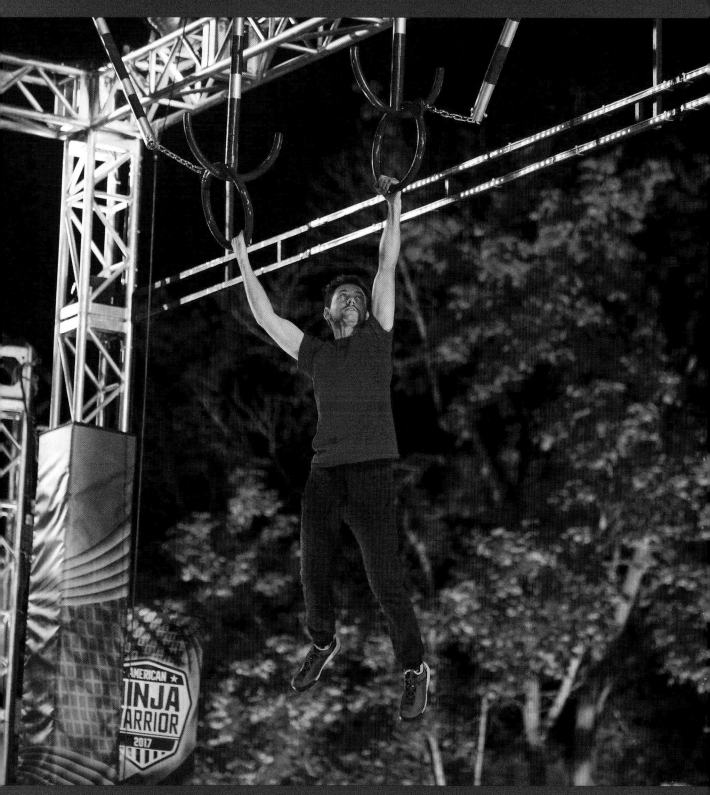

In an emotional run during Season 9's Denver Finals, Dalton Knapp, who had watched *American Ninja Warrior* from his hospital bed for years while he was battling cancer, competed alongside his brother, Drew. Dalton, shown here on the Ring Swing, made it all the way to the Salmon Ladder.

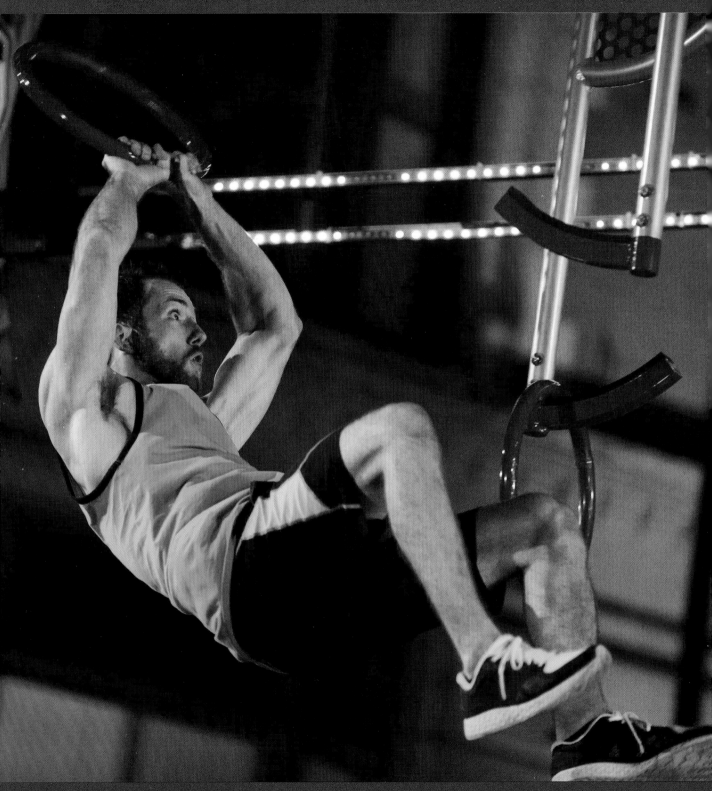

Nico Gentry, who was born with nystagmus, a neurological disorder, and is legally blind, takes on the obstacle course during Season 9's San Antionio Qualifiers.

Storm. "The appeal of *American Ninja Warrior* is that the competitors are everyday people, relatable to the viewers. By sharing their stories, we give the audience a reason to root for them on their journey."

Executive producer Brian Richardson notes that once the hundred or so competitors are selected for each city's Qualifying round, "we start thinking about stories for each of them," he says. "Our producers review submission tapes, do phone interviews weeks before the competition, and then do interviews on-site the day before competition begins. All of this is to see who has a great story to tell and to get viewers invested in the athlete's run."

"We root for these people. We care about them," adds executive producer Arthur Smith. "We fall in love with them, and that's what makes the run so much more exciting. The runs are exciting in themselves but when you feel something and you care for something, it affects you differently."

THE HEART OF A NINJA

Some ninjas who compete on *American Ninja Warrior* are fighting more than an obstacle course:

- Grand Rapids, Michigan student Steven Moul, who is autistic and also a super-fan of *American Ninja Warrior*, competed in Kansas City in Season 7. He made it past the Quintuple Steps, the first obstacle, before succumbing to the Big Dipper.
- Dalton Knapp, who used to watch *American Ninja Warrior* from his hospital bed during his cancer treatments, competed in Season 9 in Denver alongside his brother, Drew.
- Nico Gentry, who first appeared in Season 9 during the San Antonio Qualifiers, was born with a neurological disorder called nystagmus, which affects the muscles behind his eyes, rendering him legally blind.
- Zach Gowen, who lost a leg to cancer when he was only eight years old, competed without his prosthesis in the Indianapolis Qualifying round of Season 8, making it halfway through the course.

> Submission videos are incredibly hard to make. You have to sell yourself in two to three minutes. I've always followed the same formula—starting with a cool shot that hopefully makes a producer want to see more, followed by a talking intro, a story about me, and ending with a fun action edit showing off some strengths of mine.
> —Geoff Britten

- Jimmy Choi of Season 9 battles young-onset Parkinson's Disease off the course when he's not taking on the obstacles on the course.

Others compete for a cause. K9 Ninja Andrew "Roo" Yori of Season 8 dedicated his runs on *American Ninja Warrior* to raising awareness of dog adoption. Sarah Poulin, who lost her five-year-old son Jacob to brain cancer in 2016, competed on *American Ninja Warrior*—a show he loved—in Season 9 in his honor.

In Season 8, construction worker Kenneth Niemitalo competed in Atlanta and shared the story of his daughter Hazel, who was born in April 2015 and had been diagnosed with congenital nephrotic syndrome, a kidney disease that has no cure other than a donor transplant. Amy Schlee, an *American Ninja Warrior* fan, had been watching the episode

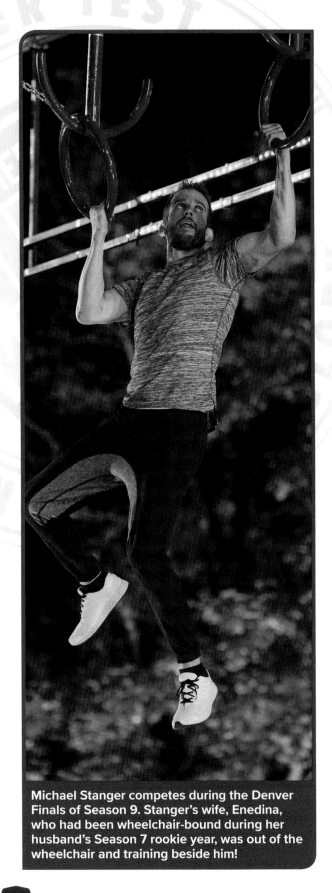

Michael Stanger competes during the Denver Finals of Season 9. Stanger's wife, Enedina, who had been wheelchair-bound during her husband's Season 7 rookie year, was out of the wheelchair and training beside him!

and volunteered to become Hazel's donor. In Season 9, Schlee was standing on the sidelines with Niemitalo's family to watch him run the course.

And then there was Michael Stanger, a walk-on in Season 7 whose wife, Enedina, was in a wheelchair due to a rare disorder, Ehlers-Danlos syndrome. Stanger drove with friends for 23 hours and waited in line for eight days to get the chance to compete and put a smile on his wife's face. Host Akbar Gbajabiamila called his performance on the course "a physical love letter to his wife." Even more remarkably, when Stanger competed in Season 9, his wife, who had begun ninja training alongside him, was out of the wheelchair!

REDEFINING SUCCESS

American Ninja Warrior competitors exemplify more than physical strength or agility—their inspiring stories show what it means to fight and to believe. "When I think of the runs that really stick in my memory," says host Matt Iseman, "for every history-making run like Kacy Catanzaro, there's a run like Sarah Poulin, a mother who was running to honor the memory of the son she lost to brain cancer only months before. I think of Michael Stanger running for his wife and family. These rounds where the athletes share their stories and share their hardships are what the audience truly relates to. Life isn't always easy, and I think if you were to watch a show and see someone battling some of the same struggles you may be facing in your life, it makes you feel not so alone. And it also gives you hope. If that person can continue to fight, maybe you can too."

Iseman adds, "It's been remarkable seeing the show really redefine what success means. Traditionally, it meant winning, going all the way, hitting the buzzer, but for so many athletes just getting on the course is a victory. And I think that's what makes the show so popular, that the obstacles the athletes conquer off the course are more impressive than the ones they conquer on the course."

> We're in the middle of a thunderstorm in Kansas City at four o'clock in the morning, and we're surrounded by thunder and lightning, and Peter Szeliga, the casting producer, comes into the booth and says, 'Kent, can we please run one more person? The guy drove 12 hours.' I go, 'Peter, I've got to shoot stand-ups with the host, I've got so much stuff that I've got to do.' He says, 'His wife also drove, she's in a wheelchair.' I say, 'Okay, we'll run one.' Now, no one expected Michael Stanger to complete the course. He was a walk-on. We had little information on him and sure enough, there he was. It's such an amazing story. He was a fan of *Ninja Warrior*. He gave so much up to his wife to support her. He literally carried her up the stairs every night. His back was killing him. He goes back to the gym. He gets in good shape. He's watching *Ninja Warrior* on television. His wife turns to him and says, you need to go on this show, and so he does. He waits in line, and then he's the last runner of the night and he completes the course. We are very, very blessed because these stories happen again and again and again and again.
> —Executive Producer Kent Weed

WARRIOR WORDS

NEXT-GEN NINJA: An athlete who has grown up watching *American Ninja Warrior* season after season, training and waiting until they are old enough to compete. The phrase is short for Next-Generation Ninja.

NEXT-GEN NINJAS

Many of *American Ninja Warrior*'s fans were kids when they first started watching—they were under the age limit and too young to compete on the show. However, over the years, many of them trained in their backyards and on playgrounds and at their local gyms, emulating the moves they saw on the show, watching how to clear the obstacles, training for the day when they, too, could show their stuff on the obstacle course. Now, many of those kids have come of age and can legally compete on *American Ninja Warrior*. They are the Next-Generation Ninjas.

"What we're seeing now is the next generation of the *Ninja Warrior* athlete," says host Matt Iseman. "They've grown up training for this sport since they were 12 or 13 or 14 years old. This is their sport. And I think they're going to take *American Ninja Warrior* to the next level."

"They scare me," says host Akbar Gbajabiamila of this emerging crop of atheletes. "These new competitors have years and years of film to watch, and they have been training for a long time. They're like metahumans—they can do super-crazy things. They're young, they're strong, and they don't have

a lot of fear. Young kids just do whatever comes to mind. They don't think about stuff. So when they step on the *Ninja Warrior* course, they just go straight for it no matter how hard or how long the obstacle is, and the producers and ATS have been designing some crazy and diabolical obstacles!"

And with the growth of ninja gyms across the country, Next-Gen Ninjas have more access to obstacle training than the show's competitors before them. "Sometimes you'd have to go cross-country just to be able to train at a place that had some of the facilities," Gbajabiamila says. "Now, within two to three hours of a major city, you can find a ninja gym. They're all over. It's literally a movement."

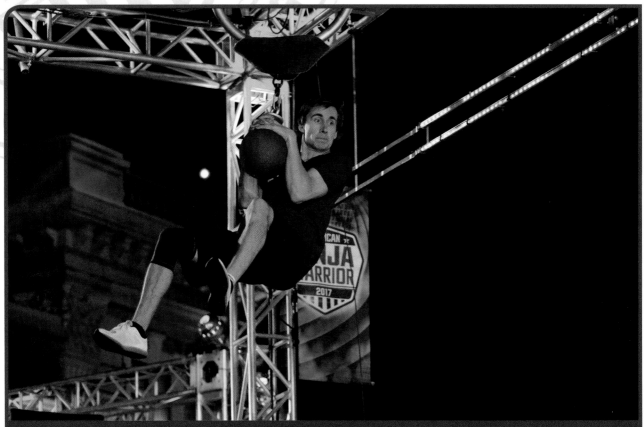

Next-gen ninja Charlie Andrews made his debut in a *Ninja Warrior* broadcast when he represented MIT in *Team Ninja Warrior: College Madness* in 2016. Andrews, who entered regular competition in *American Ninja Warrior*'s Season 9 in Los Angeles, is shown here on Cannonball Drop in the City Finals.

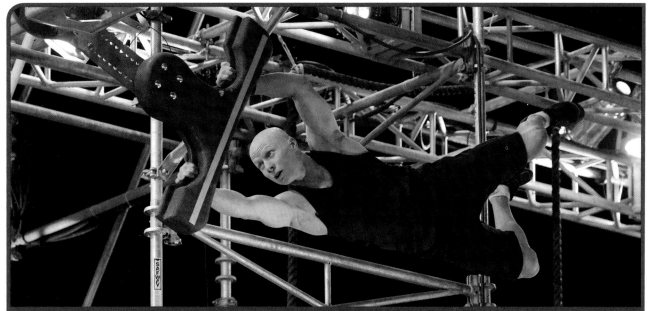

A walk-on in Season 6, Kevin Bull—shown here on Wingnut Alley in Stage Two of Season 9's National Finals—would go on to become one of the most competitive and consistent ninjas in *American Ninja Warrior* history.

WARRIOR WORDS

WALK-ON: A competitor who, although not invited to appear on a season of *American Ninja Warrior*, waits outside the course at any of the Qualifying cities during shooting in hopes of getting a shot at running the course. Athletes have been known to sleep in tents for a week or more, hoping to get first dibs, almost like a Black Friday sale. Since there is usually only time to run 20 to 30 people from the walk-on line, there is no guarantee that a walk-on candidate will appear on the show.

WALK-ONS

Approximately 100 people are selected to run the course in each of the cities that the *American Ninja Warrior* production is visiting. If would-be ninjas are not chosen for the show, they can try their luck on what's called the walk-on line. In each city, just outside the course, potential competitors line up, and the show producers pull a few extra competitors from this line to round out the group of athletes. Although being a walk-on doesn't guarantee athletes a slot on the show, casting director Angelou Deign says the show executives like to see 15 to 25 walk-on competitors run the course in each city.

"The number of walk-on competitors varies per city, based on several factors ranging from how many booked competitors there are in that city to weather-related issues that may cause technical delays," Deign says. "If it's pouring rain on shoot day, we may be limited on the amount of time we have to film—in which case, we focus on getting the scheduled/booked competitors on the course." Some notable ninja legends have come from the walk-on line, such as Kevin Bull.

Walk-ons have been known to camp out for as long as a month for the chance to run the *American Ninja Warrior* course! Kevin Carbone, the designer

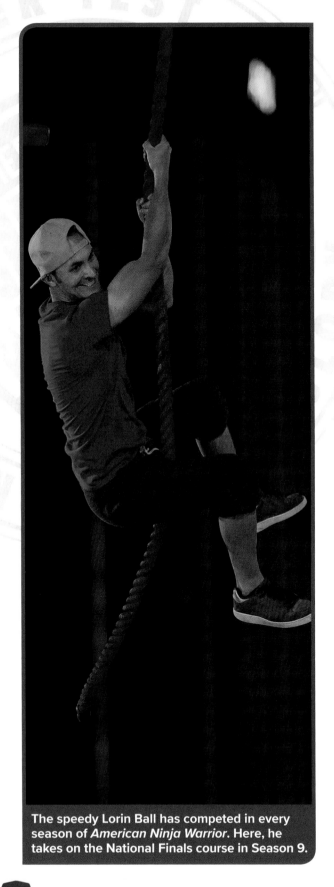

The speedy Lorin Ball has competed in every season of *American Ninja Warrior*. Here, he takes on the National Finals course in Season 9.

of the Wingnuts obstacle, was a walk-on in Season 9 and made it all the way to the National Finals his rookie year. When he didn't get a call to compete on the show after submitting his application and video, "the guys at my gym suggested I could be a tester or wait in the walk-on line," Carbone says.

"I packed up my Jeep and headed south. My parents thought I was crazy! We didn't even know where the *American Ninja Warrior* course was going to be set up, so John Brown started the line at a nearby park. We hung out all day, exercising together, and the line began to grow. It felt like the best day camp I ever attended, we had so much fun. On the Sunday before the show started, we moved the line to the speedway, and there were about 35 guys and girls!"

Carbone got his chance and finally stepped up to the starting line. "I had such a mix of emotions," he says, "a happy combination of excitement, fear, and wanting to throw up! The countdown started, and I took my first steps and stopped thinking and started doing."

THE NICKNAMES

So many of the ninjas have become recognizable simply by their nicknames—"Real Life Ninja" (Drew Drechsel), "Island Ninja" (Grant McCartney), "The Godfather" (David Campbell), "Captain NBC" (Jamie Rahn). According to executive producer Arthur Smith, the nicknames didn't happen by chance. They were an intentional aspect of the show.

"We're all about branding, and when you brand people—"Cowboy Ninja," "Mighty Kacy"—it's easier to remember them," he says. "The branding comes from a lot of sources. Sometimes it's from Matt Iseman and Akbar Gbajabiamila, who are phenomenal. Sometimes it comes from the producers. And we all work together on that, and once we have a good handle it becomes part of the vernacular of the show. It is a concerted effort to brand people so that they become memorable and stand out."

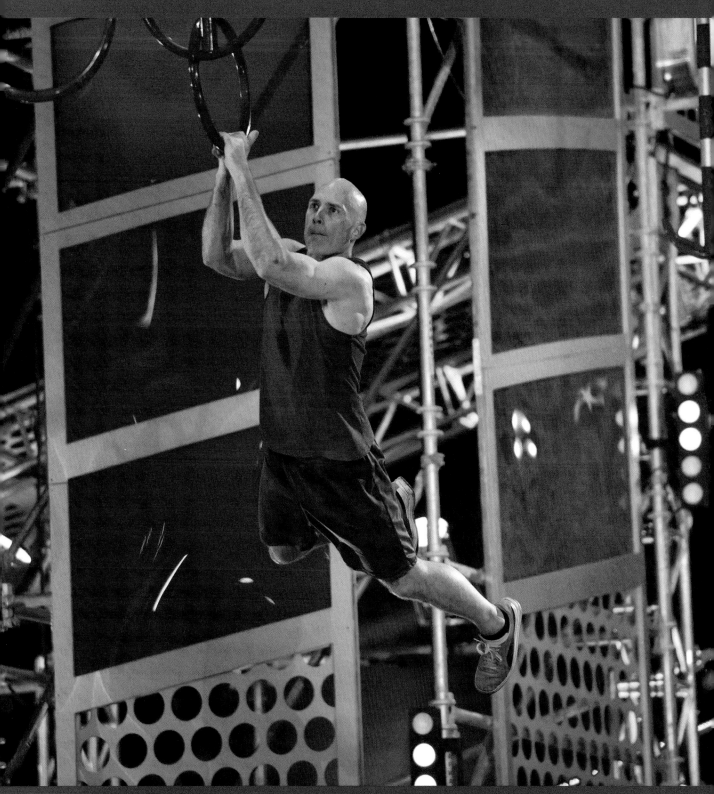

Many *American Ninja Warrior* competitors are known by their ninja nicknames, such as "The Godfather" David Campbell, shown here on the Giant Ring Swing during Stage Two of the Season 9 National Finals in Vegas.

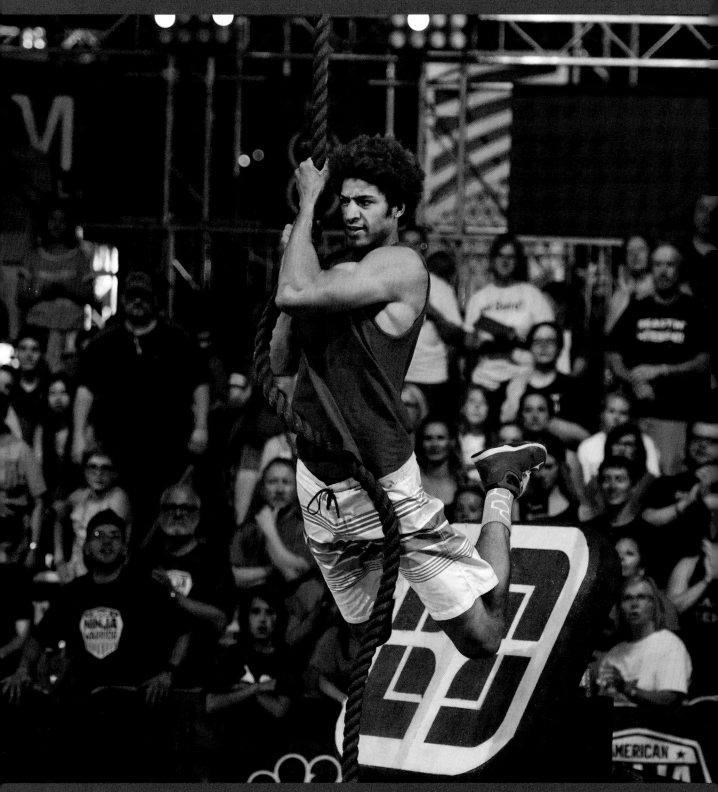

Six-foot-six Jon Alexis Jr., known to fans as "The Giant," competes in the National Finals in Las Vegas in Season 9.

FAN FARE

THE VETERANS

Each season of *American Ninja Warrior* brings back familiar faces. They're the ninjas that fans of the show have come to know and love. They're from all over the United States, they have diverse backgrounds, but they all have one thing on their mind—crushing the course. Here's a roundup of some of *American Ninja Warrior*'s fan favorites and those who made history.

JON ALEXIS JR.

Known as "The Giant," Jon Alexis Jr., a carpenter from Newton, Massachusetts, stands at 6-foot-6 and is one of the tallest competitors ever to appear on *American Ninja Warrior*. He first competed in Orlando in Season 7—alongside his father, Jon Alexis Sr.—and put up the fastest time in the Qualifiers, but did not make it to the National Finals. Alexis returned in Philadelphia in Season 8 and put up the second fastest time in the Qualifiers and placed high enough in the City Finals to move on to Vegas. He returned to the National Finals in Season 9. Alexis also competed in *Team Ninja Warrior* as part of Jesse "Flex" Labreck's team, Labreckfast Club. In Season 9, Alexis hit his first buzzer in Vegas on Stage One.

BRIAN ARNOLD

Brian Arnold has been one of the most consistent competitors on *American Ninja Warrior*. In his first five seasons, he never failed to reach Stage Two. In Season 5, he reached the Flying Bar obstacle, which was the farthest that any American had ever gone. Following his success in Season 5, Arnold was selected to compete in *USA vs. Japan*, where he won both his Stage Two and Stage Three heats, again reaching the Flying Bar on Stage Three. Following Season 6, Arnold was selected to represent America in *USA vs. The World*. Again, he won both his Stage Two and Stage Three heats, but this time he was able to complete Stage Three—a feat that no American had been able to do. Arnold's team "Party Time," featuring Jake Murray and Jennifer Tavernier, were the winners of the inaugural *Team Ninja Warrior* competition. Following Season 5, Arnold, who is a member of the Wolfpack Ninjas, left his job as a nursing home maintenance director to focus on family and *Ninja Warrior*. He currently has the longest streak of Stage One finishes among ninjas—six in a row!

LORIN BALL

Denver's Lorin Ball, a gym owner who has appeared on every season of *American Ninja Warrior*, is known as a "go fast or go home" competitor. He either dominates the course—often clearing it with the fastest time of the night, as he did in the Season 9 Denver Qualifiers—or he takes a shocking fall.

WOLFPACK NINJAS
The Wolfpack Ninjas are Brian Arnold, "Wolfpup" Ian Dory, "Ninjadoc" Noah Kaufman, and "SheWolf" Meagan Martin. They train together in Colorado and are dedicated to using their skills and influence to motivate others to enjoy a healthy life.

ALLYSSA BEIRD

Allyssa Beird—affectionately nicknamed "Ms. Beird," because she's a schoolteacher from Marlborough, Massachusetts—helped make *American Ninja Warrior* history in Season 8, her rookie year, when she was one of four women to qualify for the Philadelphia Finals (she later received a Wild Card spot to the National Finals). In Season 9, she became the first woman to clear an *American Ninja Warrior* course that season when she hit a buzzer—her first!—during the Cleveland Qualifiers. (She was also the first competitor to clear the I-Beam Gap obstacle that night.) Additionally, she became just the sixth woman ever to scale the Warped Wall and the fifth woman ever to complete a Qualifying course. Her performance was so inspiring that host Akbar Gbajabiamila tossed this teacher an apple from the host stand—she earned it! Plus, in the National Finals of Season 9, she became only the second woman—behind Jessie Graff—to ever hit a Stage One buzzer. Talk about an A+!

MIKE BERNARDO

Washington, D.C., firefighter Mike Bernardo has competed in every season of *American Ninja Warrior* since Season 2. In the St. Louis Qualifiers in Season 6, he shocked fans when he failed to get across the Bridge of Blades, slipping on one of the platforms. However, in the 2016 *American Ninja Warrior All-Star Special: Skills Challenge* Bernardo performed an epic climb up the Super Salmon Ladder, igniting the audience and his fellow ninjas on the sidelines.

GEOFF BRITTEN

Maryland professional cameraman Geoff Britten took a turn in front of the cameras for a shot at *American Ninja Warrior* glory in Season 6, and in Season 7 he shot to ninja fame when he became the first competitor ever to complete all four stages of the National Finals. However, moments later, Britten saw that $1 million prize slip away when Isaac Caldiero scaled Mount Midoriyama just

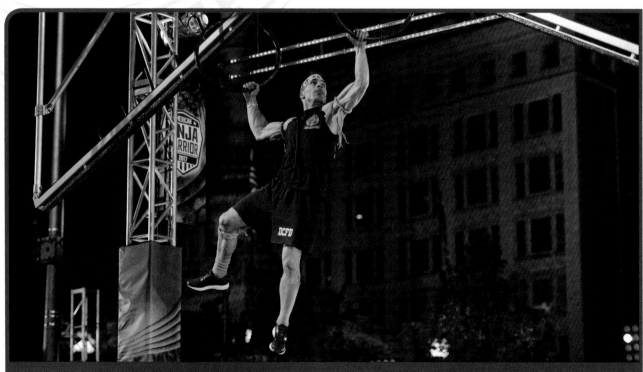

Firefighter Mike Bernardo has competed in every season of *American Ninja Warrior* since Season 2. Here, he masters the Ring Jump during the Cleveland Finals in Season 9.

BECOME AN AMERICAN NINJA WARRIOR: THE ULTIMATE INSIDER'S GUIDE

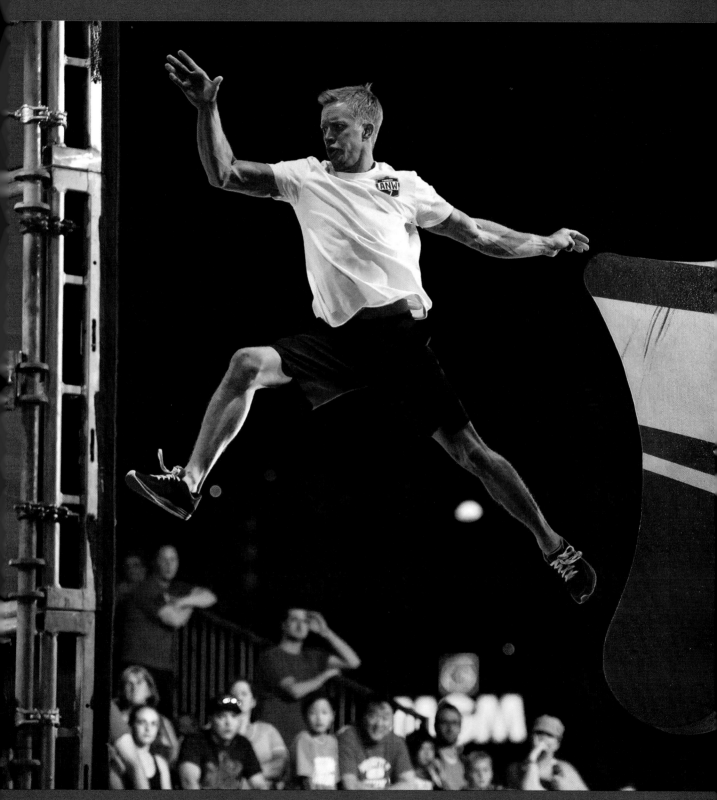

In Season 7, Geoff Britten, shown here completing the Butterfly Wall in Stage Two, became the first competitor in *American Ninja Warrior* history to complete all four stages of the National Finals in Las Vegas.

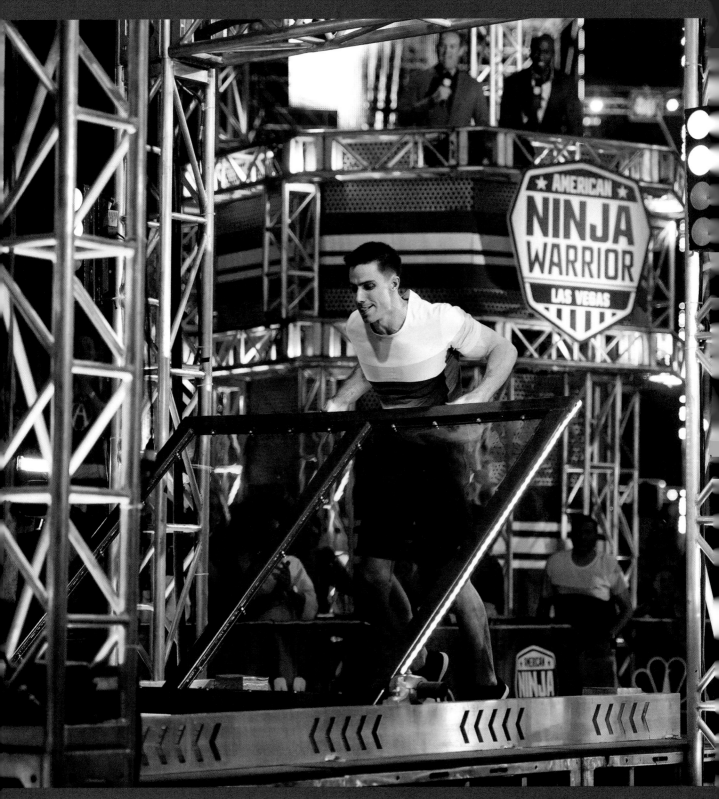

"Papal Ninja" Sean Bryan crushes the Wall Flip in his Stage Two run in Season 9. Bryan was one of three ninjas (along with "Philly Phoenix" Najee Richardson and "The Weatherman" Joe Moravsky) to go on to Stage Three that season.

seconds faster! Britten, who earned the nickname "Popeye" because of his massive forearms, remains the only competitor to ever have a perfect season, completing all six obstacle courses and hitting all six buzzers. After an early exit in the Season 8 National Finals, Britten announced in 2016 that he was taking time off from *American Ninja Warrior*, but fans hope he'll return one day (for more on Britten, see page 246).

SEAN BRYAN

Known as "Papal Ninja," Sean Bryan has competed on *American Ninja Warrior* since Season 8. He received his bachelor of arts degree from UC Berkeley, where he studied physics and was on the men's gymnastics team. In 2015, he completed his master of arts in theology at the Dominican School of Philosophy & Theology. He currently serves as the animating director of the Lay Mission Project. He was one of only three ninjas (along with Najee Richardson and Joe Moravsky) to make it to Stage Three in Season 9.

> I was definitely a fan of both *American Ninja Warrior* and the original Japanese show, although I didn't follow closely enough to know who everyone was at first. My fascination was mostly with the obstacles. I had wanted a competitive obstacle course sport since I was a little kid, and the *Ninja Warrior/SASUKE* shows looked like it.
>
> —Kevin Bull

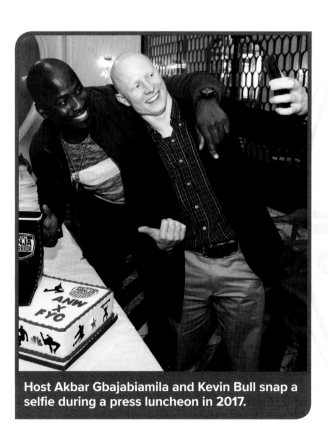

Host Akbar Gbajabiamila and Kevin Bull snap a selfie during a press luncheon in 2017.

KEVIN BULL

In Season 6, stock trader Kevin Bull first appeared on *American Ninja Warrior* as a walk-on and finished the Los Angeles Qualifying course with the fourth-fastest time. One of the fastest and most consistent ninjas, Bull is probably most known for using an unorthodox approach to complete the Cannonball Alley obstacle—using his feet to grab the third cannonball, rather than his hands—and he would eventually be one of only two competitors to complete the LA Finals course that season. Bull, who lives with a condition called alopecia, which causes his distinctive hairless look, has also appeared on *Team Ninja Warrior* as a member of "Team Grit."

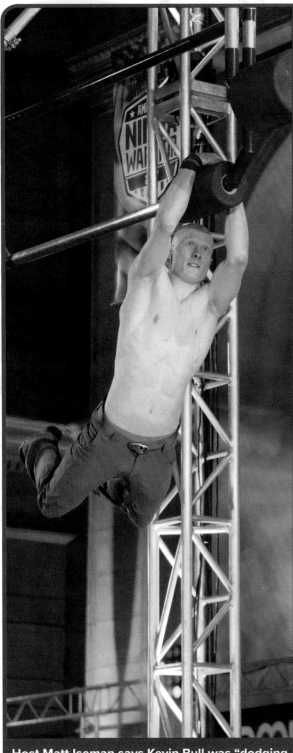

Host Matt Iseman says Kevin Bull was "dodging bullets" when he nearly lost his grip on the Battering Ram in Season 9's Los Angeles Qualifier. However, the veteran ninja was able to recover and complete the course with one of the fastest times of the night.

> No one could figure out Cannonball Alley, and Kevin Bull improvised. He was going outside the box, went upside down, inverted, and was able to complete the obstacle.
> —Host Akbar Gbajabiamila

> A lot of our ninjas run the course to bring more attention to causes that are important to them. For example, one of our well-known competitors, Kevin Bull, has alopecia. He's used the show to bring more awareness to those with the condition. When you look at Kevin out there on the course, and then you see twenty-five young kids with alopecia out there cheering alongside him, it's amazing to see – he's running for them.
> —Executive Producer Arthur Smith

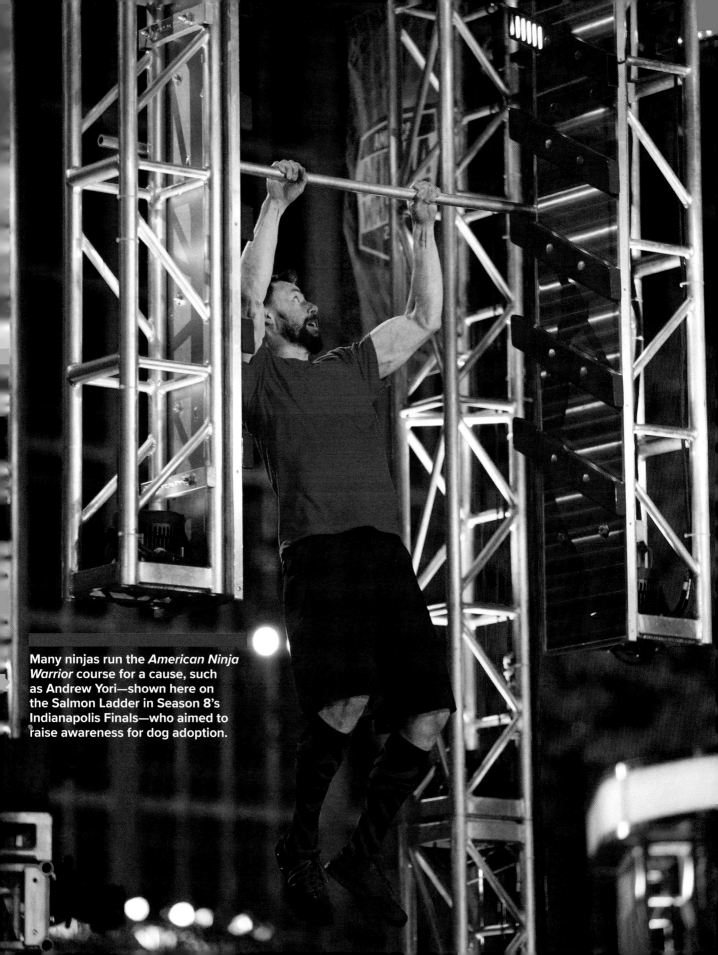

Many ninjas run the *American Ninja Warrior* course for a cause, such as Andrew Yori—shown here on the Salmon Ladder in Season 8's Indianapolis Finals—who aimed to raise awareness for dog adoption.

NINJA SPOTLIGHT:

ISAAC CALDIERO

Former busboy and professional climber Isaac Caldiero had been a big fan of *SASUKE*, and after seeing it come to America was immediately interested. "But I had no insight or clue how to actually participate in a show," he says. "I was pretty consumed by my climbing career, but after speaking with a close friend whose friend had competed, I got the info for how to submit a video to the casting agency."

Caldiero's submission video showcased his life and skills as a pro climber, juggler, biker, and slackliner, to name a few of his interests. "I thought my video was awesome and that there was no chance of the producers denying me," he says. "Unfortunately, I uploaded the video a few minutes too late and I was bound to the infamous and dreadful walk-on line."

But Caldiero's first appearance on the show in Season 5 has gone down as one of the most memorable in *American Ninja Warrior* lore as he walked to the starting line wearing a Jesus costume. "I wanted to do something to make myself stand out among the masses of people in the walk-on line," he says. "I just so happened to have a spare Jesus costume lying around from a past Halloween, and, thus, 'Ninjesus' was born!"

Caldiero took the competition by storm and made it all the way to Vegas in his rookie year until the Jumping Spider took him out. The following year, he made it to Stage Two when he fell on the Salmon Ladder, but by Season 7 he was determined to go all the way and cleared Stage Four with the fastest time, becoming the first and only winner of *American Ninja Warrior* to date!

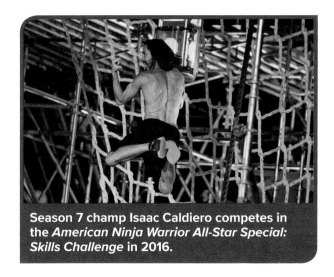

Season 7 champ Isaac Caldiero competes in the *American Ninja Warrior All-Star Special: Skills Challenge* in 2016.

DAVID CAMPBELL

Nicknamed "The Godfather," David Campbell has appeared on every season of *American Ninja Warrior*. He started his ninja career during *American Ninja Challenge*, earning a place in *SASUKE* 22, 26, and 27, making it to Stage Three in the latter two. He climbed his way to Total Victory in *SASUKE* Vietnam in 2016. Today, a lot of people build *Ninja Warrior*-style obstacle courses, but Campbell is known as the very first ninja to build a large-scale course in his backyard.

NINJA SPOTLIGHT:

KACY CATANZARO

Petite powerhouse Kacy Catanzaro, nicknamed "Mighty" Kacy, is a woman of firsts. She was the first woman to conquer the 14-foot Warped Wall on *American Ninja Warrior*'s Season 6, becoming the first woman to complete a Qualifying course. That same season, she went on to become the first woman to hit a buzzer in a City Finals course and earn a spot in the Las Vegas National Finals. To date, she is still the only woman who has ever completed a City Finals course!

The New Jersey native and former gymnast, who defied expectations and inspired fans around the globe, announced in Season 9 that she would be retiring from *American Ninja Warrior* competition and moving to wrestling (she signed with World Wrestling Entertainment). Yet, she returned for one final time to the ninja spotlight, taking on the epic Mega Spider Climb in the 2018 *American Ninja Warrior All-Star Special: Skills Challenge*.

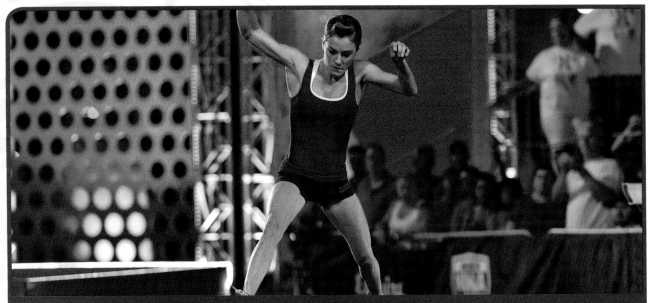

"Mighty" Kacy Catanzaro negotiates Piston Road while competing in the National Finals in Season 7, the year following her history-making runs.

> Oh, boy, Kacy Catanzaro—5 feet tall, just under 100 pounds. She redefined strength for me. When she had her epic run on Season 6, in the back of my mind I was thinking, *Oh, good, she's coming out*, but if I'm honest with myself, I judged her. I looked at her and thought, *No way she can do this, but it's good that she's been training. It's fun, good spirit, just being here is a big deal and just going on the course.* She rewrote everything—she rewrote my hard drive. But then the very next time she competed in the City Finals, I thought, *Boy, what she did in Qualifying was amazing, but I don't know if she'll do it in the Finals. If she falls anywhere in the back half of the course, she'll be a beast.* And then she goes out and runs the table, and I lost it. From that point on, I never judged another competitor.
>
> —Host Akbar Gbajabiamila

IAN DORY

Farmer Ian Dory, a Wolfpack Ninja known as the "Wolfpup," is one of the most consistent ninjas in *American Ninja Warrior* history. First competing in Season 6, Dory has never failed to hit a buzzer in any Qualifying and City Finals course in which he has competed. In Season 9's Denver Finals, he came close to a fall and was nearly out of steam on the final obstacle, the Elevator Climb. However, he managed to flip his legs over the ledge and drag himself to the buzzer to become the only finisher of the course that night.

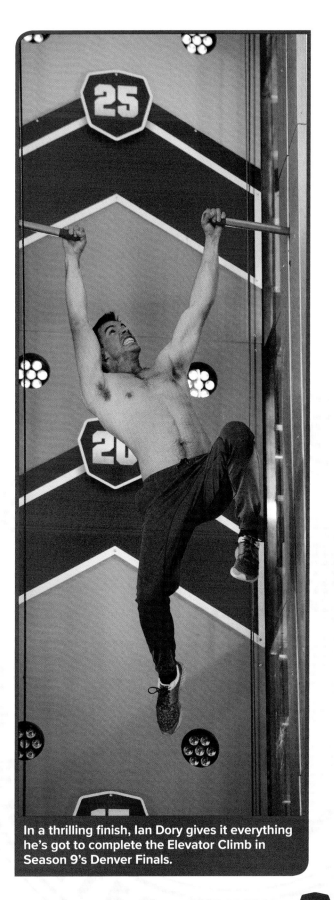

In a thrilling finish, Ian Dory gives it everything he's got to complete the Elevator Climb in Season 9's Denver Finals.

NINJA SPOTLIGHT:

DREW DRECHSEL

"Real Life Ninja" Drew Drechsel is an American gym owner, *American Ninja Warrior* competitor, and one of the most successful foreigners ever to compete on *SASUKE*. He first appeared in *SASUKE 27* in 2011 as one of the 10 *American Ninja Warrior* finalists and has made appearances in every *SASUKE* after *SASUKE 30*, making him known as a "Third Stage Regular" among Japanese fans. He has been competing on *American Ninja Warrior* since Season 3–the year he reached Stage One but had to withdraw from the competition due to a knee injury on Half-Pipe Attack. In Season 8, Drechsel–who was the captain of the Real Life Beasts in *Team Ninja Warrior* Seasons 1 and 2–obliterated the Atlanta Qualifying course with the fastest time of the night and would go on to become the Last Man Standing that season.

NATALIE DURAN

A rookie in Season 5, YouTube personality Natalie Duran didn't make the City Finals that season but returned with a vengeance in Season 8, making it all the way to the Warped Wall. Although she failed to climb it, she was still able to make it to the City Finals, placing 19th among the night's ninjas (she went on to compete as a Wild Card in Vegas). Additionally, Duran participated in *Team Ninja Warrior* as part of Team Golden Hearts with "Island Ninja" Grant McCartney and team captain Neil Craver, and also appeared on *Celebrity Ninja Warrior*, coaching actress Mena Suvari.

DANIEL GIL

Known as the "Kingdom Ninja" for his devotion to his faith, Daniel Gil is a professional ninja athlete and a three-time National Finalist on *American Ninja Warrior*–in Season 8, he was one of only two competitors to beat Stage Two in the National Finals. Gil was also selected to compete in the *All-Star Special: Skills Challenge* and was chosen to be a team captain on Season 1 of *Team Ninja Warrior*. In 2013, he began working at Iron Sports Gym, in his hometown of Houston, Texas, where he is now director of the home-school program and trains for *American Ninja Warrior*.

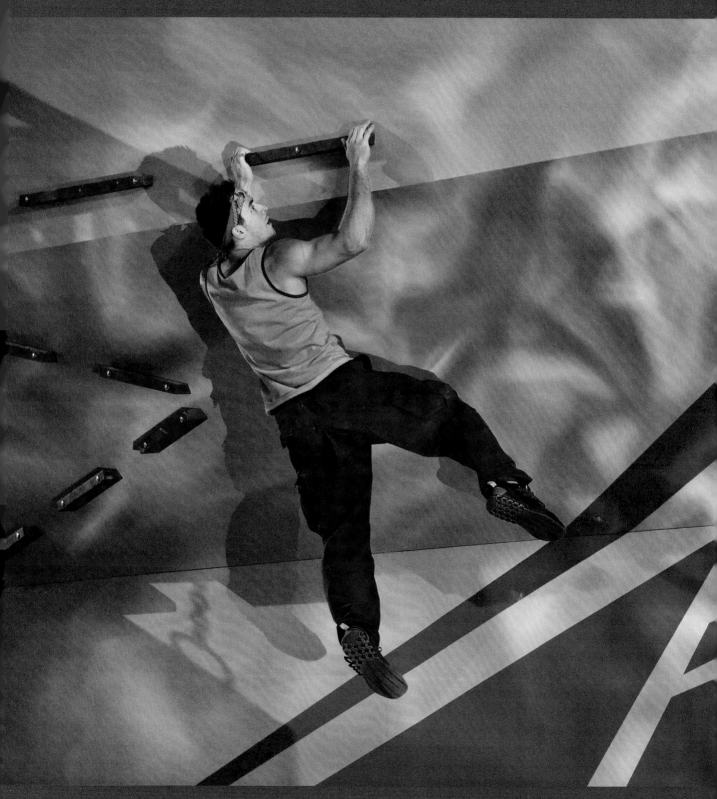

Over the years, "Real Life Ninja" Drew Drechsel has proven to be a beast on the *American Ninja Warrior* course. Here, he conquers the Ultimate Cliffhanger on Stage Three of the National Finals in Season 7.

NINJA SPOTLIGHT:

TYLER GILLETT

Next-gen ninja Tyler Gillett of Newman, Georgia, has been watching *American Ninja Warrior* since he was 14 years old, and he has been training to be a competitor for just as long. He built a course in his backyard, and as soon as he was old enough, he applied and got the call that he was going to compete in Season 9. Gillett completed the Daytona Beach Qualifying course and scored well enough at the City Finals to punch his ticket to the National Finals, all in his rookie year.

When he went to his home in Georgia in the time between the City Finals and the National Finals, "one of the hurricanes had destroyed his whole course," says executive producer Kent Weed. "He had nothing left. And then he got poison ivy. When he finally got to Vegas, he said, *Okay, I've got to get through this course.*"

And, with an inspirational run, Gillett completed Stage One in Vegas. "The moment was unbelievable," says executive producer Arthur Smith. "He's got a whole big group waiting for him. His parents are there. When Tyler gets interviewed by Kristine Leahy, he's crying. Seven years. Seven years of his life, and Kristine asks, 'Is it worth it?' And he goes, 'Oh my God, yes.' She asks, 'Did you ever think you'd be here?' And Tyler answers, 'The day I watched the very first show I knew I was going to be here one day.' We love that this is a show that you could watch and someday be on, and we know that right now there are a lot of teenagerswho are training, who are getting ready."

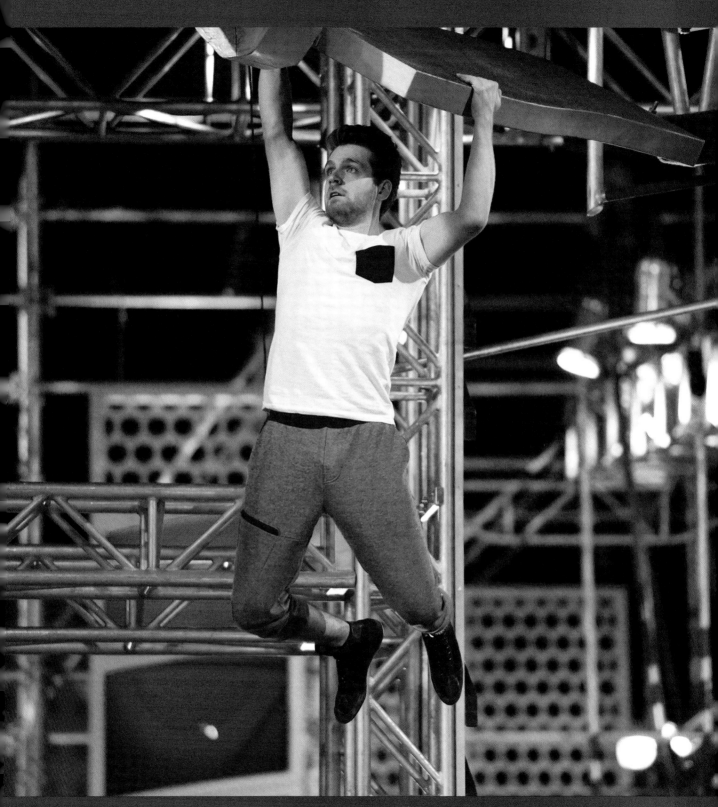

Next-gen ninja Tyler Gillett, shown here on the Wave Runner, made it all the way to Stage Two of the National Finals in his rookie year, but his inspirational run would end there.

NINJA SPOTLIGHT:

JESSIE GRAFF

This superhero can fly! Professional stunt woman Jessie Graff is one of the most popular competitors on *American Ninja Warrior*. Breaking both stereotypes and records, she came onto the ninja scene at the Los Angeles Qualifiers in Season 5, and in her rookie year made history by becoming the first woman to qualify for a City Finals course. In the City Finals that season, she became the second woman to reach the Warped Wall, and although she failed to climb it, she went on to Vegas as a Wild Card and became one of two women to reach the Jumping Spider.

In Season 7, she clinched sixth place in the Finals, earning her ticket to Vegas and becoming the second woman behind "Mighty" Kacy Catanzaro in *American Ninja*

Warrior history to qualify for the National Finals. She would go on to become the second woman behind "SheWolf" Meagan Martin to reach the Warped Wall, and although she timed out this time around, she wasn't done yet.

In Season 8's LA Qualifiers, Graff, five-foot-eight and a pole vaulter in college, made history once again when she blazed through all six obstacles, making her not only the first woman that season to complete the Qualifying course, but also the first woman to complete the newly modified 14.5-foot Warped Wall, and she ultimately finished the course in eleventh place. In Season 8's National Finals, Graff put on a historic performance by not only becoming the first woman to get over the Warped Wall in Stage One but by becoming the first woman to conquer Stage One in *America Ninja Warrior* history. Additionally, she became the first female Team USA member, and along with Jake Murray, Josh Levin, "Kingdom Ninja" Daniel Gil, "Real Life Ninja" Drew Drechsel, and Brian Arnold represented the United States in the third *USA vs. the World*, becoming the first woman ever to clear Stage Two.

In *American Ninja Warrior*'s Season 9, she again punched her ticket to Vegas, making it the third year in a row that she qualified for the National Finals. However, she had a shocking exit when she fell on the Flying Squirrel just before she could complete Stage One.

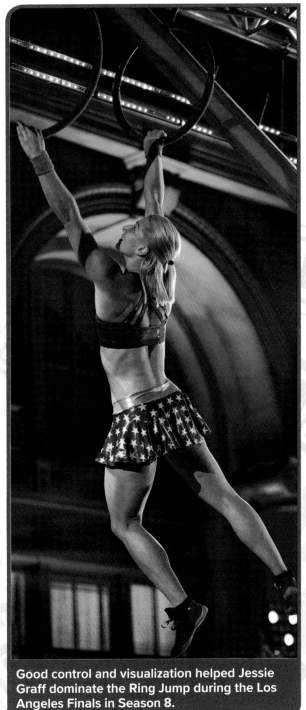

Good control and visualization helped Jessie Graff dominate the Ring Jump during the Los Angeles Finals in Season 8.

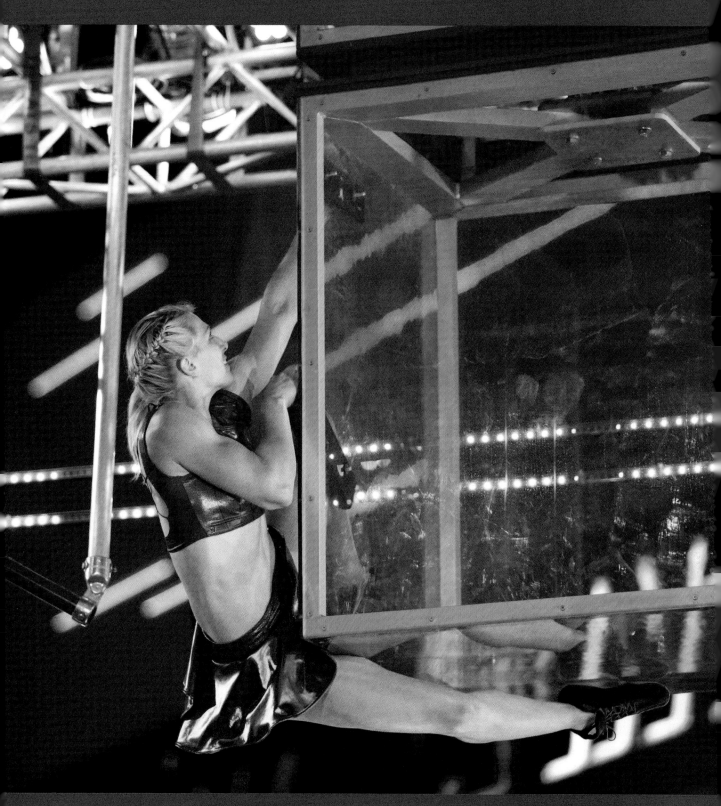

Competing strategically is what has helped Jessie Graff crush the ninja course each year. She used a creative move to clear the ninja-killing Giant Cubes, shown here, during the Daytona Beach Finals of Season 9.

> Jessie Graff was one of the smartest athletes on our show. She was determined to conquer Stage One, which she did in Season 8. The season before, however, she didn't make it because she ran out of gas at the Warped Wall, and she said, 'You know what, I need to do exercise that's going to increase my stamina and make my legs stronger,' so she started focusing specifically on that, and she would do lunges and plyometrics, and she would practice getting her stamina so that by the time she got to that Warped Wall she wouldn't be tired. It was something that Meagan Martin also had when she got to the Warped Wall, but Jessie was different. Rather than just go back to the routine, she analyzed it. She got scientific about it. I really applaud her for it, and, sure enough, it worked the next year. She trained perfectly and knew exactly what she needed to do to complete the course.
>
> —Executive Producer Kent Weed

> Drew Drechsel and Jessie Graff have both been so good for so long. And what I truly love about them is how supportive they are of other athletes. What I think makes them great is that they rise to the occasion. As the stakes get higher, they seem to perform better.
>
> —Host Matt Iseman

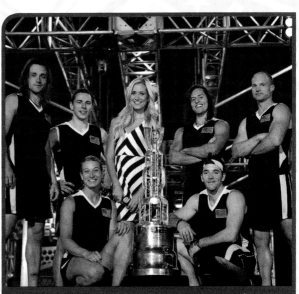

Sideline reporter Kristine Leahy poses with 2017's *USA vs. The World* champs (pictured left to right) Jake Murray, Josh Levin, Jessie Graff, Daniel Gil, Drew Drechsel, and Brian Arnold.

NINJA SPOTLIGHT:

JESSE "FLEX" LABRECK

Typically, the elite women of *American Ninja Warrior* have backgrounds in gymnastics, pole vaulting, or rock climbing. Jesse Labreck didn't fit that mold. She was a track star from the University of Maine.

"The way track translated for me was the fact that it's an individual sport, and *American Ninja Warrior* is very individual," Labreck says. "It's just you up there on that starting platform. It's you running through that course. That helped. Plus, I worked on power and explosion for 12 years of my life in track, and for everything but the upper-body obstacles, it helps a lot. The Warped Wall, any trampoline jump, or any kind of running between obstacles, my track always translates."

Labreck says *American Ninja Warrior* came onto her radar when she saw the viral video of Kacy Catanzaro's history-making performance in Dallas in 2014. "I hadn't actually heard of *American Ninja Warrior*," she says. "I did track and field at UMaine, so what had taken over my life was track and field. I didn't really know about the show before that."

Labreck—who was a caregiver for a young girl named Emeline Sterpe, who has cerebral palsy—became the breakout star of Season 8, her freshman season, with host Akbar Gbajabiamila exclaiming she was a "Labreck House!" She had a solid run in the Philadelphia Qualifier, making it to the Rolling Thunder obstacle until she lost her grip.

"I don't remember the course or my run very well," she says of that first time she stepped up to the starting line. "I wasn't scared. I don't think I had stage fright, but it was so overwhelming, and it's gone. I can't remember it anymore."

Labreck still made it to the City Finals, where she managed to beat Rolling Thunder and become just the fifth woman ever to scale the Warped Wall. She made it all the way to Stair Hopper before falling but still clinched a spot in Vegas—becoming only the fourth woman in *American Ninja Warrior* history to qualify for the National Finals and the first woman to do it as a rookie.

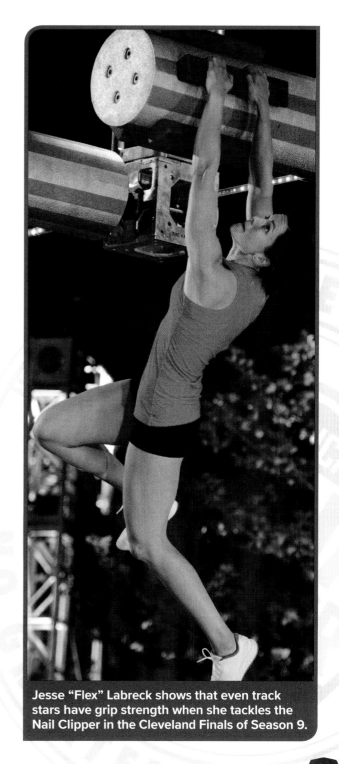

Jesse "Flex" Labreck shows that even track stars have grip strength when she tackles the Nail Clipper in the Cleveland Finals of Season 9.

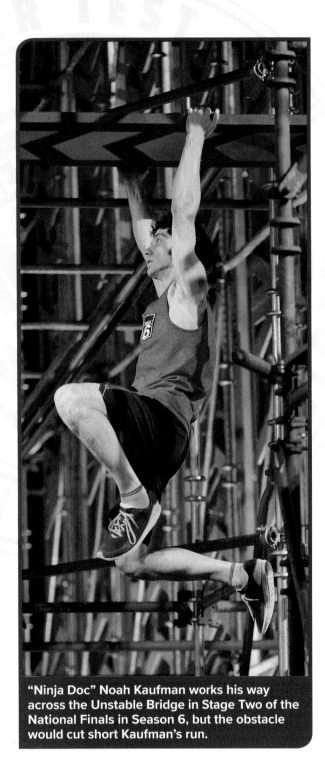

"Ninja Doc" Noah Kaufman works his way across the Unstable Bridge in Stage Two of the National Finals in Season 6, but the obstacle would cut short Kaufman's run.

to the City Finals—he was so close, placing 31st!—he returned for Season 8. That season, he cleared the Qualifying course and also turned in a solid performance in the City Finals that earned him a spot in the Top 15, punching his ticket to the National Finals. He made his second trip to Vegas in Season 9.

NOAH KAUFMAN, M.D.

Noah Kaufman, M.D., known as the "Ninja Doc," has dedicated his life to emergency medicine and is also an avid rock climber of over 25 years. He first appeared on *American Ninja Warrior* in Season 5—fans may remember his one-armed hang from the Warped Wall coupled with a victory fist-pump during the Los Angeles Qualifiers (he made a similar move on the Warped Wall the following season in the Denver Qualifiers). He is also a two-time National Finalist, completing Stage One both times.

WHY DID YOU TRY OUT FOR *AMERICAN NINJA WARRIOR*?

"I had a friend who was on the show, Jon Alexis Jr., who was trying out, and I was helping him with his submission video. I ended up having a really good time helping him, and then he asked me to go to a local competition with him. I met Michelle Warnky and Jamie Rahn, and I had a really good time, so it kind of just went from there. I really like doing local competitions, so I decided to apply."
—Jesse "Flex" Labreck

GRANT McCARTNEY

Grant McCartney, a flight attendant for Hawaiian Airlines, danced onto the *American Ninja Warrior* scene in Season 7 in the Los Angeles Qualifying round. Known as the "Island Ninja," McCartney was a fan of the show growing up, when it was on the G4 network.

NICK HANSON

"Eskimo Ninja" Nick Hanson—a coach who hails from Unalakleet, Alaska, which sits along the Bering Sea—first competed in the Los Angeles Qualifiers in Season 7. Although he just missed out on advancing

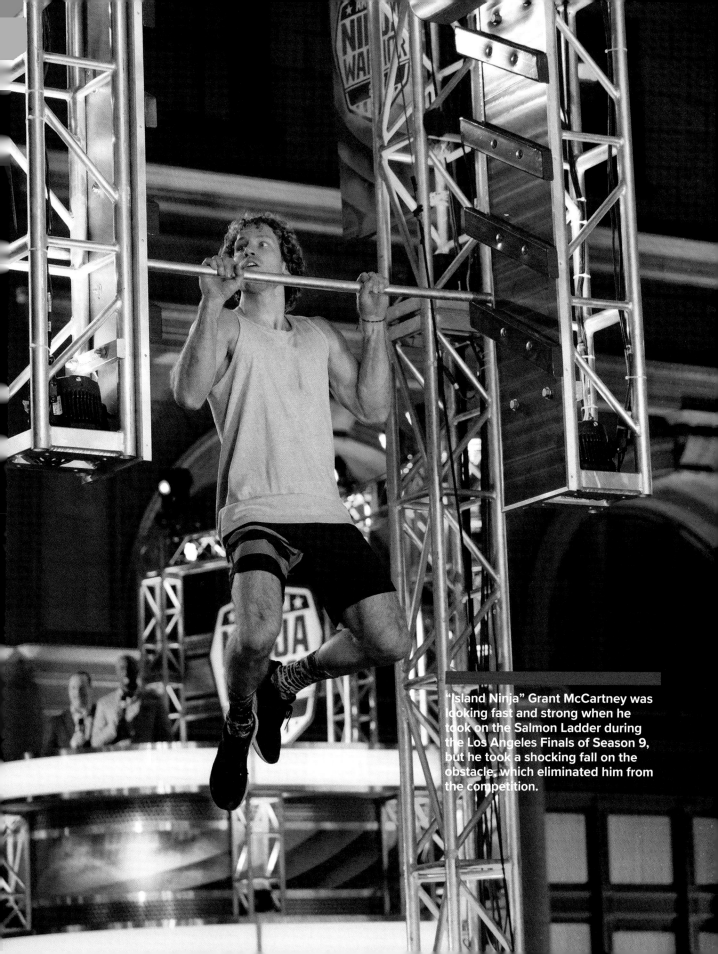

"Island Ninja" Grant McCartney was looking fast and strong when he took on the Salmon Ladder during the Los Angeles Finals of Season 9, but he took a shocking fall on the obstacle, which eliminated him from the competition.

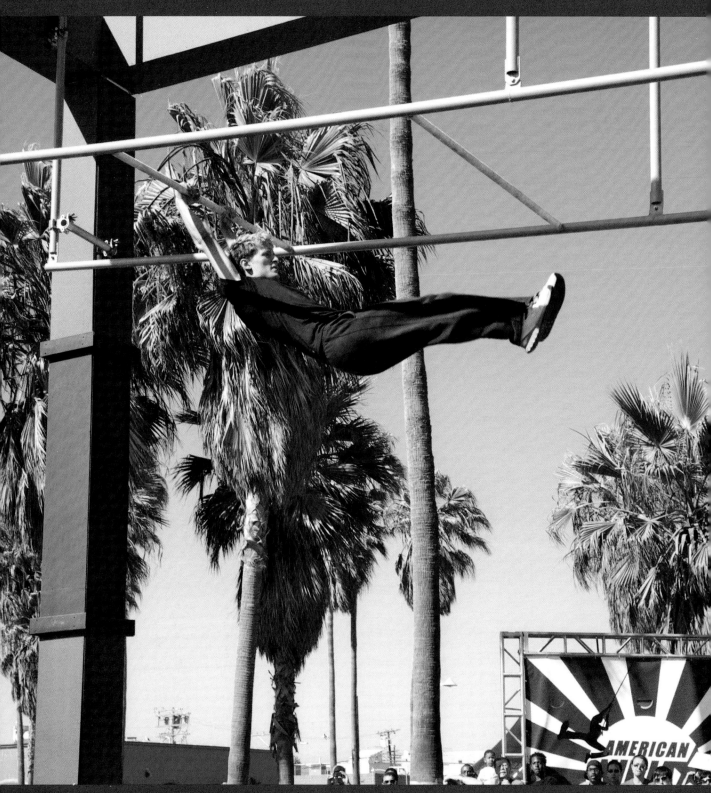

Levi Meeuwenberg, shown here in Season 2, became a breakout star during the early seasons of *American Ninja Warrior*.

"I've always had the mentality of 'I could do that, I could do that,'" McCartney says. "I told myself 'I'm gonna do that one day' as a kid, I grew up, and put it on the back burner. In college, I saw *American Ninja Warrior* and told my family, 'I'm gonna do that!' Then my mom passed away unexpectedly, followed by my grandmother a couple of months later and my great-grandmother a little bit after that, plus my stepdad. I lost a lot of people in my family, and it was the season of death where I realized life is very short, so I set out to do multiple things I'd said I was going to do. The first thing on the list was to do the Running of the Bulls in Spain. The second was to do *American Ninja Warrior*."

McCartney made it to Vegas his first two seasons, but fell short in Season 9 when he failed to complete the Salmon Ladder.

JAMES McGRATH

James "The Beast" McGrath has competed on *American Ninja Warrior* eight times. In Season 3, he was a walk-on who slept in his aunt's van the night before the competition who would go on to become a star of the ninja world, making it to the National Finals six times.

LEVI MEEUWENBERG

A professional freerunner and stunt man, Levi Meeuwenberg was one of the standout competitors in the early days of *American Ninja Warrior*. He was a number one qualifier for the second *American Ninja Challenge*, and on his first appearance became the Last Man Standing—he was the only one to move on to Stage Three.

Grant McCartney is the most memorable at the buzzer. He has all of the up-to-date dances. I've seen him Whip, I've seen him Nae Nae, I've seen him do the Cat Daddy, I've seen him do the Running Man Challenge, and I think he's thrown a couple of throwback dances in there as well. I think he even tried to do the Kid 'n Play, but it didn't work out because he didn't have anybody to do it with.

—Host Akbar Gbajabiamila

NINJA SPOTLIGHT:

MEAGAN MARTIN

Meagan Martin, known as the "SheWolf," from Lake Mary, Florida, is a professional rock climber who appeared on *American Ninja Warrior* first in Season 6. She was the first woman to complete Qualifying rounds in two back-to-back seasons, and she has hit more buzzers than any other woman in ninja history. She also was the first woman to beat the Rail Runner, and she has scaled the Warped Wall five times—more than any other woman in *American Ninja Warrior* history.

Martin's love for climbing began in her childhood when she liked to climb trees. When her mom made her read for an hour each day, Martin chose to climb up in a tree with her book to do her reading. "I just love the constant challenge that climbing creates," she says. "Even when you are successful, it's only for a moment, and then you are on to your next challenge, so I create this never-ending cycle of pushing yourself always to be better."

Martin started climbing at age 11 and was competing in gymnastics at a very early age. She tried pole vaulting in January of her freshman year of high school, and while she wasn't interested in the sport at first, she got hooked. She credits both gymnastics and climbing with helping her transition to pole vaulting—gymnastics gave her the body awareness, speed, strength, and acrobatic skills she needed, and climbing helped to keep her strong after quitting gymnastics. At the end of her junior year of college, Martin realized that she wanted to pursue climbing competitively as well as make it her career following college graduation. She currently lives in Boulder, Colorado, and is a coach at ABC Kids Climbing Gym.

"Climbing has taken me to some of the most beautiful places, which I am thankful for," says Martin, who is a member of the Wolfpack Ninjas.

> I watched the original Japanese version of the show from time to time when I was in high school, but I didn't watch it religiously. I never watched the American version before applying for the show, ironically. There was an email going around the climbing community about the show wanting more female climbers to participate, so I thought I might as well send in an application, and if they picked me that would be cool!
>
> —Meagan Martin

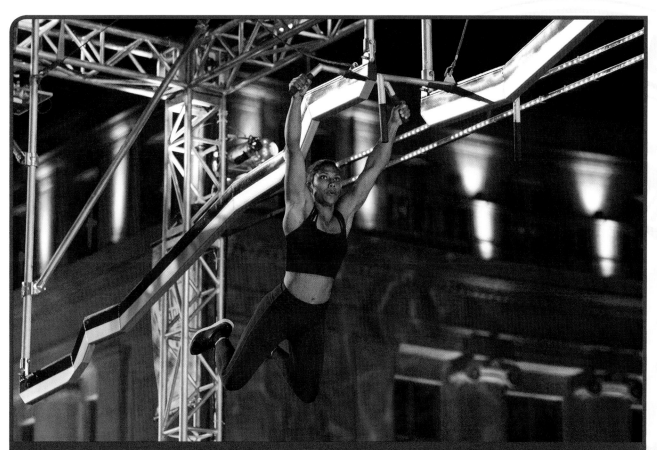

Meagan Martin may have gotten wet on the Rail Runner in the Denver Qualifiers of Season 9, but she came back more determined than ever in the City Finals and became the first woman to conquer the obstacle.

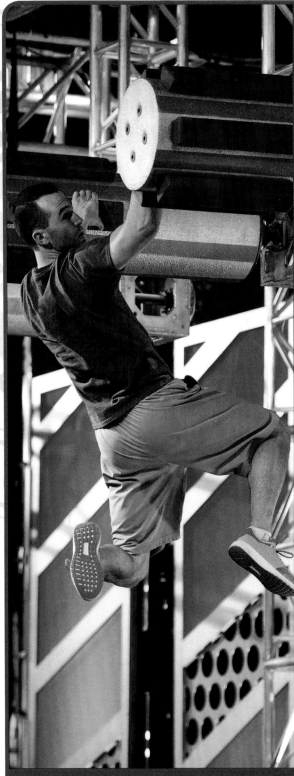

"The Weatherman" Joe Moravsky breezes through the Nail Clipper during Stage Three of the Season 9 National Finals. He would go on to become the Last Man Standing.

> Joe Moravsky doesn't look like an athlete, he really doesn't, but he's got something else in him. I need to sit him down and figure out what it is with Joe Moravsky that makes him so good.
> —Host Akbar Gbajabiamila

JOE MORAVSKY

"The Weatherman" Joe Moravsky stormed onto the *American Ninja Warrior* course for the first time in Season 5 and has become one of the most consistent competitors on the show. A five-time National Finals competitor, he has made it past Stage One in every season and was the Last Man Standing in both Season 6 and Season 9.

> Joe Moravsky is one of the strongest competitors. He may not be the most physically gifted ninja, but I don't know that anyone has more competitive drive than "The Weatherman."
> —Host Matt Iseman

JAKE MURRAY

Looking for the unexpected? Jake Murray is your ninja. Just before Season 7, Jake Murray became an internet sensation when his *Footloose* parody submission video went viral. Who could forget the ninja who backflipped up the Warped Wall in Season 8 at the Indianapolis Finals? Or, later in that same season, when he ran Stage One at the Las Vegas Finals with a fanny pack? What was inside? A corn dog and goggles, of course, for a quick bite to eat before his plunge into the water below to celebrate clearing Stage One.

MY FIRST SUBMISSION VIDEO

CHRIS WILCZEWSKI:

"My original submission video consisted of a lot of homemade obstacles. To be honest, I didn't really talk much. I think I said one awkward line and hoped they would pick me for what I could do on my course."

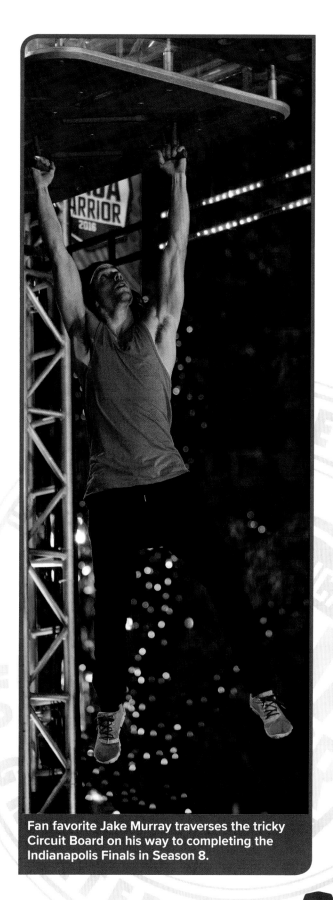

Fan favorite Jake Murray traverses the tricky Circuit Board on his way to completing the Indianapolis Finals in Season 8.

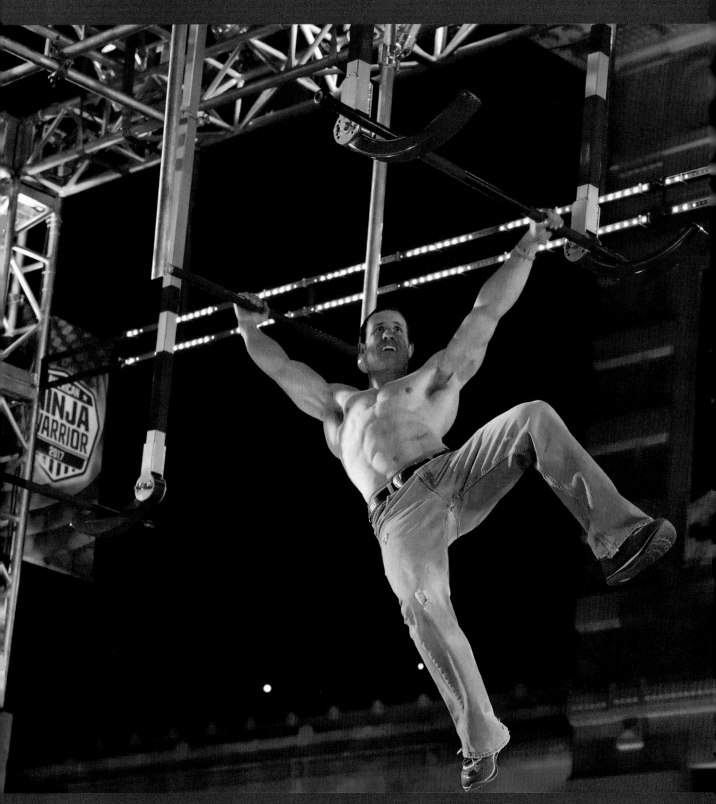

In Season 9, "Cowboy Ninja" Lance Pekus, shown here on the Bar Hop, made it through the Kansas City Qualifier with the fastest time of the night.

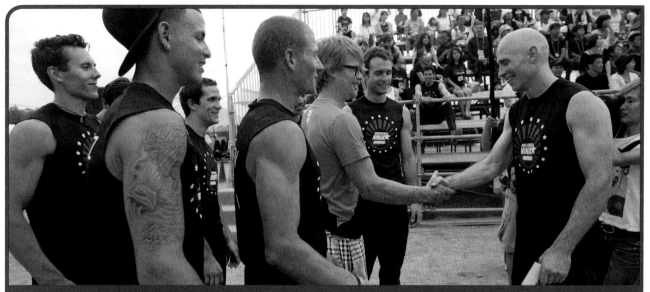

In the Season 3 Finals in Japan, American competitors (pictured left to right) Travis Rosen, Flip Rodriguez, Jake Smith, Brent Steffensen, Brian Orosco, Travis Furlanic, and David Campbell enjoy some downtime.

MAKOTO NAGANO

Although he hasn't made an appearance on *American Ninja Challenge* or *American Ninja Warrior*, fisherman Makoto Nagano is a *Ninja Warrior* legend around the globe. This charismatic figure achieved the fastest times on Stage One and Stage Two on *SASUKE* and made the most appearances in the Final Stage—a total of five times. He achieved Total Victory in *SASUKE 17*.

BRIAN OROSCO

A freerunner and real estate agent, Brian Orosco competed in *American Ninja Challenge* and *American Ninja Warrior* multiple times. He also represented the United States in *SASUKE* five times, making it to both Stage Two and Stage Three twice.

LANCE PEKUS

Known as the "Cowboy Ninja," Lance Pekus made his *American Ninja Warrior* debut in Season 4. Pekus, who lives in isolated Salmon, Idaho, works seasonally for the Forest Service and on his father-in-law's ranch. He had an early exit in Season 8 but took time between seasons to refocus and rediscover his ninja passion. With his trademark

MY FIRST SUBMISSION VIDEO

MEAGAN MARTIN:

"My first submission video consisted of me climbing, coaching climbing, and then playing around at a parkour gym. I actually think that the parkour gym portion was my first time at a parkour gym, which is kind of funny!"

cowboy hat and jeans, Pekus was back in the saddle in Season 9, hitting the buzzer with the fastest time at the Kansas City Qualifiers and going far enough in the City Finals to punch his ticket to Vegas. During the National Finals, it was revealed that Pekus's wife, Heather, has multiple sclerosis, and when Pekus hit the Stage One buzzer with 45 seconds left, it wasn't only the fastest run of the night but also the most emotional.

Jamie Rahn, known as "Captain NBC," strategizes on the Floating Monkey Bars during Season 7's Pittsburgh Finals.

JAMIE RAHN

Nicknamed "Captain NBC" and usually sporting some seriously cool-colored hair, Jamie Rahn has competed in seven seasons of *American Ninja Warrior*, beginning with Season 2. He has made it to the National Finals five times. He is part owner of Pinnacle Parkour Academy (PPK), founded in 2010, which was the first facility on the East Coast dedicated solely to parkour and freerunning. He runs PPK's Cherry Hill location and has a background in various sports including football, skateboarding, racquetball, weight lifting, and bodyweight training. Rahn was born with a four-inch brain cyst, which can cause debilitating migraines that he constantly balances with diet, exercise, and sleep.

NAJEE RICHARDSON

Known as the "Philly Phoenix," Najee Richardson is a former elite competitive gymnast who had his career cut short because of a knee injury. In Season 8, his sophomore season on *American Ninja Warrior*, Richardson advanced all the way to Stage Two of the National Finals. Richardson, who was a member of Team Matt in the Season 8 *All-Star Special: Skills Challenge*, has dedicated himself to becoming one of the best ninja warriors and travels across the country, inspiring others to overcome obstacles. Richardson advanced to Stage Three in Season 9.

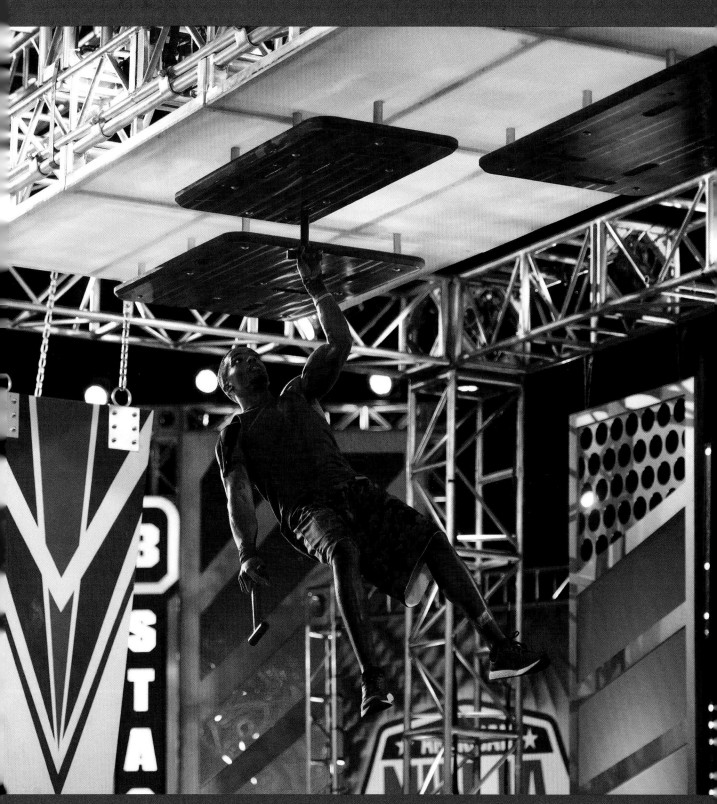

"Philly Phoenix" Najee Richardson made it all the way to Stage Three in the Season 9 National Finals. Here, he takes on the challenging Key Lock Hang obstacle.

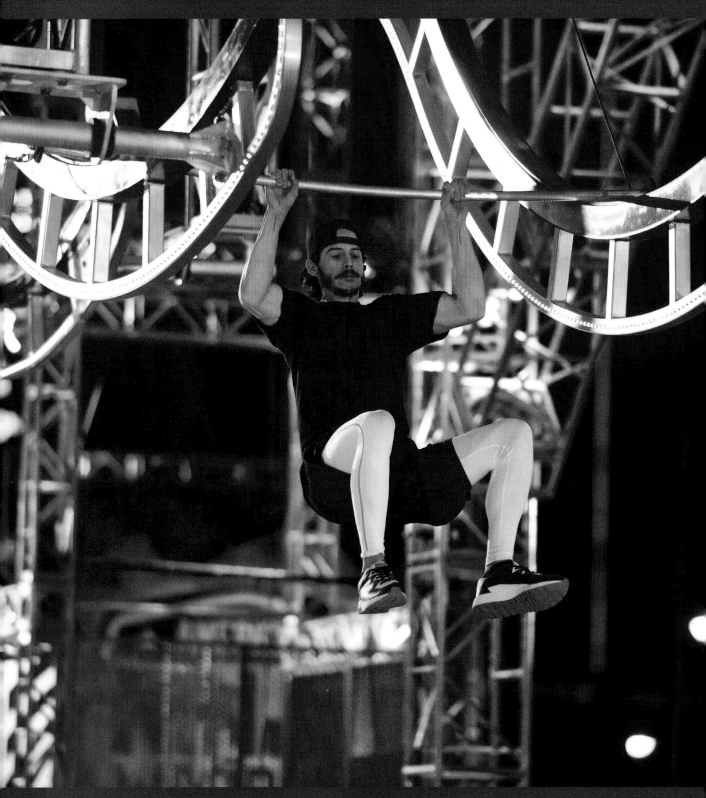

In Season 7, fan favorite Flip Rodriguez did away with his trademark black-and-white face mask. He is shown here competing in the National Finals of Season 9.

DAVID "FLIP" RODRIGUEZ

With seven seasons under his belt, stunt man Flip Rodriguez started out on *American Ninja Warrior* as a 21-year-old rookie and over the years would go on to wow audiences with his speed and agility. Until Season 7—and in *SASUKE 27*, as one of the US representatives—he wore a variety of black-and-white face masks that had become his trademark. While he often said that the mask was to protect himself, in Season 8 he revealed he had suffered sexual abuse from ages 9 to 15. This brave admission, he has said, was meant to inspire others in similar situations to talk about what was happening to them and help end the abuse and pain. Rodriguez is a parkour and ninja coach at Tempest Free Running Academy in Los Angeles.

LUCI ROMBERG

A champion gymnast, stunt woman, all-conference soccer player, and freerunner, Luci Romberg became one of the three Qualifiers representing the United States in the third *American Ninja Challenge* and

> " Flip told us he was going to do this, that he thought he felt comfortable using *American Ninja Warrior* as a platform or a venue to air this very, very difficult thing for him to face in his life. The outpouring of support from the community and other people who said, 'Hey, I couldn't say anything either until I saw your story,' is crazy. There have been so many inspiring stories to come out of the show. It's like Oprah meets the Olympics.
> —Executive producer Kent Weed "

became the first woman ever to clear the Jumping Spider in Stage One during *SASUKE 21*. She has competed several times on *American Ninja Warrior* and *Team Ninja Warrior*, for the latter as one of the members of Kevin Bull's Team ExpendaBulls.

TRAVIS ROSEN

A familiar face on *American Ninja Warrior*, Travis Rosen has competed in the last eight seasons and is a seven-time National Finals competitor—at 42 years of age, he is the oldest competitor to ever clear Stage One. What's more, he also competed in *SASUKE 27* and got to taste Stage Four in *American Ninja Warrior: USA vs. The World*. A busy family man, Rosen still finds time to train and keeps coming back to get the chance to conquer Stage Four on *American Ninja Warrior*.

SAM SANN

Sam Sann is a longtime ninja competitor who made his first appearance on *American Ninja Warrior* in Season 4. After succumbing to his nemesis, the Giant Cycle, in back-to-back seasons (Seasons 5 and 6), Sann came back with a vengeance in Season 7, completing both the Houston Qualifying and City Finals courses, qualifying for the National Finals. Sann founded his own gym, Iron Sports, in Houston, Texas, and also trains ninjas such as "Kingdom Ninja" Daniel Gil and Jody Avila.

BRETT SIMS

Brett Sims was the first runner-up in the very first *American Ninja Challenge* and became one of the two first US athletes, along with Collin Bell, in *SASUKE 19*. He also participated in *SASUKE 20*, all *American Ninja Warrior* seasons except 3, 5, and 7, and *Team Ninja Warrior*'s Season 2 as a member of Travis Rosen's Team TNT.

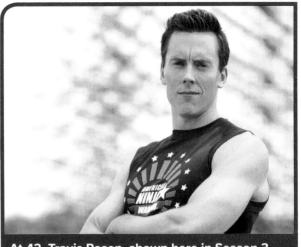

At 42, Travis Rosen, shown here in Season 3, became the oldest *American Ninja Warrior* competitor to ever complete Stage One.

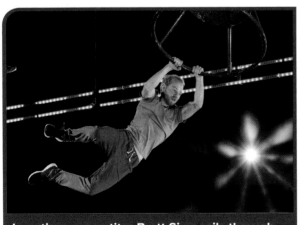

Longtime competitor Brett Sims sails through the Spin Cycle during Season 8's Atlanta Finals, becoming one of the few ninjas to finish the course and marking Sims's first appearance in the National Finals.

> We've seen world-class athletes from other sports come here and not experience the success they expected. But we've also seen athletes who never had great accomplishments in the past discover that they could have great success here by working harder than I ever thought possible. I think it's what makes the show so great: the harder you work, the better you do.
>
> —Host Matt Iseman

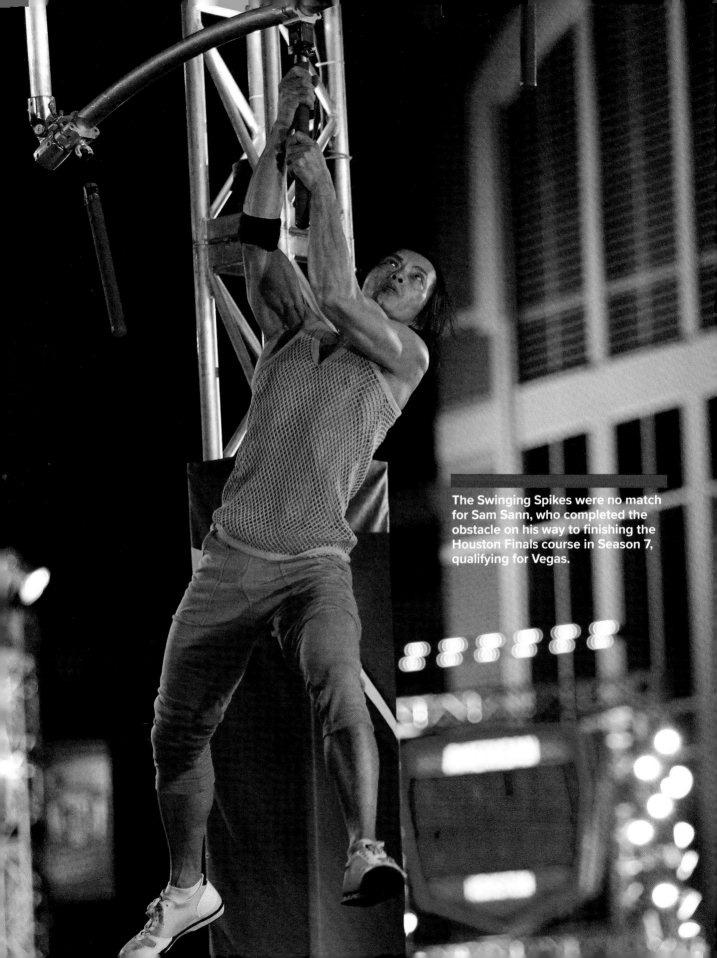

The Swinging Spikes were no match for Sam Sann, who completed the obstacle on his way to finishing the Houston Finals course in Season 7, qualifying for Vegas.

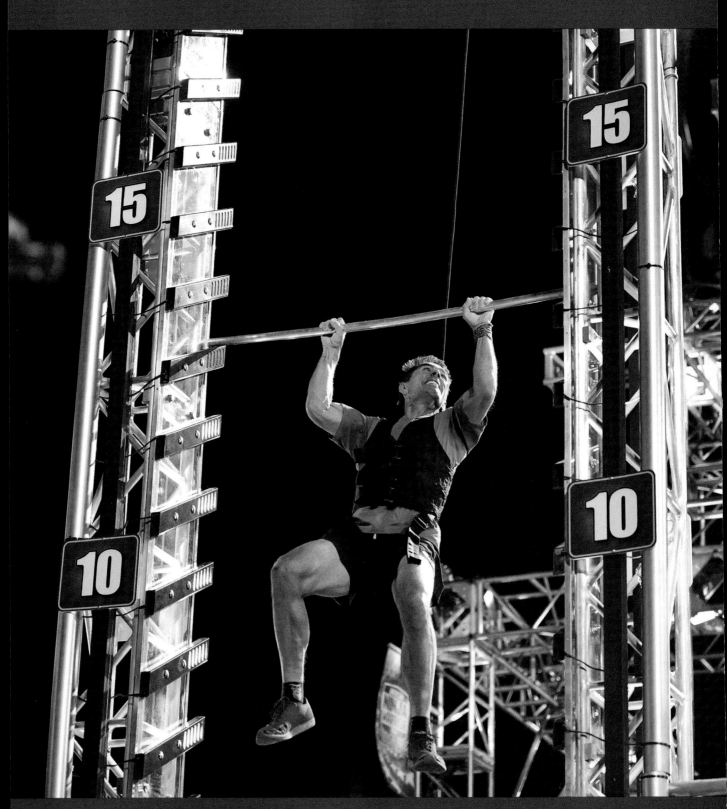

Grandfather Jon Stewart makes his way up the grueling Double Salmon Ladder in 2016's *American Ninja Warrior All-Star Special: Skills Challenge*.

BRENT STEFFENSEN

Brent Steffensen from San Antonio, Texas, represented the United States in *SASUKE 26, 27,* and *32,* and is an eight-year veteran of *American Ninja Warrior*, making it to the National Finals many times. In Season 4, he was the only competitor to reach Stage Three and became the first American to defeat the Ultimate Cliffhanger. He is a managing partner/athlete at Alpha Warrior, based in San Antonio.

JON STEWART

Jon Stewart is a father, grandfather, and construction manager who first hit the ninja scene in Season 5. He failed to climb the Warped Wall in the Denver Qualifying round and again in the Qualifier of Season 6 but he placed 27th that season and was able to move on to the City Finals. This time, he scaled the Warped Wall on his third and final try and continued to rouse the crowd as he tackled the next four obstacles of the Back Half, becoming, at age 52, the oldest competitor to finish a City Finals course, prompting host Akbar Gbajabiamila to say, "I want to see Jon Stewart's birth certificate!" Two years later, in the Oklahoma City Finals, he broke his own record by becoming the oldest man, at 54, ever to qualify for Vegas.

RYAN STRATIS

Ryan Stratis grew up in the small town of Putney, Georgia, and played sports in high school—he wrestled, swam, and played soccer. He was active with the JROTC program, which led him to North Georgia College to pursue a commission as an

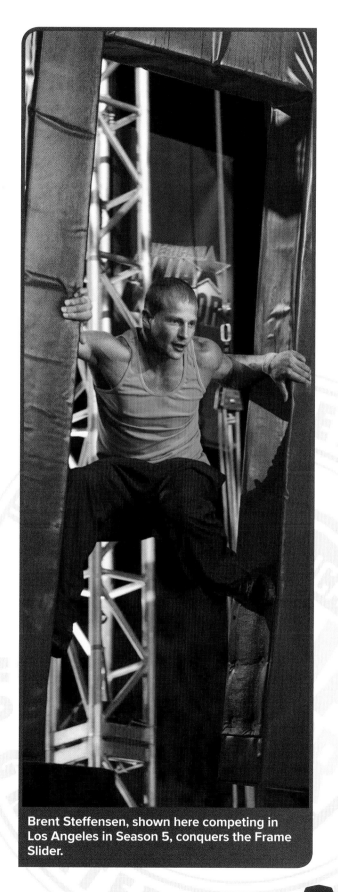

Brent Steffensen, shown here competing in Los Angeles in Season 5, conquers the Frame Slider.

DID YOU KNOW?

In 2017, John Loobey, at age 65, became the oldest ninja ever to complete an obstacle—beating his own record from the year before—at the Daytona Beach Qualifiers. In Season 9, he completed two obstacles, the Floating Steps and the Rolling Pin, but fell on the Wingnuts.

NINJA SPOTLIGHT:

TOWERS OF POWER

American Ninja Warrior's Towers of Power consist of Chicago-area firefighters Brandon Mears and Dan Polizzi, both of whom made their debut on the show in Season 5. Interestingly, this dynamic duo has never made it to the National Finals together! In Seasons 6 and 8, Polizzi moved on to Vegas, while six-foot-five Mears advanced to Vegas in Season 7, becoming the tallest competitor at that point ever to clear Stage One.

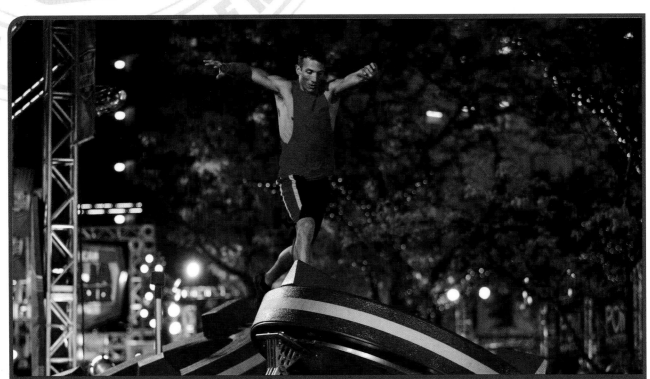

On his way to the National Finals in Las Vegas, firefighter Dan Polizzi shows his agility on the Disk Runner during the Indianpolis Finals in Season 8.

Army Officer in the Georgia Army National Guard. Military obstacle courses sparked his interest in *Ninja Warrior*, and he tried to get onto *American Ninja Challenge*, but was not selected. However, Stratis would go on to make his mark on *American Ninja Warrior*. He has appeared on all nine seasons of the show—in Season 3, he traveled to Japan as one of the 10 US athletes in *SASUKE 27*—and made it to Mount Midoriyama many times, including Season 8, which took place approximately four months after he underwent shoulder surgery.

MAGGI THORNE

Maggi Thorne is known for her tremendous support of her fellow ninjas and is often seen on the sidelines cheering them on. She and Jessie Graff were both college roommates and teammates on the University of Nebraska track team—Thorne was a two-time captain, running sprints and hurdles. A mother of three, Thorne made it to the City Finals for the first time in Season 9 and became the first woman to clear Crank It Up, which earned her a spot in the National Finals.

MICHELLE WARNKY

A personal trainer, Michelle Warnky is one of the first women to open a ninja-style training gym—Movement Lab Ohio, in Columbus. She first came on the *American Ninja Warrior* scene in Season 5, was the second woman to scale the Warped Wall, and has made it to the National Finals four times.

CHRIS WILCZEWSKI

Chris Wilczewski is a longtime competitor on *American Ninja Warrior* who competed on six seasons of the show, making it to the Finals three times (for more on Wilczewski, see page 256).

JARED "JJ" WOODS

Miami stunt man JJ Woods began his *American Ninja Warrior* career in Season 4 and has proven to be a solid competitor over the years, making the National Finals four times. In Season 9, during the Daytona Beach Finals, he revealed he was dedicating his run to an eight-year-old girl named Zoey, who had been diagnosed with Stage Four Neuroblastoma.

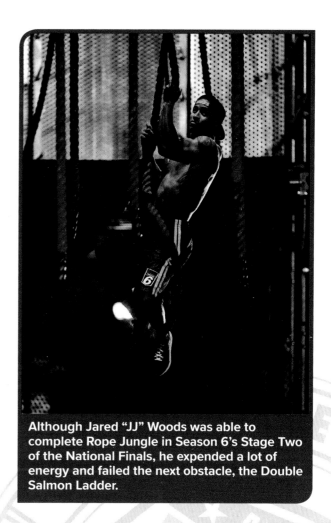

Although Jared "JJ" Woods was able to complete Rope Jungle in Season 6's Stage Two of the National Finals, he expended a lot of energy and failed the next obstacle, the Double Salmon Ladder.

DID YOU KNOW?

In nine seasons, only eight women have made it past the Warped Wall in competition on *American Ninja Warrior*:

- Kacy Catanzaro
- Michelle Warnky
- Meagan Martin
- Jessie Graff
- Jesse Labreck
- Allyssa Beird
- Barclay Stockett
- Rebekah Bonilla

Nika Muckelroy was the first woman to make it past the fifth obstacle and to the Warped Wall in Season 5's Denver Qualifiers, but she failed to make it over.

THE NINJA COMMUNITY:

FEELING THE LOVE

Ninjas are a tight-knit bunch—they have a bond that extends beyond the course and the cameras—and often pack the sidelines for one another as they run the *American Ninja Warrior* obstacle course.

"The camaraderie is so different than any other sport," says Chris Wilczewski. "Ninjas are incredibly supportive and willing to help each other. I have never seen anything like it before. The overwhelming challenge of taking down the course has brought us all together. I think most ninjas would agree when I say we just want one of us to beat it! It doesn't matter who! As a result you get very close friendships that develop both on and off the course."

"It's always nice to be in a sport where you can be friends with the competition and supportive of one another—it's actually a lot like that in climbing, too," notes "SheWolf" Meagan Martin. "It's a rarity and one of my favorite things about *American Ninja Warrior*."

"When you're on set and on location, you—I'm sorry for being corny—kind of feel the love," says executive producer Arthur Smith. "You really, really, do. When Kevin Bull, who's now one of the stars of the sport, was a walk-on with alopecia, no one's ever heard of him, and he comes on during a night when everyone is struggling with one obstacle, Cannonball Alley. No one's completed it yet, and everyone's doing the eighth obstacle the traditional way and this guy that no one's ever heard of comes on, does it backward, and completes it. And the ninjas celebrate it. They're going crazy. The guys who couldn't do it before Kevin Bull celebrate. The guys who are coming up after Kevin Bull celebrate. Everyone's celebrating, and that's what *Ninja* is about."

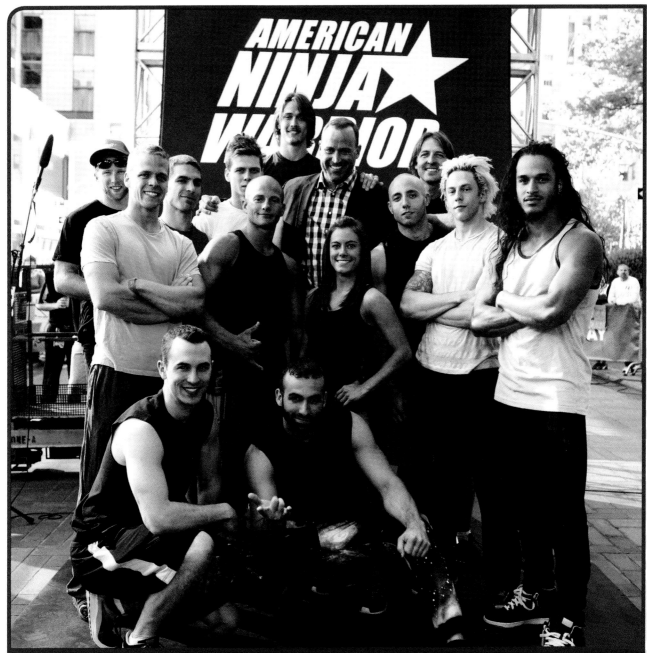

American Ninja Warrior host Matt Iseman (center) stops by NBC News' *Today* show with competitors, including (left to right) Chris Wilczewski, Mike Bernardo, Joe Moravsky, Brian Wilczewski, Brent Steffensen, Heriberto "Reko" Rivera, Rob Moravsky, Kacy Catanzaro, Noel Reyes, Jamie Rahn, and Luciano Acuna Jr.

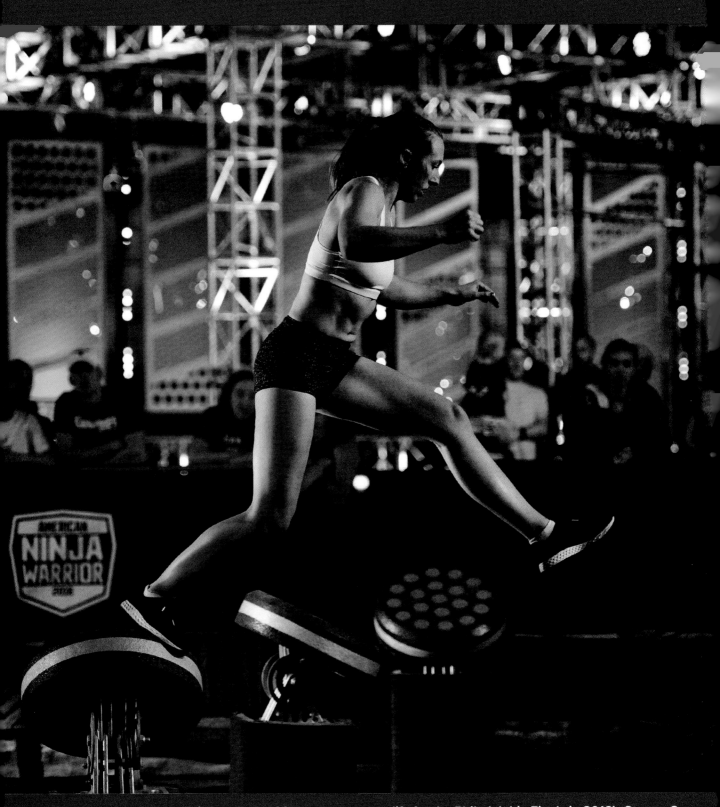

Schoolteacher Allyssa Beird was one of four women to qualify for the Philadelphia Finals in 2016's Season 8, her rookie year. She later received a Wild Card spot in the National Finals. She is shown here on Snake Run, the first obstacle of Stage One that year.

CHAPTER 4

THE TRAINING

Staying fit is certainly no sweat for ninjas, but crushing obstacles takes something more—something beyond the typical regimen. *American Ninja Warrior* success requires speed, agility, balance, upper-body strength, grip strength, a strong core, and more. At times, it requires impeccable timing, stamina, and explosive movement. Therefore, ninja training varies widely. Here, veteran competitors reveal how they work out to up their obstacle game.

OBSTACLE WORK

For many ninjas, a core part of ninja training involves upper-body obstacle work, which has been a mainstay of *American Ninja Warrior*'s challenge, particularly in the later seasons. "As the show has grown, upper-body training sessions have become more and more important," says Chris Wilczewski. "In the early years, it was more important to be strong on trampolines and other lower-body obstacles."

"There was one competitor on *Ninja Warrior* who was a weight room warrior but refused to train ninja-style," says host Akbar Gbajabiamila. "He wouldn't do any of the obstacles. He'd just think, *Well, if I can do X amount of workouts in the gym, I'll be a* Ninja Warrior *beast*. Well, he was wrong. He was never able to go that far."

CLIMB TIME

While there's no single athletic background that can guarantee success on the obstacle course, many ninjas will say rock climbing has been invaluable to their workout regimen. The upper-body strength, grip strength, and core stability needed on the

> " I don't know that anyone has an advantage. We've seen rock climbers who made it to the top of Stage Four. Gymnasts like Kacy Catanzaro have great body awareness, but Drew Drechsel and Daniel Gil don't really come from traditional athletic backgrounds—they're just amazing athletes who happened to discover *America Ninja Warrior.*
>
> —Host Matt Iseman "

obstacle course are employed by rock climbers every day. Additionally, climbers have developed the ability to swing and throw their bodies and also problem-solve on the spot, both of which can come in handy on an obstacle course that has been created to surprise competitors at every turn.

Of all the aspects of her training, Jesse "Flex" Labreck says rock climbing has become the single most important element. "I rock climb probably three days a week," she says. "I ninja train two days a week, and I do a little bit of weight training and track stuff in there. As it gets closer to competition, I swap those. I do ninja training three days a week and rock climb maybe one or two times a week. Just so I can get more obstacle training in right before the show."

Surprisingly, Labreck hadn't started rock climbing until after she started training for *American Ninja Warrior*. "I was struggling with the Cliffhanger, so I asked for advice from some fellow ninjas, and they suggested rock climbing. Then I just fell in love with rock climbing, and I became addicted to it. I like that it's a problem every time you go up on the wall, and it's super challenging. And there are different levels—you can work your way up, and you can see yourself getting better by the grades you're doing."

CARDIO

Cardio training—running, swimming, biking, anything that raises the heart rate and gets the muscles moving—provides several benefits for ninjas. Mostly, it helps to strengthen the heart and lungs, which improves endurance on the obstacle course. While "SheWolf" Meagan Martin climbs five to six times a week for about three to four hours a day, she added cardio to her training before Season 8. Now, she does cardio two to three times a week for an hour. And while she believes that her climbing background has been advantageous to her on *American Ninja Warrior*, she says that cardio, at this point in her career, is most helpful.

> Climbing—and bouldering, specifically—has been the most important training tool for me, as a ninja warrior. The body control, grip strength, and mental toughness you need for *Ninja Warrior* is very similar to high-level bouldering.
> —Geoff Britten

Surprisingly, Martin does not train obstacle-specific very much. "I usually start training about a month before the Qualifying episode is filmed," she says. "When I train obstacles, it's usually once a week, but for Season 9 I was able to consistently train twice a week one month before the Qualifier." On obstacle training days, she usually climbs in the morning and does obstacles in the late afternoon or evening.

DAILY TO-DO LIST

CHRIS WILCZEWSKI:

1. Obstacles in the morning
2. Climbing midday
3. Conditioning in the evenings

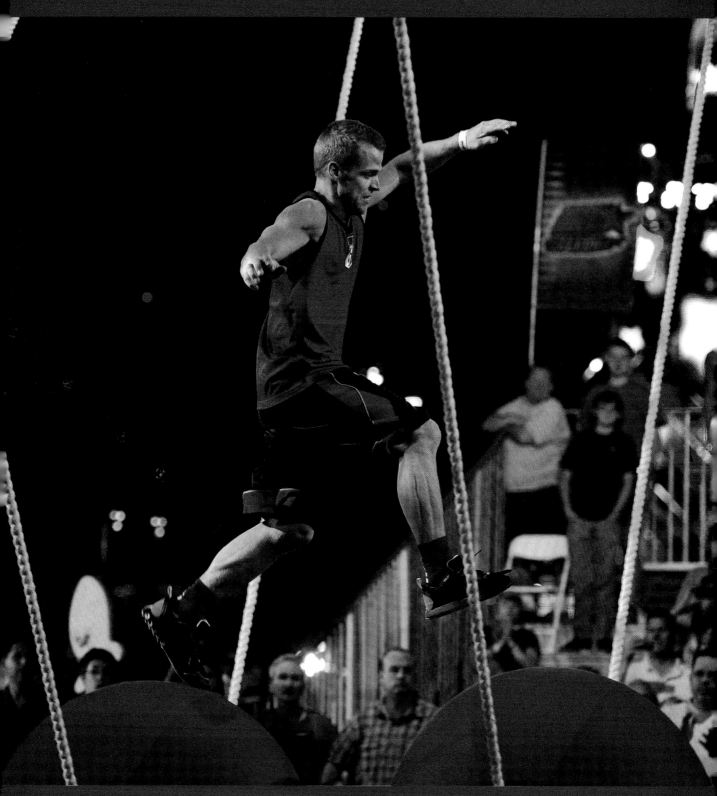

Chris Wilczewski conquers the Spinning Bridge right before clearing the final climb in Stage One of the Las Vegas National Finals in Season 6.

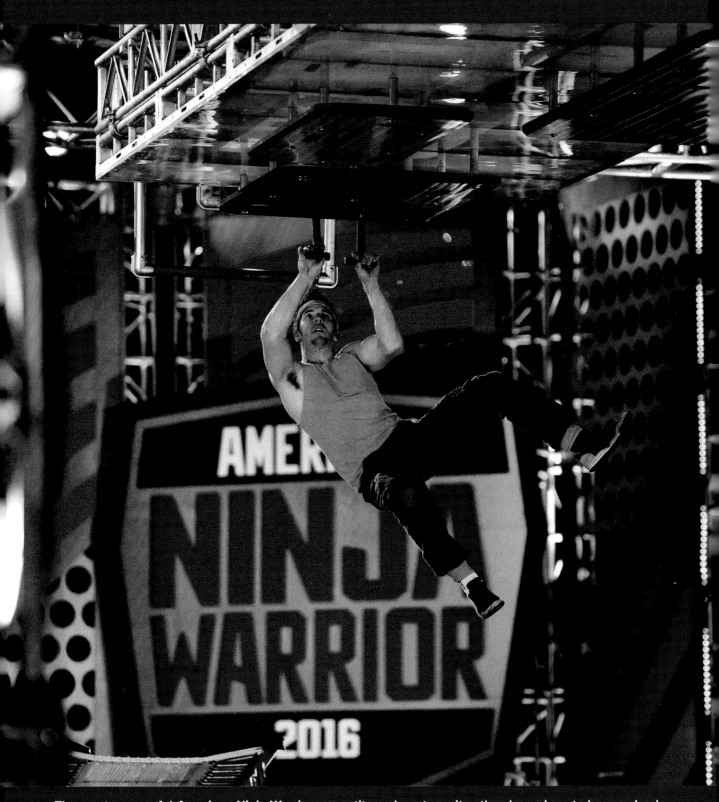

The most successful *American Ninja Warrior* competitors show tenacity—they know how to bounce back from a tough fall. In Season 6, "Real Life Ninja" Drew Drechsel missed the rope on the Downhill Pipe Drop and went out in the Miami Finals. However, Drechsel, shown here in the Season 8 National Finals, came back stronger than ever, making it to Stage Three the next two seasons.

Everybody falls on *American Ninja Warrior*. Everybody. Even when Isaac Caldiero took home the million dollars he fell in the Kansas City Finals. Geoff Britten is the only one to have a perfect season, six for six on the buzzers—and then the next year in Vegas, he fell on the very first obstacle on Stage One. That's because it is so hard. *American Ninja Warrior* is unlike any other show in that only two people have ever finished. Every other athlete who has set foot on the course fell. That's why I think they need to have an incredible determination, and a drive to succeed. For so many athletes, failure can crash their drive. But ninjas just see it as a challenge. It drives them to work harder. I love when we see someone fall on the course and then the next year we see their submission video that they filmed immediately after falling. Their thoughts didn't turn to pity. They turned to perseverance.

–Host Matt Iseman

CIRCUIT TRAINING

Circuit training—with its fast pace of various movements—targets strength building and muscle endurance for athletes. Kevin Bull trains approximately five days a week, with two easy or rest days. "Most of that time is strengthening and conditioning your body, but working on skills and body awareness is also very important and can be time-consuming," he says. "The backbone of my training is both rock climbing and circuit training with weights."

Bull says the circuit training provides strength, injury prevention, and cardio, and the rock climbing provides upper-body endurance and grip—basics that are needed to get past most of the obstacles. "But at the end of the day, the course tests for weaknesses," he says, "and it's your biggest weakness that will probably eliminate you, so an activity that improves a personal shortcoming is the best activity for any athlete attempting the course."

MIX IT UP

Many ninjas will say that they don't just settle on one type of training to prepare for *American Ninja Warrior*. They like to mix it up. Isaac Caldiero's training/climbing routine changes depending on the season and the weather. "When it's go time versus work time, I train every day, preferably mid-afternoon—mostly by myself or with my girlfriend Laura. It varies day to day from more intense to less intense workouts."

"Island Ninja" Grant McCartney's training regimen is a steady and varied mix of movement. "I train calisthenics three days a week—rock climbing, pull-ups, obstacle training, push-ups, dips," he says. "I run two to five days a week, between two to six miles a day, and I do CrossFit workouts once to twice a week. I always take Sunday off. Sunday is for the Lord and just for rest."

CORE STRENGTH

Core strength training works the lower back and the abdominals in unison. When ninjas have a solid base, their limbs can move powerfully and under control. In fact, all athletic movements incorporate the core in some way, and when the muscles of the trunk and torso are stabilized, ninjas have better body control, better balance, and more power.

While some ninjas might use medicine balls or balance boards to build their core, others find climbing is able to replicate those same moves and work those same muscles. "The entire sport of rock climbing works on so many different things that help you with *Ninja Warrior*," says Jesse Labreck. "Your body control, your grip strength, your core control, all of that really helps."

TO-DO LIST

JESSIE GRAFF:
1 WEEK BEFORE COMPETITION

1. Take a trip to APEX NorCal (a six-hour drive) to train on actual obstacles for two days.
2. Taper off to four relative rest days

READY, SETS, GO!

Pull-ups are the single most important exercise for "The Weatherman" Joe Moravsky. His regimen:

- **Do as many as possible in ten minutes**

- **Do as many as possible without assistance, followed by assisted pull-ups**

PASSION

When talking about skills and competencies needed for success on the obstacle course, it's easy to quantify how many hours of training ninjas put in or the number of sets or reps of a specific athletic movement. What's not so easy to quantify, however, is the heart of a ninja.

Passion for this sport is not something that can be logged into an app, but it's evident in ninjas' eyes when they step onto the course. It's the thing that drives them to train every day, multiple times a day, to sacrifice, to want more from their bodies when their bodies are telling them there is nothing left.

"Focus and preparation get you through the course," says Jessie Graff, "but heart and passion get you through the preparation. It takes way more heart to do your ninth set of max-out pull-ups on a random day at home alone in December than it does to give a Herculean effort in front of all the cameras. It's the determination to get through all nine sets every three days all year that gets you farther on the course."

THE MENTAL GAME

"I had a really good coach in college that prepared us in mental toughness," says Jesse "Flex" Labreck, "so for me I think that translates to *Ninja Warrior* because it's just you out there. It's just you telling yourself that you want this so badly, and sometimes you do have

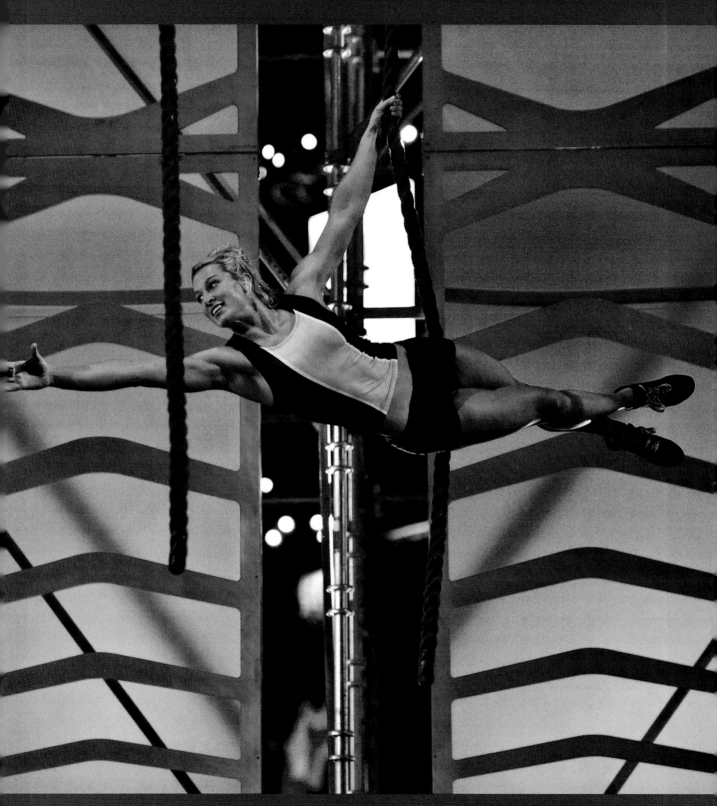

"Focus and preparation get you through the course," says Jessie Graff, shown here competing in Season 7's *American Ninja Warrior All-Star Special: Skills Challenge*.

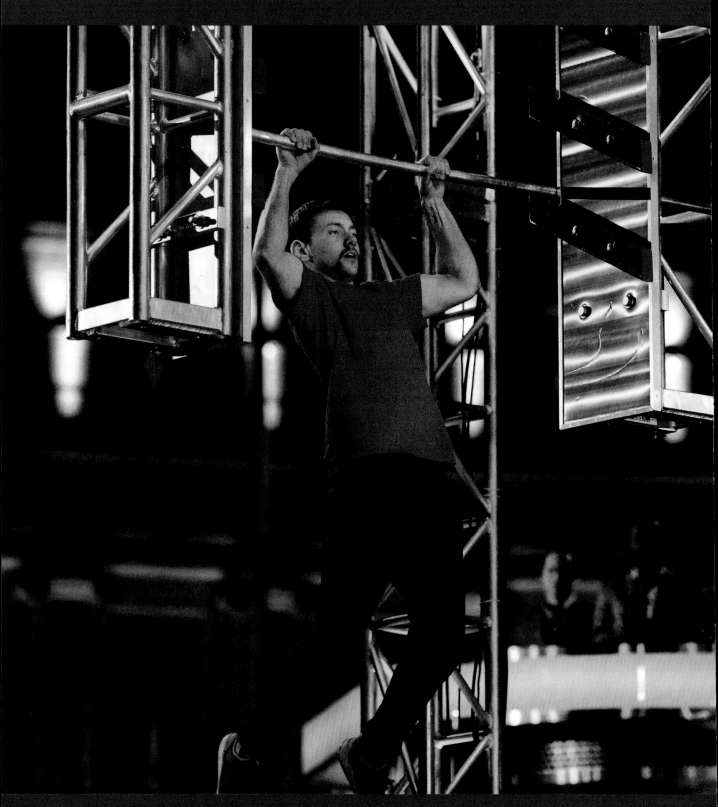

Mental toughness drove Dalton Knapp, who battled cancer off the course in order to compete on the *American Ninja Warrior* course. Here, he takes on the Salmon Ladder in the Denver Finals of Season 9.

to remind yourself how bad you want it. Honestly, I like to push myself, and I like to win. I think that helps drive me mentally when it gets tough."

"Mental toughness will get you through long hours of boring training or distance OCR [obstacle course racing], like a long and grueling mud run," notes Jessie Graff, who warns that proper training is integral to a successful run. "*Ninja Warrior* will buck you sideways off the course before you know you're in trouble. You're either prepared, or you're not. If you get to a point where you're fighting with every last ounce of strength to hold on, you've kinda won."

Graff adds that mental toughness is paramount when, for example, ninjas fall or slip on a simple balance obstacle and are eliminated before they get the chance to test their limits. "Fighting to come back from that disappointment requires immense mental toughness," she says.

"The mental game is most important in *Ninja Warrior* because the consequences of a mistake are so high," says Kevin Bull. "One slip, and your

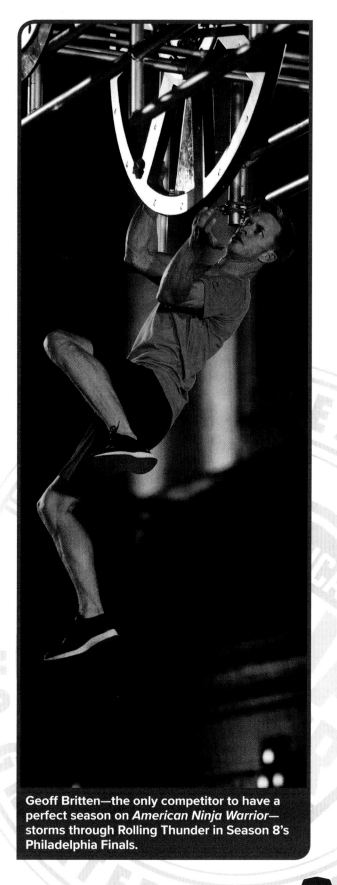

Geoff Britten—the only competitor to have a perfect season on *American Ninja Warrior*—storms through Rolling Thunder in Season 8's Philadelphia Finals.

> " Heart is important. You've got to want it! When you see someone on the course and their body sags or they look down, they are done. You can't do that on *Ninja Warrior* if you want to succeed. You have to fight, and dig deep.
>
> —Geoff Britten "

season is ended. It's kind of unique in the sporting world and very stressful for us as athletes. What helps me is finding ways of eliminating the self. I focus on objectives and goals while on the course. By thinking only of the goals, I have been able to push myself past things that would normally have stopped me, like exhaustion or fear."

"The mental side of being on *American Ninja Warrior* is by far the most important aspect," notes Isaac Caldiero. "There is so much more going on beside the physical challenges on the show. I specifically do a lot of breathing exercises mixed with positive visualization techniques that I have taught myself through the extensive years of being a free solo rock climber where my life is literally in my own hands and where failure is not an option. New challenges dubbed as impossible are what drive me."

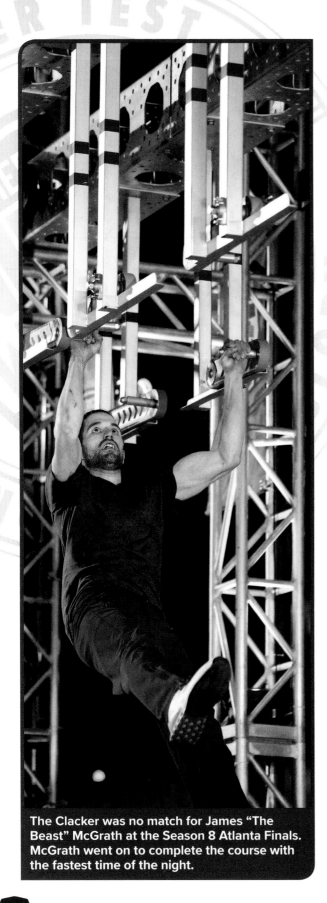

The Clacker was no match for James "The Beast" McGrath at the Season 8 Atlanta Finals. McGrath went on to complete the course with the fastest time of the night.

DID YOU KNOW?

It is not in the official rules, but there is an unspoken rule that *American Ninja Warrior* gives "a limited amount of equal time" to ninjas to rest in between obstacles, according to executive producer Kent Weed. "Although," he says, "if you are going for the fastest time—which we see many times—then it's irrelevant."

FINDING THE TIME

With life pulling us in so many directions, it can sometimes be difficult to find the time to train, but ninjas say it is imperative that athletes find a way if they are serious about competing. "Training has always been hard for me," says Geoff Britten. "I don't like to train! I've found that keeping it fun works best. Things like climbing or doing challenges with friends in ninja gyms has always worked for me. I've never lifted weights or worked out in regular gyms. Working a lot, it's hard to find the

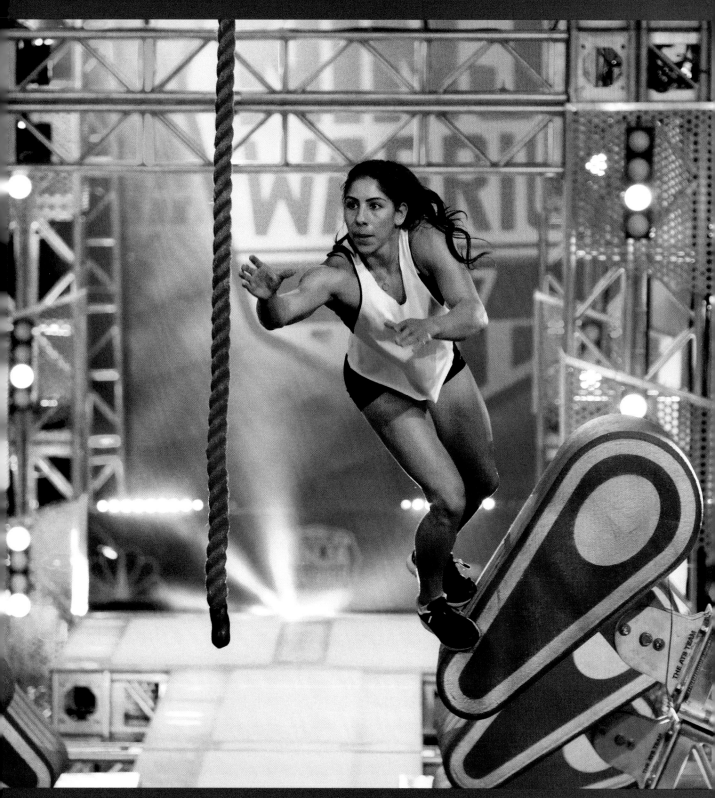

Ninjas know that even the slightest break in concentration can lead to getting wet on *American Ninja Warrior*. Here, Tiana Webberley focuses on getting past the Floating Steps in Los Angeles during Season 9.

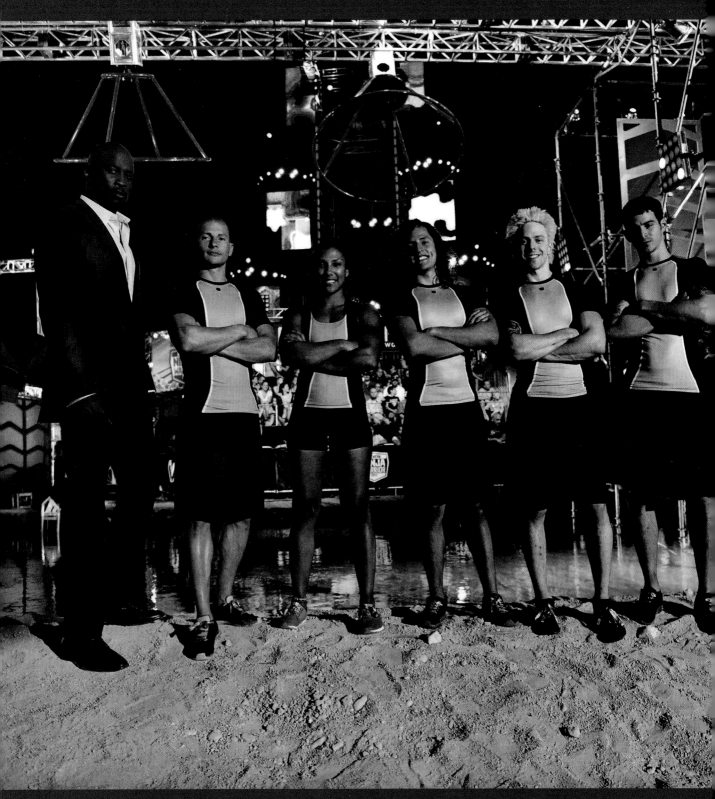

Host Akbar Gbajabiamila (left) stands with 2016's *American Ninja Warrior All-Star Special: Skills Challenge's* Team Akbar: Brent Steffensen, Meagan Martin, Daniel Gil, Jamie Rahn, and Flip Rodriguez.

For me, having played football, with the nicks and bruises that I've gotten over the years, I have a lot of joint issues, so I try to do things that are a bit more controlled. I'm trying now to step out and do things that are more explosive. I call it the 'Ninja Workout.' I've worked out with people like Flip Rodriguez and Jessie Graff, and they've inspired me to get out of my comfort zone. I'm a natural weight room guy. I do my weight room, I do my cardio. I do a few box jumps here and there, and pat myself on the back thinking I'm explosive, and I'm not.

—Host Akbar Gbajabiamila

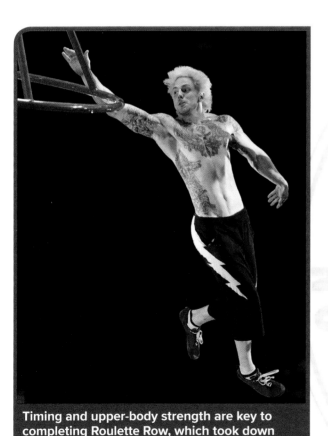

Timing and upper-body strength are key to completing Roulette Row, which took down "Captain NBC" Jamie Rahn during Stage Two of the Season 7 National Finals.

READY, SETS, GO!

"For pull-ups, my overall workout will revolve around the '30 Seconds Rest' the show allows you in between obstacles. On different days this can mean different things. Early in the off-season when I am just getting back into training, I'll do 10 sets of 10 with 30 seconds rest in between. As I become more conditioned, I will start doing more reps per set. For example, I will do 4 sets of 25 reps with 30 seconds rest in between. The goal is to be capable of recovering in 30 seconds or less. This helps prevent me from getting tired as the course builds in difficulty with each obstacle."

—Chris Wilczewski

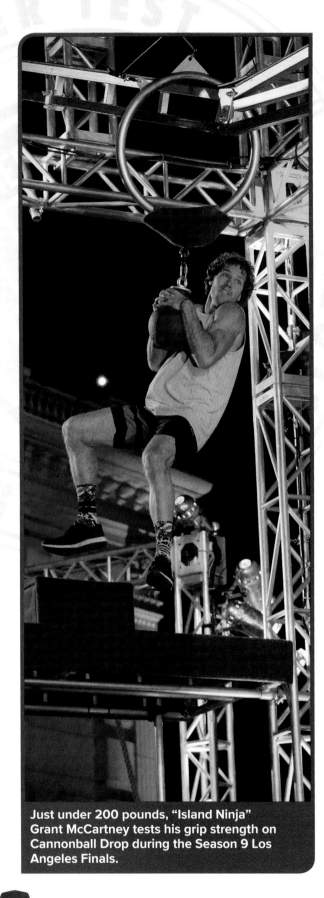

Just under 200 pounds, "Island Ninja" Grant McCartney tests his grip strength on Cannonball Drop during the Season 9 Los Angeles Finals.

time to train, but I've found out that if you don't watch TV, play games, or laze around you can accomplish so much!"

"Originally, I did no training," says "Island Ninja" Grant McCartney. "I hopped off the couch, did some pull-ups that day they told me they wanted me to come, and I just got as ready as I could."

Even with little training, McCartney made the National Finals his rookie year, but that incredible showing prompted him to start training more in the months before he appeared in Vegas. "Once I made the National Finals that year, I trained for three months," he says. "I never really was a rock climber, so I started doing that. Now, going into the second and third year, I train a lot. Now I'm training every day, including CrossFit and body training stuff."

Even while working as a flight attendant for Hawaiian Airlines, he squeezes in time for training during layovers, visiting ninja gyms, camps, and other venues.

"I don't train any heavier than what I already weigh, because I'm about 195, which is about 30 to 40 pounds heavier than most of the ninjas," he says. "So I don't need to gain weight—I just need to gain muscle density."

NINJA KNOW-HOW

DO NINJAS TRAIN TOGETHER?

KEVIN BULL: "It's very difficult for ninjas to train as partners because we are so spread out and a lot of us are very busy on crazy schedules. Since moving down to Southern California, though, I have been able to train fairly regularly with Jessie Graff and Tiana Webberly."

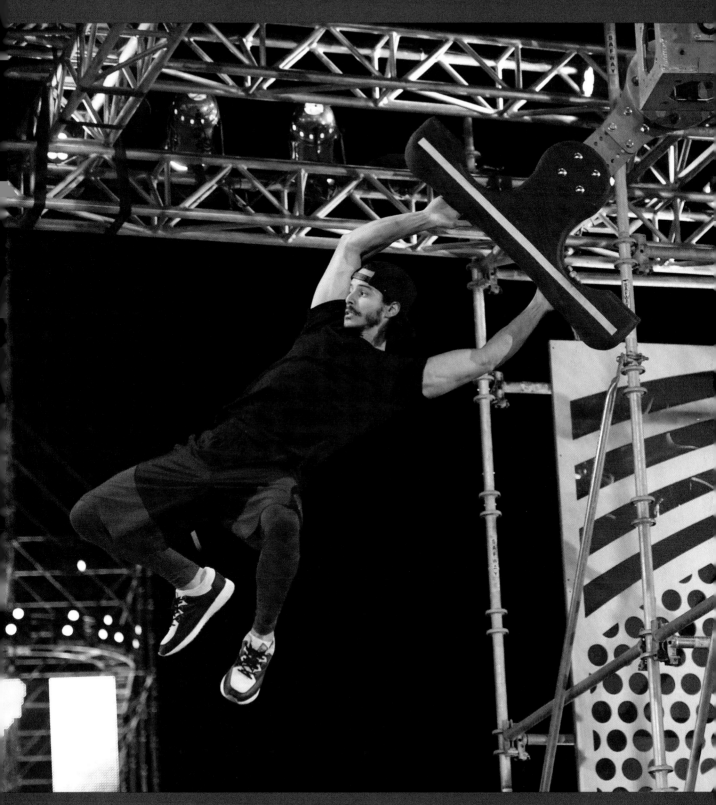

Flip Rodriguez takes on Wingnut Alley in Stage Two of the National Finals in Season 9, but the Ninja Killer did in the fan favorite, who ended his run there.

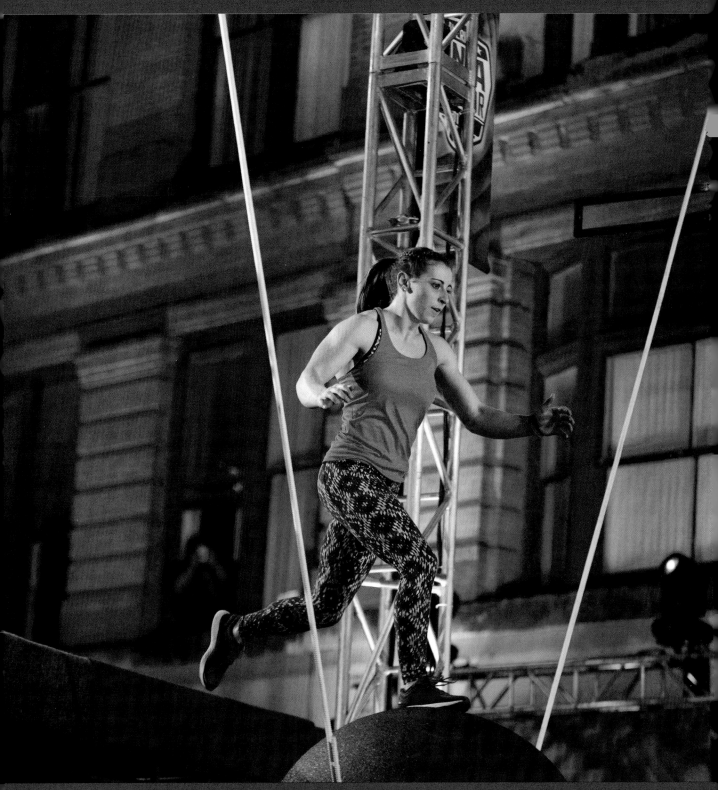

Barclay Stockett steadies herself across the Spinning Bridge during the San Antonio Qualifier in Season 9. Stockett landed the top spot in the Women's Top 5.

READY, SETS, GO!

In her weight training, Jesse "Flex" Labreck does some heavy legs—squats, power clean, deadlift. Three by six is usually as much as she does, because, she says, "I do it pretty heavy." Then she gets down to three by three, depending on the weight, and then does "something explosive" right after to keep her power in her legs, followed by ab work. "I typically stay away from upper body in the weight room," Labreck says, "because I get so much upper body in the rock climbing and the ninja training."

NINJA KNOW-HOW

DESCRIBE YOUR TRAINING IN ONE WORD:

GEOFF BRITTEN: "Exhausting."
KEVIN BULL: "Varied."
ISAAC CALDIERO: "Focused."
MEAGAN MARTIN: "Hectic."
JOE MORAVSKY: "Focused."
CHRIS WILCZEWSKI: "Dedicated."

WEEKLY TO-DO LIST

"THE WEATHERMAN"
JOE MORAVSKY:
Monday: Rock climb
Tuesday: Ninja gym
Wednesday: Rest
Thursday: Ninja gym
Friday and/or Saturday:
   Rock climb
Sunday: Rest

TECH TALK

While some ninjas use some technology in their training—for example, Chris Wilczewski uses the Climbing 30/30 app to track interval times on his dead hangs and Jessie Graff uses an Under Armour training mask—many prefer to go tech-free. "The body's ability to push itself varies from day to day, and your trackers can't measure that," says Kevin Bull. "I like to listen to my body to maximize my effort in any given training session."

> *American Ninja Warrior* is one of the most difficult sports. In the history of the show, only one individual has made it a full season without failing. It's important for athletes to accept failure, be able to learn from it, and come back stronger.
>
> –Chris Wilczewski

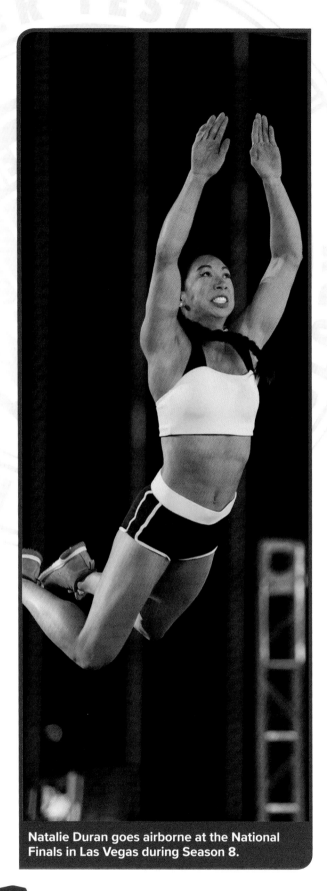

Natalie Duran goes airborne at the National Finals in Las Vegas during Season 8.

> I always am conscious of what I eat, but I definitely step it up about a month prior to competition. No fast food, low carbs, low sugar! A few cheat days, too.
> —"The Weatherman" Joe Moravsky

WHAT DO NINJAS EAT?

It's no secret that good, clean fuel provides better mileage and—in the case of ninjas—better performance and mood. To maintain focus, strength, and stamina, many ninjas opt for balanced meals with healthy helpings of protein, fruits, and vegetables, but, overall, ninja diets tend to be as diverse as their training.

Two or three months prior to go time, Isaac Caldiero says he eats very healthy and light—"very little meats and mostly vegetarian with no alcohol or caffeine. My training is extensive and nonstop up until about a week before I perform." A week before Competition Day, he tones down the intensity of the training, for recovery, but keeps up the healthy eating.

Grant McCartney admits he's not the healthiest eater. "I eat crap. I've changed it up a bit, but I still like my sweets, like candy, but I challenge myself to do better. I do a lot of running, and, depending on the season, I'm training five or six days a week with upward of 10 miles a day. And if you eat crappy, that mile two or three is when your body goes 'all right, all right' and gives up on you."

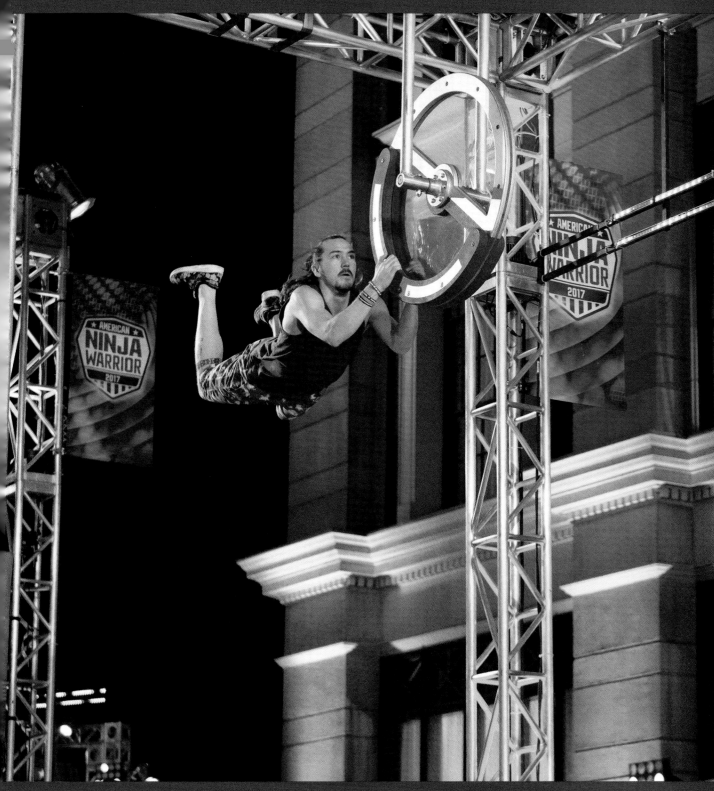

"Eskimo Ninja" Nick Hanson exhibits stone-cold focus on the Fly Wheels during the Los Angeles Finals of Season 9.

> I'm not a real big diet guy. Some ninjas eat next to nothing. I know a guy who eats one meal a day, and it's four to five scoops of ice cream. It's crazy. Another one is super healthy–he's a vegetarian, and it blows my mind when he goes to a restaurant and orders only sides. I didn't even know you could do that!
>
> –"Island Ninja" Grant McCartney

NINJA FUEL:

ISAAC CALDIERO'S NINJA POWER SMOOTHIE

Ingredients:
2 cups almond milk
1 banana
1/2 cup frozen blueberries

1 spoonful almond butter or
   peanut butter
1 spoonful plain yogurt
1 tsp. chia seed

Directions: Add all ingredients into a blender, cover, and puree on high speed until ingredients are combined.

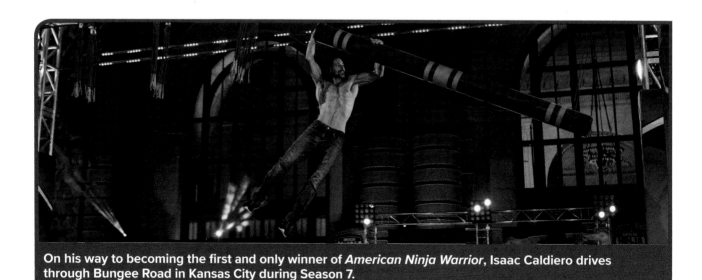

On his way to becoming the first and only winner of *American Ninja Warrior*, Isaac Caldiero drives through Bungee Road in Kansas City during Season 7.

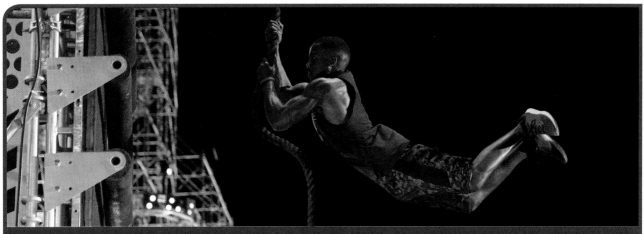

"Philly Phoenix" Najee Richardson soars while taking on the Swing Surfer during his Stage Two appearance in the National Finals of Season 9.

NINJA FUEL:

WOLFPACK ROASTED VEGETABLES

The Wolfpack Ninjas—Brian Arnold, "Wolfpup" Ian Dory, "SheWolf" Meagan Martin, and Noah Kaufman—have banded together to help fight child obesity and reduce the sugar in kids' diets. Their recipe for roasted vegetables is a healthy replacement for french fries or any other sides with unhealthy fat levels or high calorie counts.

Ingredients:

1 tbs. thyme
2 tbs. rosemary
4 tbs. California olive oil
2 tbs. vinegar
$1/4$ tsp. garlic salt

Pepper to taste
4 cups assorted veggies
(brussels sprouts, asparagus, zucchini, broccoli, peppers, whatever you love!)
$1/4$ c. lemon zest

Directions:

1. In a bowl, stir together thyme, rosemary, California olive oil, vinegar, garlic salt, and pepper.
2. Toss with your favorite vegetables until they are coated.
3. Spread evenly on a large roasting pan.
4. Roast for 35 to 40 minutes in a preheated oven (475° F), mixing every 10 minutes or until vegetables are cooked through and just slightly browned.
5. Ten minutes before finishing, add the lemon zest (a Wolfpack secret!), and mix one final time.

COUNTDOWN TO COMPETITION DAY

As Competition Day nears, ninjas tend to ease up on their training. Chris Wilczewski says he lets his body recover and concentrates only on technique with the obstacles. "I try to focus on obstacles like the Salmon Ladder, Flying Bar, or Slack Ladder," he says. "I pick the Salmon Ladder because I know this obstacle will almost always be in a City Finals course. The obstacle is very easy to make a mistake on. Therefore, I like to practice the technique over and over again. This way, I feel comfortable I won't miss."

Even though the Flying Bar typically isn't in a Qualifying course, Wilczewski says there are a few obstacles that require similar hip coordination. "This type of coordination can be difficult to master, so I like to train it right before competing," he says. "The Slack Ladder is a significant obstacle for building full body awareness."

"As the competition gets closer, it is important to taper your training a bit so that you are fresh enough to compete," says "SheWolf" Meagan Martin. "I actually don't change my diet at all."

NINJA KNOW-HOW

"As the show gets closer, I try to eat healthier and lose a pound or two. The day before, I've always gone out and had a giant bacon burger. Let me tell you, having group ninja dinners and watching everyone eat salads while you order bacon burgers is quite a treat. The looks I've gotten!"

—Geoff Britten

Charlie Andrews pumps his way up the Elevator Climb in what was hailed as the run of the night during Season 9's Los Angeles Finals.

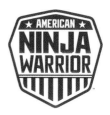

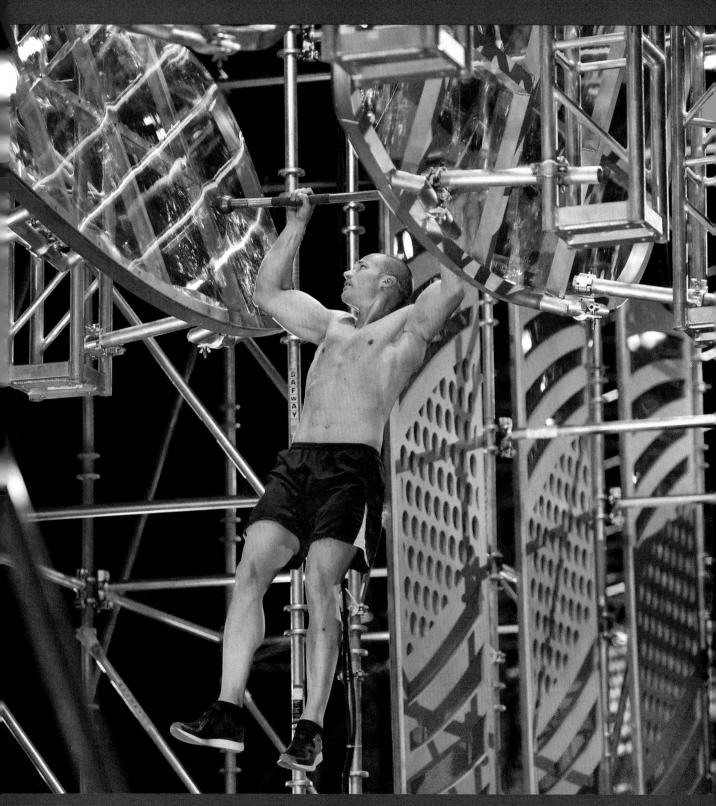

Brian Arnold made it all the way to Stage Two of the National Finals in Season 8, but the veteran competitor gassed out on the Double Wedge, shown here.

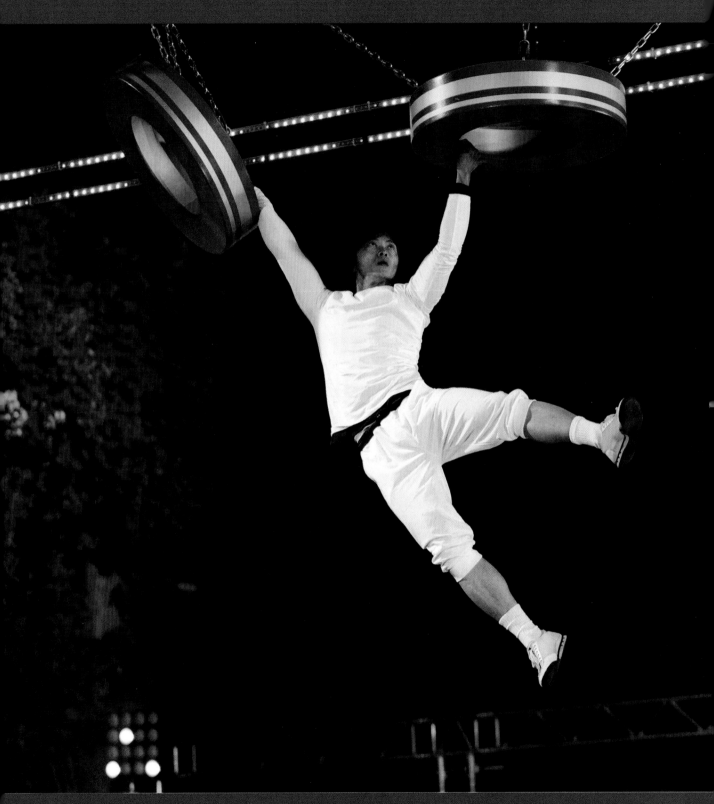

Sam Sann looked strong on the Tire Swing in the Qualifying round of Season 8 in Oklahoma City, but the veteran ninja had a surprising fall on the dismount, knocking him out of the competition.

CHAPTER 5

GO TIME

It's the Big Day. Comp Day. Go Time. The day ninjas have been training for all year long. When ninjas step up to that Qualifier starting line they are composed and ready. But what goes on before then? How do they warm up? Who do they bring with them? How do they feel? Are they nervous? Self-assured? In this chapter, *American Ninja Warrior* athletes share their competition day activities.

> A lot of competitors aren't accustomed to operating under that amount of pressure. It's a huge amount of pressure when you know there's a million dollars on the line, there are millions of people watching at home, and there are thousands in attendance. Not to mention that if you mess up, you don't get another opportunity until next year. There are 365 days until the next opportunity, so that's a lot to process. And oh, by the way, you have to run the course. That's hard.
> —Host Akbar Gbajabiamila

CALMING NERVES

Ninjas may sometimes seem like they're superhuman, but they are not impervious to nerves. For many athletes, even those who are accustomed to participating in races, meets, or other athletic events, competing on *American Ninja Warrior* is very different from what they're used to. There are the cameras, the audiences, the pressure.

"I usually haven't slept very well and am extremely nervous," says Jesse "Flex" Labreck. "On Competition Day, the nerves are so crazy that you don't always feel ready, but you know the training that you've done before has prepared you well. I just think about all of the training I've done and know that everything's going to be fine."

"I definitely get butterflies when competing on *American Ninja Warrior*," says Chris Wilczewski. "When you are at home there isn't as much pressure. If you fall, you can try again right away. Competition Day is tough because any veteran will tell you that anything can happen on the course. I find confidence only when I know I have done everything I can to prepare for the course. Then I can walk to the course willing and ready to accept any outcome, because I have prepared to the best of my ability."

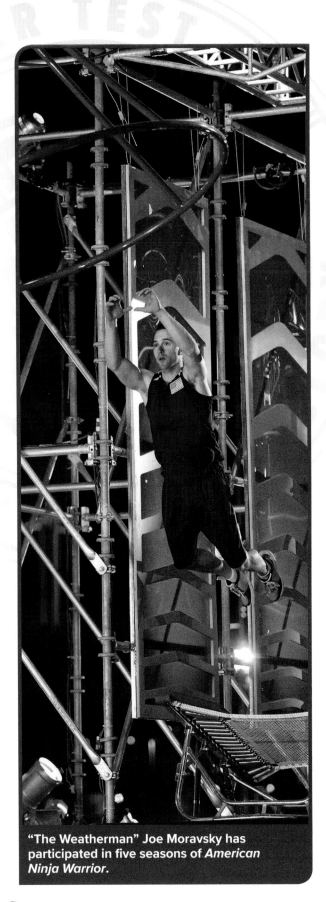

"The Weatherman" Joe Moravsky has participated in five seasons of *American Ninja Warrior*.

On Competition Day, I'm always nervous but ready to remind myself that fear exists only in my mind. I can control that fear if I so choose.
–"The Weatherman" Joe Moravsky

Mental toughness is definitely underestimated. At the end of the day, it all comes down to how mentally strong you are. That is something I feel like I have to constantly work on. Since I compete in big competitions in climbing a lot, I think I have a good base competitive mindset, but *American Ninja Warrior* is way more nerve-racking for me than climbing is. I usually just try to remind myself that it's all about having fun!
–Meagan Martin

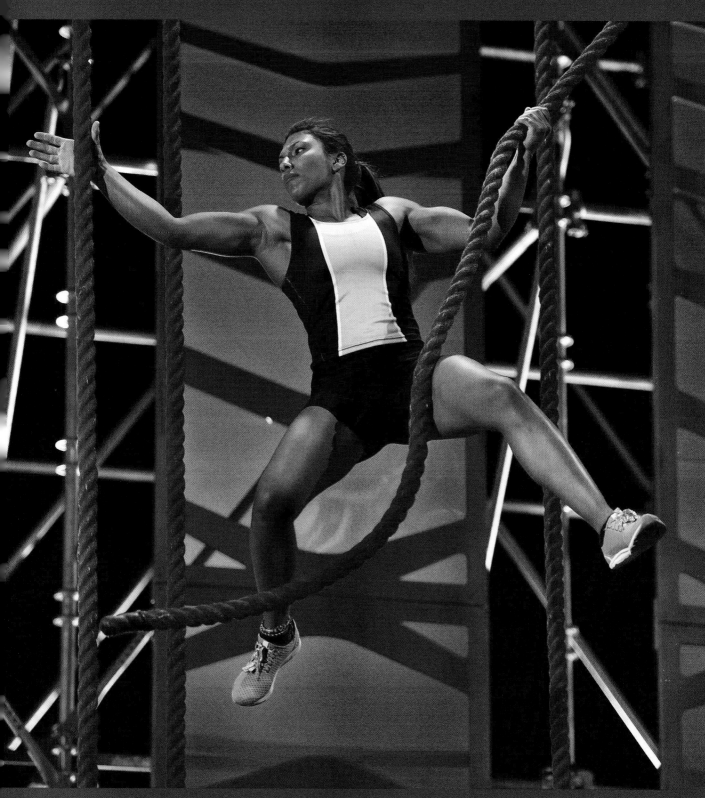

Meagan Martin competes in the 2016 *American Ninja Warrior All-Star Special: Skills Challenge.*

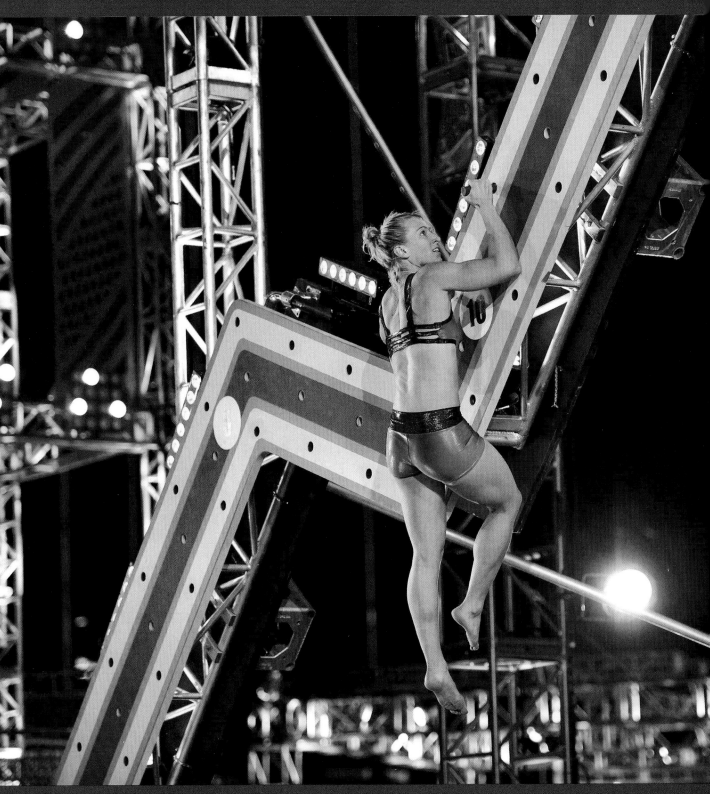

Jessie Graff concentrates on the new Thunderbolt in the 2017 *American Ninja Warrior All-Star Special: Skills Challenge.*

STAYING FOCUSED

On Competition Day, Jessie Graff likes to sleep in and tries to eat a "real" breakfast, but will eat some seaweed and a protein bar if she's in a rush. "It's about being focused and alert, so you can harness everything you have to do your absolute best on that day," she says.

"My regimen revolves around not getting too excited and controlling my emotions," notes Isaac Caldiero. "Anybody can train physically and be more than strong enough to complete the *American Ninja Warrior* course. It's not that hard physically."

Caldiero believes his mental toughness is what helped him dominate the course in Season 7.

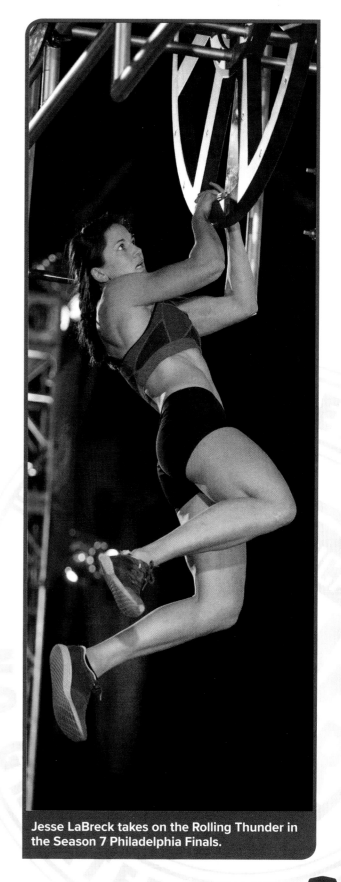

Jesse LaBreck takes on the Rolling Thunder in the Season 7 Philadelphia Finals.

"Having all the pressure to win and become the first *American Ninja Warrior* champion on top of the audience, the cameras, and the fact that you're competing during the middle of the night had made it a nearly impossible feat for so many years. With my mental fortitude, I was able to break the spell."

> "I actually don't feel any stage fright. I am very used to competing in front of crowds, so I usually am just in the zone and focused.
> –Meagan Martin

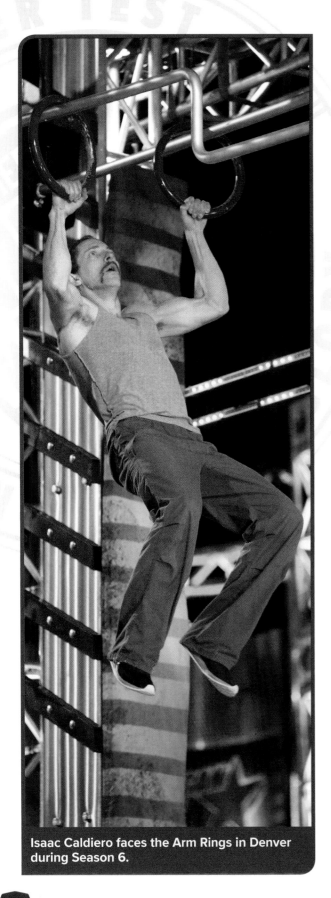

Isaac Caldiero faces the Arm Rings in Denver during Season 6.

DE-STRESSING

"When I wake up on Competition Day, I like to relax," says Chris Wilczewski. "I take my motorcycle out or play video games—anything to take away my stress. I think this helps me come in relaxed and ready to go."

"On Comp Day, the day-to-day life events and emotions do not exist—even my family, friends, and loved ones are all temporarily put on hold," notes Isaac Caldiero. "I'm feeling relaxed, confident, and in control."

WHO NEEDS SLEEP?

Because the runs take place in the middle of the night, it can be an adjustment for rookies. Many are not accustomed to walking up to a starting line at three o'clock in the morning. Even veteran ninjas have to readjust to the overnight competition.

"It's definitely hard competing overnight," says Jesse "Flex" Labreck. "Your sleep schedule hasn't really

Chris Wilczewski finished ninth in the Season 6 National Finals.

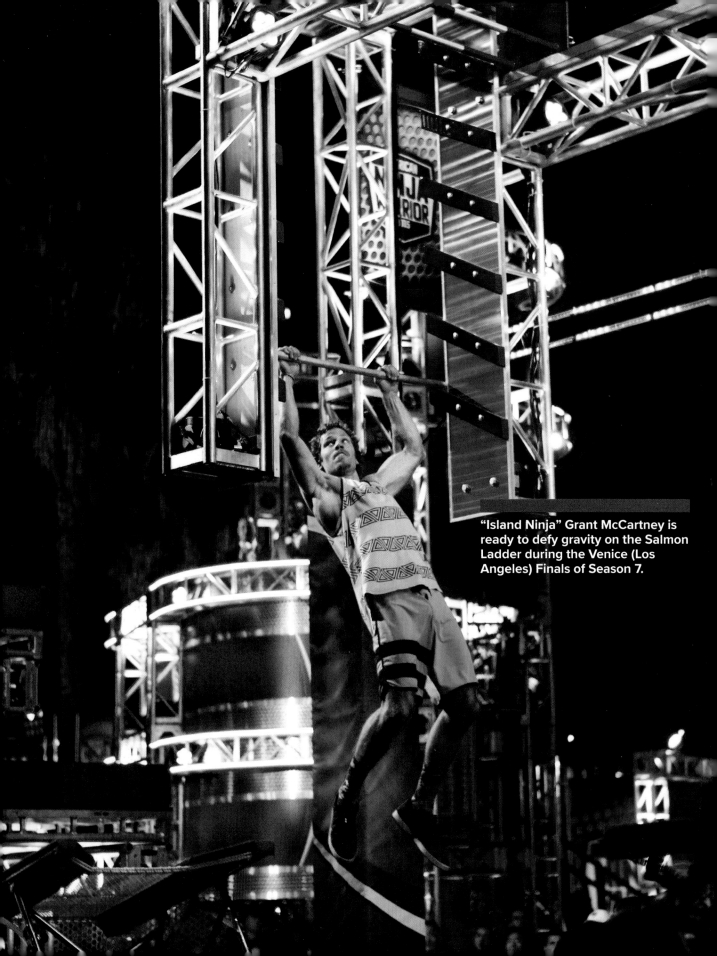

"Island Ninja" Grant McCartney is ready to defy gravity on the Salmon Ladder during the Venice (Los Angeles) Finals of Season 7.

changed, you're tired but have so much adrenaline. That's one of the biggest changes. And there's the atmosphere of how much energy there is—it's crazy. In track and field it's not quite so crazy."

"People always tell me, 'Oh, I could do that, I could do that,'" says "Island Ninja" Grant McCartney. "Okay, come try it at 3 or 4 A.M. after you've been up all night in some time zone you're not normally in."

LAST-MINUTE TRAINING

If there is time before his run, Kevin Bull likes to do some parkour/balance work to prepare his mindset. "My strategy on the course is almost always to be aggressive," he says. "I want to perform at my best, and I can't get there if I'm being tentative."

> Most of Competition Day I feel highly stressed and nervous. I don't really feel ready until I get my first foot on the course, and after that, things are okay.
>
> —Kevin Bull

NINJA KNOW-HOW

COMP DAY MUST-HAVES
JESSIE GRAFF:

1. A blanket to stretch on
2. Foam roller and lacrosse ball
3. Protein bars
4. Chocolate espresso beans
5. Adhesive heating pads
6. Sweats and a coat

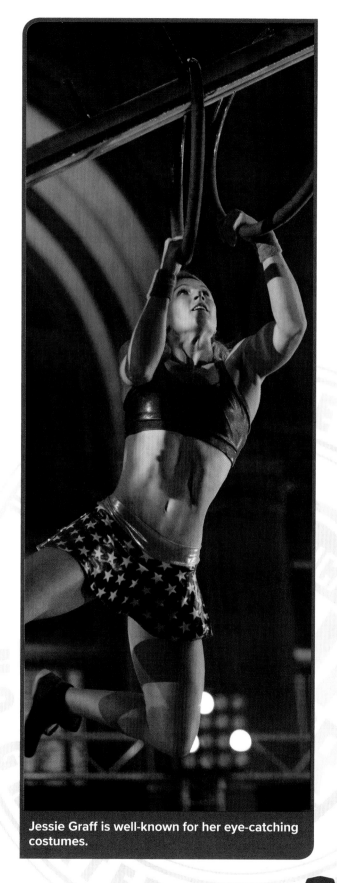

Jessie Graff is well-known for her eye-catching costumes.

Ninjas will also watch fellow athletes run the course, hoping to pick up additional tips that will help them attack the obstacles. "We definitely watch each other," says Jesse Labreck. "I don't watch every single run, because you have to mentally prepare yourself, too. Also, just because someone does it a certain way doesn't mean that it'll work for you. I typically watch people that I know I move similarly to, or have similar height, or strength."

Geoff Britten says that once he arrives on the course and gets checked in, it's time to start going over the course mentally. "I go over every move I want to make, over and over again," he says. "I also try to come up with crazy Plan Bs and Plan Cs if something goes wrong on any obstacle. I'm a big believer in warming up, more than most. My goal is to be sweaty, tired, and out of breath 20 to 30 minutes before my run. Then I'll relax and watch the runners in front of me. I retie my shoes a lot—I want them as tight as possible! I also make sure the soles are squeaky clean as I step up onto the starting platform."

> A lot of these ninjas, before they get on each obstacle, will visualize themselves completing it, and I always love that. As a former professional football player, that was something that I utilized. I could see the play happening—I could see everything breaking down and how I would be a part of that play.
>
> —Host Akbar Gbajabiamila

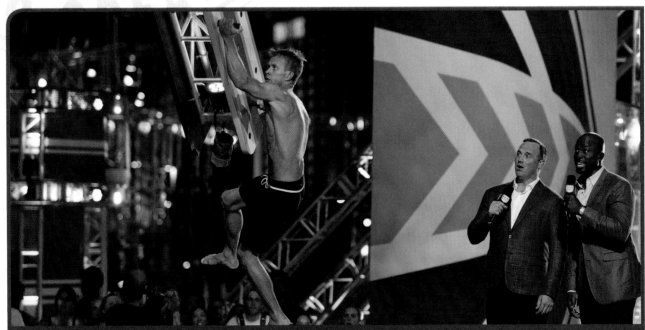

Hosts Matt Iseman and Akbar Gbajabiamila watch Geoff Britten—also known as "Popeye"—ascend the Thunderbolt in Season 8.

COMP DAY MUST-HAVES

CHRIS WILCZEWSKI:
1. Caffeine
2. Proper warm-up music!

MORAL SUPPORT

Many of the athletes who appear on *American Ninja Warrior* come with posses—spouses and/or significant others, moms, dads, friends, children, grandparents, and training partners who are often seen smiling and cheering along the sidelines. "I bring my family with me. It helps to be surrounded by people who love you and understand the work and dedication you put into your training," says Chris Wilczewski.

When Kevin Bull steps onto the course, he knows he has an extra-special group of supporters cheering for him on the sidelines—children with alopecia. "When I choose people to cheer me on, I try to pick people who will enjoy watching and who will add their excitement to the atmosphere," Bull notes. "The alopecia community has been my biggest supporter since I started, and the kids bring more excitement at competition time than anyone else."

NINJA KNOW-HOW

WARMING UP

JESSIE GRAFF: "I do a light warm-up about five hours before I expect to compete and start my real warm-up about 30 minutes before—arm circles, leg swings, kicks, pull-ups, runs, sprints, speed skaters, clapping pull-ups, uphill speed skaters, and mini-tramp."

Chris Wilczewski competed in seven seasons of *American Ninja Warrior* before a shoulder injury kept him out of Season 9.

NINJA KNOW-HOW

COMP DAY MUST-HAVES

ISAAC CALDIERO:
1. Clothes
2. Ninja shoes
3. Music that fluctuates between calm meditative chanting and upbeat techno beats.

KEEPING IT SIMPLE

Isaac Caldiero keeps his game-day warm-up simple with breathing exercises, some basic leg stretches, and pull-ups. "I mostly warm up on the course itself," he says. "The strategy is to be flawless in a calm, fluid manner that makes the obstacles look and feel effortless."

NINJA KNOW-HOW

COMP DAY MUST-HAVES

KEVIN BULL:
1. Chicken sandwich
2. Pedialyte
3. Water
4. A bag of almonds
5. Some protein bars

I've found that routines are what cause you to make mistakes. You must always be ready for the unknown.
—Isaac Caldiero

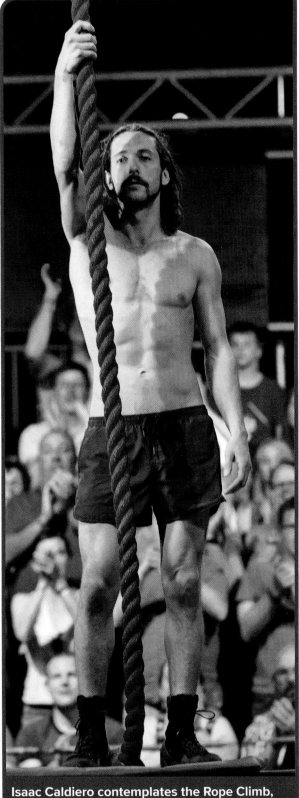

Isaac Caldiero contemplates the Rope Climb, Stage Four, just moments before becoming the fastest *American Ninja Warrior* champion.

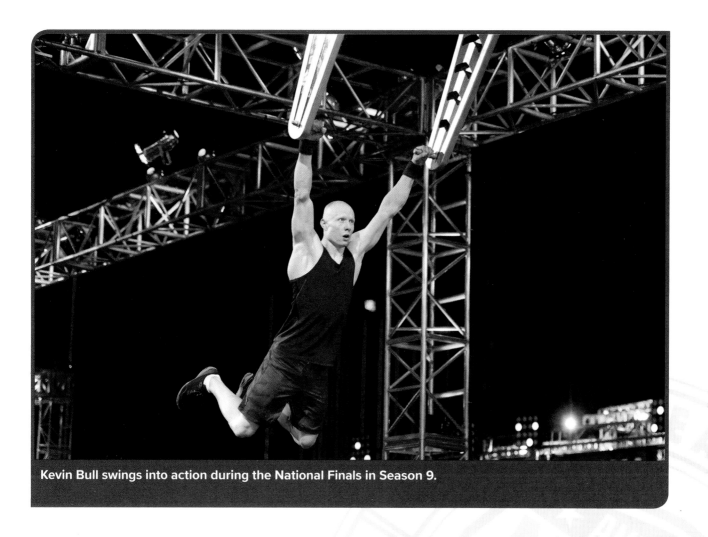

Kevin Bull swings into action during the National Finals in Season 9.

> The mental toughness comes in because of the nerves. You're on national television, you have no time to practice, you get one go, and you're put on the spot. One mess-up, and you're out.
>
> —"Island Ninja" Grant McCartney

HURRY UP AND WAIT

There can be a lot of downtime on the set of *American Ninja Warrior*. Cameras have to be adjusted. Obstacles have to be reset. Weather delays may occur. So while most of the rounds are shown in edited two-hour blocks on television, the actual shooting can take roughly four times as long, which can be an adjustment for ninjas who are raring to go.

"They can bring you up to the starting line, and go, 'All right, you ready to go? Okay, hold on, we're going to have a lunch break,'" says "Island Ninja" Grant McCartney. "I was literally standing at the starting line, in my rookie year, first time ever, I've been waiting for hours, and then they kicked me off and I had to take a breather."

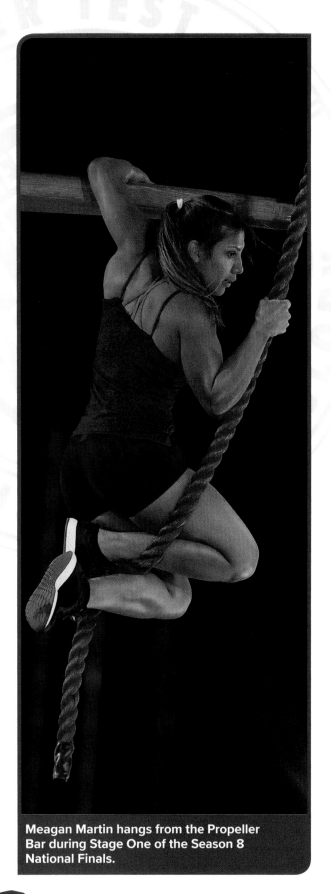

Meagan Martin hangs from the Propeller Bar during Stage One of the Season 8 National Finals.

I usually don't feel ready until I step onto the platform. In the morning, I usually am extremely nervous and just try to manage the nerves all day.

–"SheWolf" Meagan Martin

COMPETITION DAY TO-DO LIST

MEAGAN MARTIN:
"I usually make sure I have a good breakfast along with a good lunch. For *American Ninja Warrior*, I like when my parents are there, though they can't always make it. It's also comforting to have the Wolfpack there with me! I try to make sure I have a good, long warm-up so that I'm ready. I like to bring a foam roller with me!"

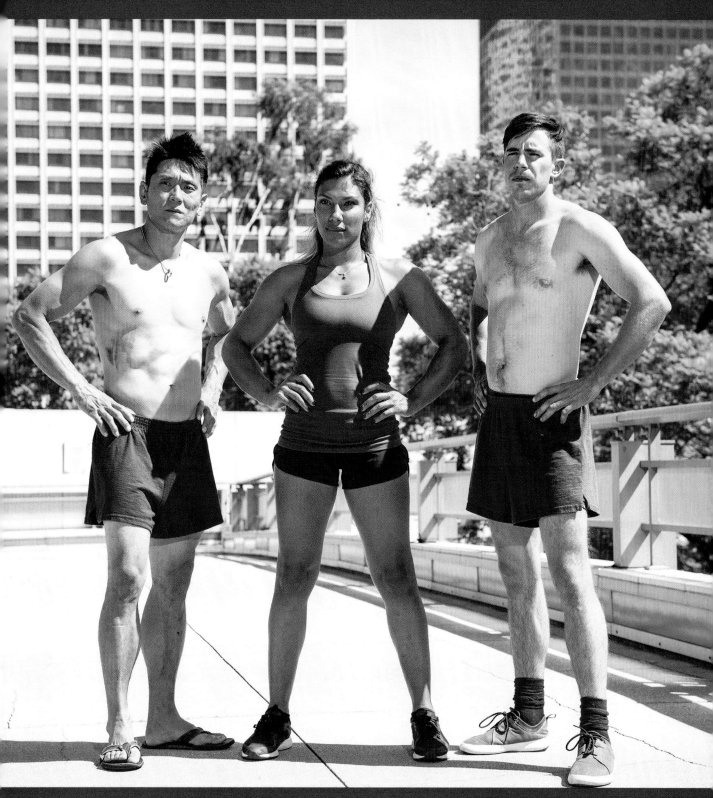

Dan Yager, Meagan Martin, and Ian Dory make up the Mega Crushers (formerly Team Midoryama) on *Team Ninja Warrior*.

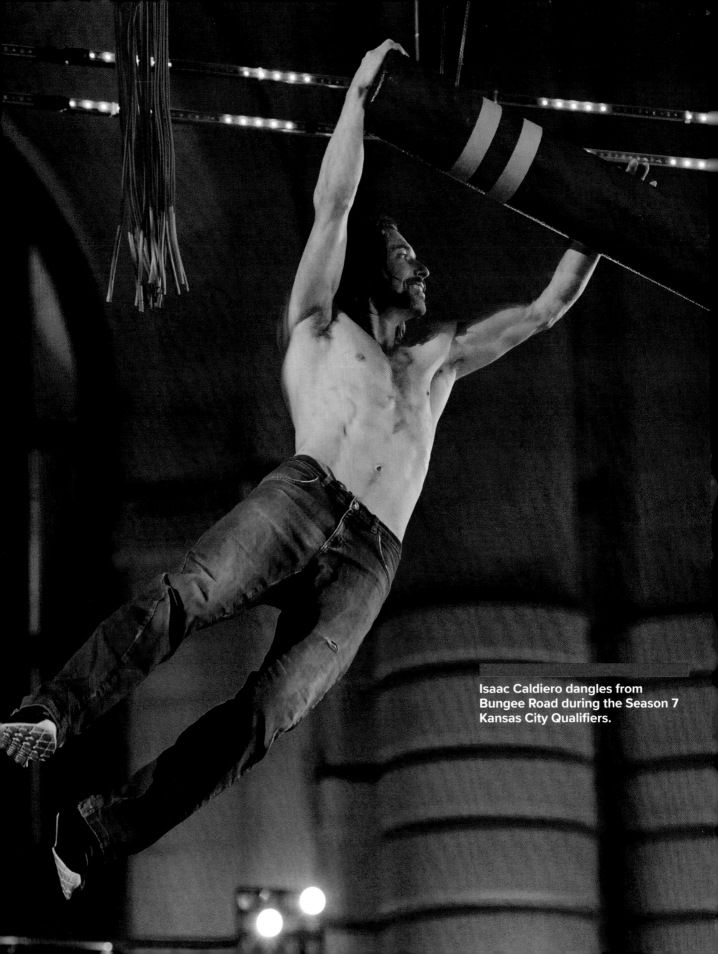

Isaac Caldiero dangles from Bungee Road during the Season 7 Kansas City Qualifiers.

COMPETITION DAY MUST-HAVES

GEOFF BRITTEN: "My outfit! My Ninja Brittens shirt, black stretchy pants, and shoes."

KEVIN BULL: "Food. Eating is always hard with the nerves, but I have to have something in my stomach."

ISAAC CALDIERO: "Calmness and hydration."

GRANT MCCARTNEY: "My dad. He's an ex-NFL player, so he's all hyped and stirs the crowd up. My brother's there as well. He's 15. He's been in Vegas with me the last couple of years and he's solid support. Also, I have my homies on the sidelines, just to get me hyped. My dad hypes the crowd, my friends hype me, and I hype my bro."

MEAGAN MARTIN: "A lot of water with electrolytes! Oh, and a chocolate power bar!"

JOE MORAVSKY: "A massive breakfast—eggs, pancakes, orange juice, bacon, and coffee."

NINJA KNOW-HOW

"I don't allow myself to get to the point where I can experience stage fright. Once that sets in, you're done."
—Isaac Caldiero

Days of competitions are roller coasters of emotion for me. It can be hard to eat enough, and my mind is racing all over the place. There is excitement, nervousness, and, of course, the realization that this is really happening!
–Geoff Britten

STAGE FRIGHT

Most ninjas don't train with cameras following them or with lights shining brightly on their every move. Therefore, running the course for the television lights and cameras can cause some ninjas to experience stage fright when they get up to that starting line.

"Mental toughness is the secret sauce," says Geoff Britten. "On the path to *Ninja Warrior* legend, you have to believe you can do it yet understand that you could fail at any moment. The lights, cameras, and crowd are all focused on you, and that scares a lot of people. It scares me! My way of dealing with that is simple. I flip the nerves. I realize I feel nervous because my body is getting ready to be so strong. There is adrenaline pumping into me, and that's okay. That's what is supposed to happen. My arm hairs will stand up before I run, and I know I'm ready to go."

For other ninjas, the lights, cameras, and action provide inspiration. "I find the cameras and crowd to be more motivating than practice situations," says Kevin Bull. "I usually get better objective performance on the course than off."

NINJA SPOTLIGHT:

GEOFF BRITTEN

"My first ever *Ninja Warrior* experience was in St. Louis in 2014. I was physically ready but had no idea how much of an impact the TV part would have on me. To put it mildly, I was terrified. Before it was my turn, I wondered whether anyone would stop me if I turned and ran away!

"It was then my time, and up I went. Working in TV, there are little things I'm aware of that others might miss—like the fact that as I walked up not all of the camera guys were 'on camera.' They were nowhere to be seen. I was getting iced out my first go! Sometimes when you get on stage, you can end up waiting forever to run, because of backstage issues, course issues, and small breaks the crew takes. I wanted to run—either away or onto the course!

"But I waited.

"A minute goes by, and I see a bunch of people walking to the starting line. It's the director of the show and a bunch of the camera guys.

"'Hey,' they said, 'you better not mess this up! You're one of us! Don't splash me!' And on and on.

"I smiled, laughed, laughed at them, and they all resumed their positions. I wasn't nervous anymore, and I cruised through the course, smiling most of the way.

"One buzzer down, the dream still alive."

> You never really know if you're ready. If you're up and you're alive and your body works, then you're ready.
> —"Island Ninja" Grant McCartney

REMEMBERING TO HAVE FUN

"*American Ninja Warrior* is a blessing that all of us have," says "Island Ninja" Grant McCartney. "I'd love to be the biggest, fastest, strongest on the course, and I'm gonna do my best every time, but if I lose track of the fact that it's fun and that I enjoy it, I've lost track of the goodness that it is. A lot of people don't have the physical capabilities that we have, and I need to remember every time that it's ultimately a fun experience."

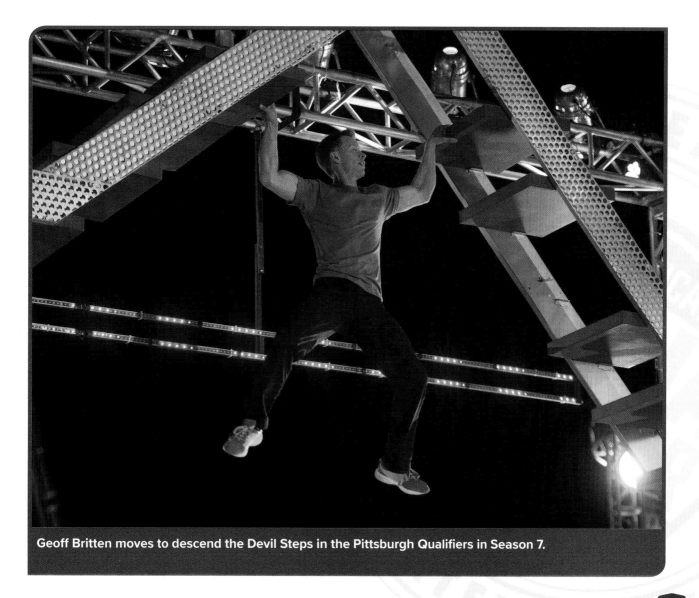

Geoff Britten moves to descend the Devil Steps in the Pittsburgh Qualifiers in Season 7.

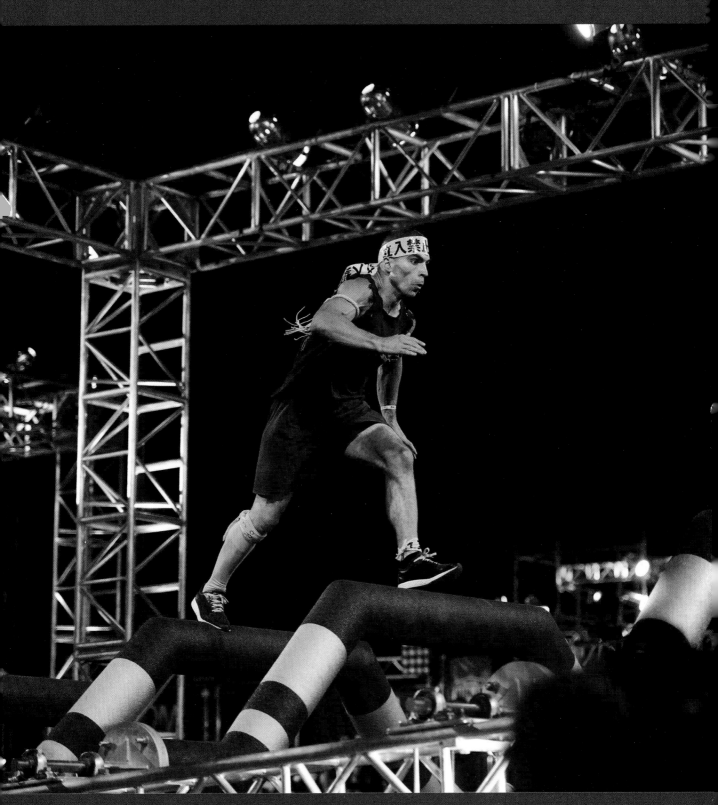

Firefighter Mike Bernardo shows his agility during the National Finals in Las Vegas during Season 9.

CHAPTER 6

NINJA NATION

Over the course of a decade, *American Ninja Warrior* has become more than a television series. What began as a show for hard-core athletes on a fledgling network has become a pop culture phenomenon and appointment television. The show has created a community of fans and ninja athletes who interact and cheer on one another, producing a positive motivational force for health in the United States.

"We've seen over the years where the edginess has been pushed on regular television," says host Akbar Gbajabiamila, a father of four. "I'm not gonna lie—as a parent, I'm tired a lot of the time, and I don't always want to have to sit there and filter what my kids are taking in: *Close your eyes. Don't listen to that. Mute that. Pause that. Go upstairs.* I can just sit back and relax and trust that *American Ninja Warrior* will be responsible and it will bring the family together.

"*American Ninja Warrior* entertains and inspires everyone," adds Gbajabiamila, who announced in Season 9 that he was in training to be a ninja on Season 10. "I think *Ninja Warrior* does a great job of telling someone's story in 90 seconds and creating a fan afterward."

GETTING OUT THERE

American Ninja Warrior is not only telling stories that inspire people but is inspiring viewers to create their own. Moms, dads, grandparents, brothers, sisters—they're heading to their backyards, their streets, their playgrounds, and their gyms to train. Ninja gyms are opening across the country—many of them managed or operated by athletes who have competed on the show. There are *Ninja Warrior* birthday parties, ninja camps, specialized *Ninja*

Warrior training programs for kids and for adults. It's a veritable *Ninja Warrior* movement! "It's a big playground, and it's fun," says executive producer Arthur Smith. "It's an extension of monkey bars and all those things you do as a kid, and that's why kids love it. We are constantly getting letters from kids."

And in a culture where many parents worry about the physical health of their children, who are often inactive due to their attachment to technology such as video games, *American Ninja Warrior* is providing the incentive for them to get outside and run, swing, and try to do all the moves ninjas do on TV.

"Everyone has a little sense of competition inside," says cohost Kristine Leahy. "We want to see people succeed and achieve lifelong goals because it makes us feel good. The difference with *American Ninja Warrior* is that the 'failures,' unlike many other competition shows, are not really failures. So many times I see a competitor fall on the course, and I expect that I am about to conduct a sad interview. Then the person quickly tells me how happy they are just that they were able to get out on the course and they're looking forward to coming back the following year. What other show allows you to keep coming back!?"

> In my training leading up to Season 7, I pushed so hard. I trained tired a lot. When we get tired, it's human nature to quit, to give in. I fought that as much as possible, knowing on the course I would get tired. It saved me, on Stage Three—at the very end, my grip was giving out. I refused to let go and screamed in my head, 'Hold on, hold on!' again and again. As I made my final bar hop, I did hang on—barely! My arms were so tired I couldn't move. Somehow, I threw myself toward the finishing platform. Matt Iseman once told me that in that moment he thought I fell, because I popped out of view for a second, and suddenly I appeared coming over the mat to complete the stage.
>
> —Geoff Britten

CHANGING LIVES

Just as *American Ninja Warrior* is affecting the lives of its viewers across the nation, it has also changed the lives of the ninjas who have appeared on the show, many of whom have been plucked from obscurity and become celebrities of the sport.

"Competing on *American Ninja Warrior* definitely changed my life," says Geoff Britten. "I work in crowded stadiums as a cameraman, and I get recognized on a daily basis, which is really cool. A lot of people tell me that I've inspired them, which is amazing. I've gotten to do a lot of cool things that would have been impossible without doing so well on the show—I've thrown out a first pitch at a baseball game and had someone start a GoFundMe for me that enabled me to fulfill a promise to my wife, that if I won I would buy her a new car. Thank you to all the incredible people who donated."

"It has been a very dramatic change for me," says Kevin Bull. "Sports competition was always important to me in life, but I didn't really have any from age 23 until 29 when I started *Ninja Warrior*. I feel much better and happier than I did then."

Like other ninjas, Bull is also recognized by fans of the show. "Literally everywhere I go," he says, "including when traveling in foreign countries, which is also a big change. It opens a lot of great doors for me, but also I am no longer an anonymous person, which presents its own challenges."

Bull says that the best thing to happen to him since competing has been connecting with the Children's Alopecia Project, an organization devoted specifically to children living with all forms of alopecia—a condition in which hair is lost from some or all areas

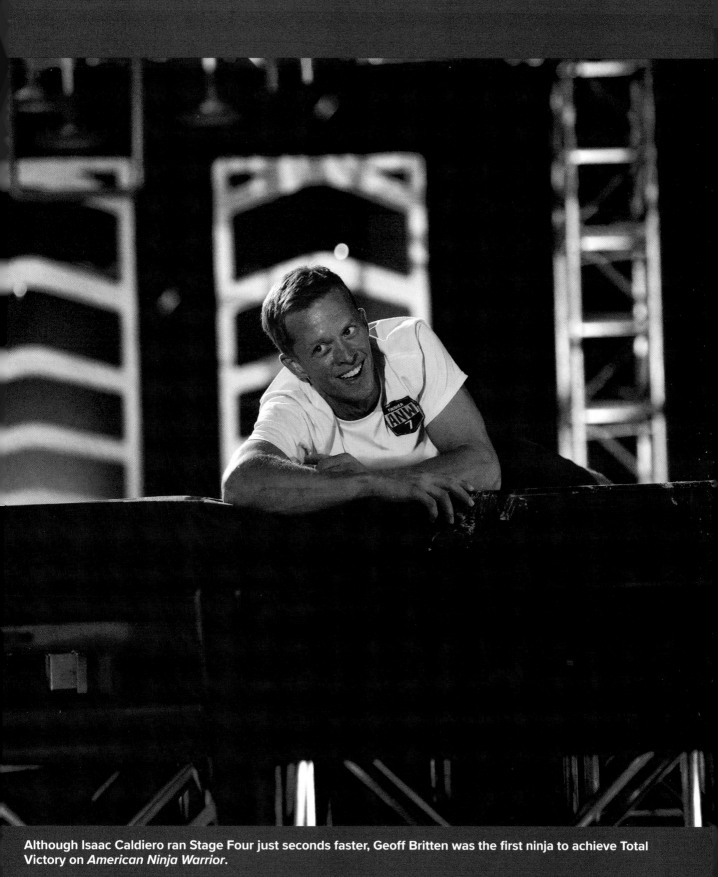

Although Isaac Caldiero ran Stage Four just seconds faster, Geoff Britten was the first ninja to achieve Total Victory on *American Ninja Warrior*.

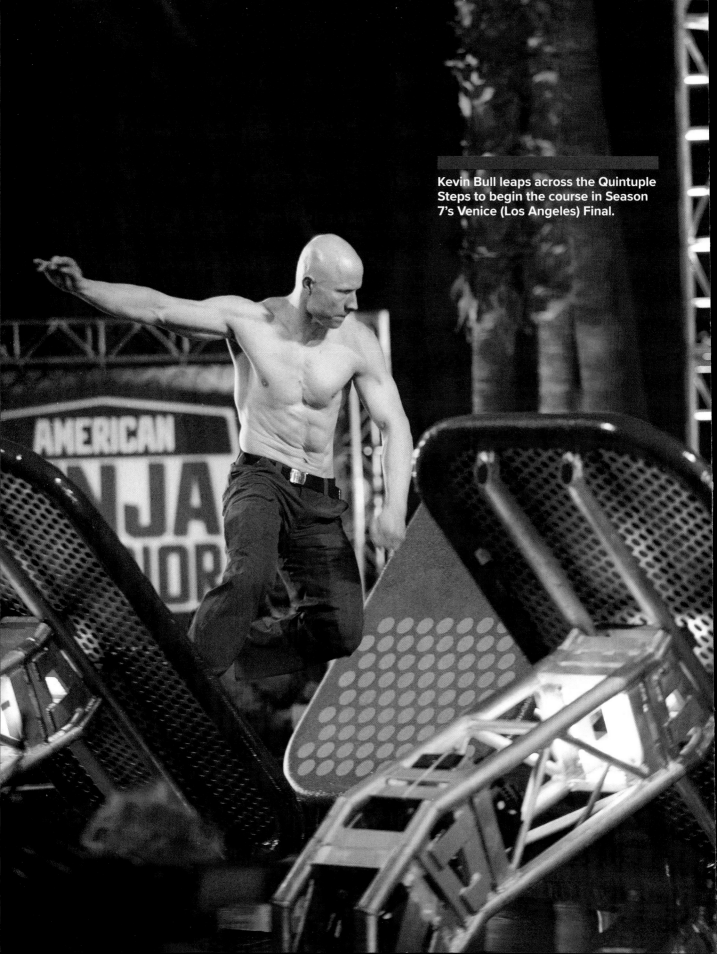

Kevin Bull leaps across the Quintuple Steps to begin the course in Season 7's Venice (Los Angeles) Final.

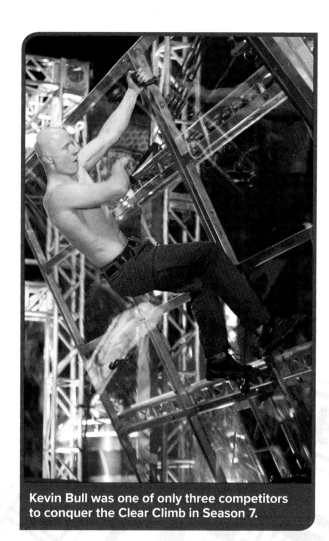

Kevin Bull was one of only three competitors to conquer the Clear Climb in Season 7.

of the body—and helping them to be comfortable in their own skin. "It was the first time I met kids who have the same hair-loss condition as I do," he says, "and I think both the kids and I have grown a lot from the events."

The organization brings kids together with peers and adult mentors. In addition to meeting Bull, kids have also met film/television/voice actors, business owners, teachers, and more. "Everyone has their own perspectives on living with alopecia, including the kids themselves," Bull says, "but the overall message is that it's okay to be different, and that having alopecia will not hold you back if you don't let it."

MAKING MOVES

Jesse "Flex" Labreck's life changed drastically over the course of the two seasons she has appeared on *American Ninja Warrior*. Three years ago, she was a teacher in Maine. "I now live in Illinois, and I'm a manager at a ninja gym," she says. "So, my life is very different. My lifestyle, my friends, my eating, everything has changed because of *Ninja Warrior*."

Her eating? "My boyfriend who I met through *Ninja Warrior* is vegetarian, and so I'm pescatarian now," Labreck says. "I eat much healthier now, and I'm much more conscious of things. I eat a lot less sugar. So, my eating has changed quite a bit."

FINANCIAL FREEDOM

Isaac Caldiero—the only competitor to win the million-dollar grand prize to date—says his life has changed very little after appearing on *American Ninja Warrior*, apart from his "living situation being a lot more comfortable."

"I have always lived a rich life," he says. "I've taught myself through my lifestyle to own very little so I don't need to make very much to survive and be happy. The biggest thing that has changed is from the adrenaline high I experienced from becoming the first American Ninja Warrior. Since this unprecedented accomplishment, there is very little in life that can give me that same feeling and excitement again."

Caldiero is currently working on a training app to teach athletes "how to become a ninja champion."

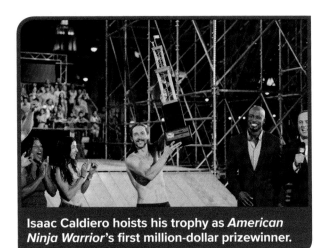

Isaac Caldiero hoists his trophy as *American Ninja Warrior*'s first million-dollar prizewinner.

> Being the first American Ninja Warrior is really a dream come true. If the prize for the show had been one dollar, I would have approached it exactly the same. For me, it was always about beating these obstacles. Lowering down from the top of Stage Four, knowing I had accomplished what I set out to do, was stunning. I remember being so shocked I could barely speak! Having my wife, my daughter, and my mom there really was important to me. I've watched the Finals a couple of times, and what I enjoy most is the emotion on my family's faces. There was no chance of my success without my wife or mom helping me along the way.
> —Geoff Britten

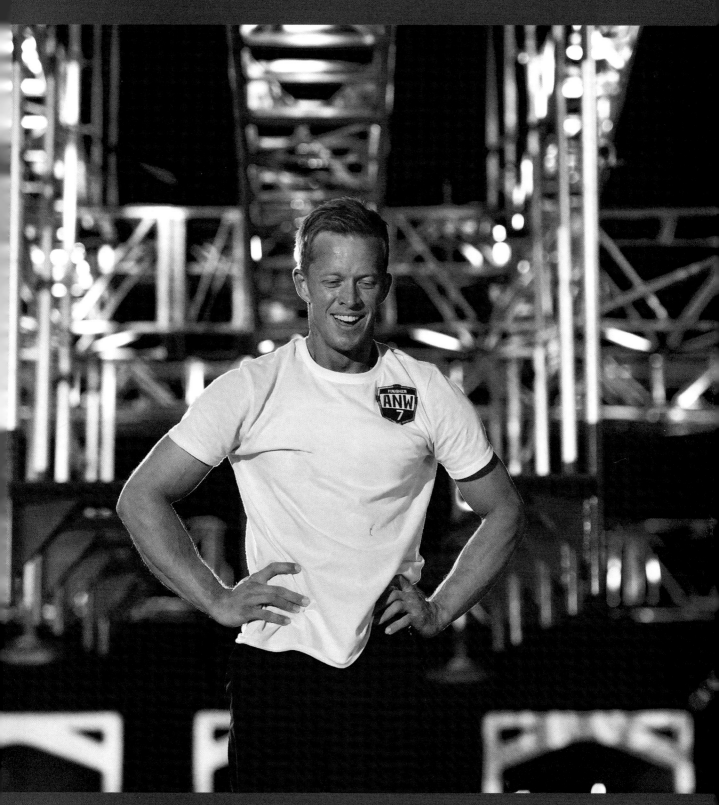

Geoff Britten completes the course with only 0.35 seconds remaining on the clock, becoming the first American to achieve Total Victory—the first American Ninja Warrior.

NINJA SPOTLIGHT:

CHRIS WILCZEWSKI

In 2011, Chris Wilczewski and his brother, Brian, a fellow ninja, built the New Jersey–based Movement Lab, one of the first Ninja Warrior training facilities in the country. Movement Lab helps bring together the top athletes of the sport and provides an opportunity for fans and future ninjas to meet the pros, train with them, and hang out with them. Wilczewski has also been involved in nonprofit work, helping to raise money for various charities, including cancer research and autism awareness.

What's more, Wilczewski has gone from the *American Ninja Warrior* National Finals to the National Ninja League, a nonprofit formed by a collective of the nation's top ninja facilities whose goal is to promote the sport of ninja obstacle courses across the United States. The League also features an elite series of annual ninja competitions across the nation that culminates with a large national competition.

"I have been able to reach youth across the nation by providing them with an opportunity to compete in a global competition," says Wilczewski, who is the driving force behind the League, which recently expanded its scope to incorporate international Qualifiers.
"I couldn't imagine what my life would be if I never competed on *American Ninja Warrior*."

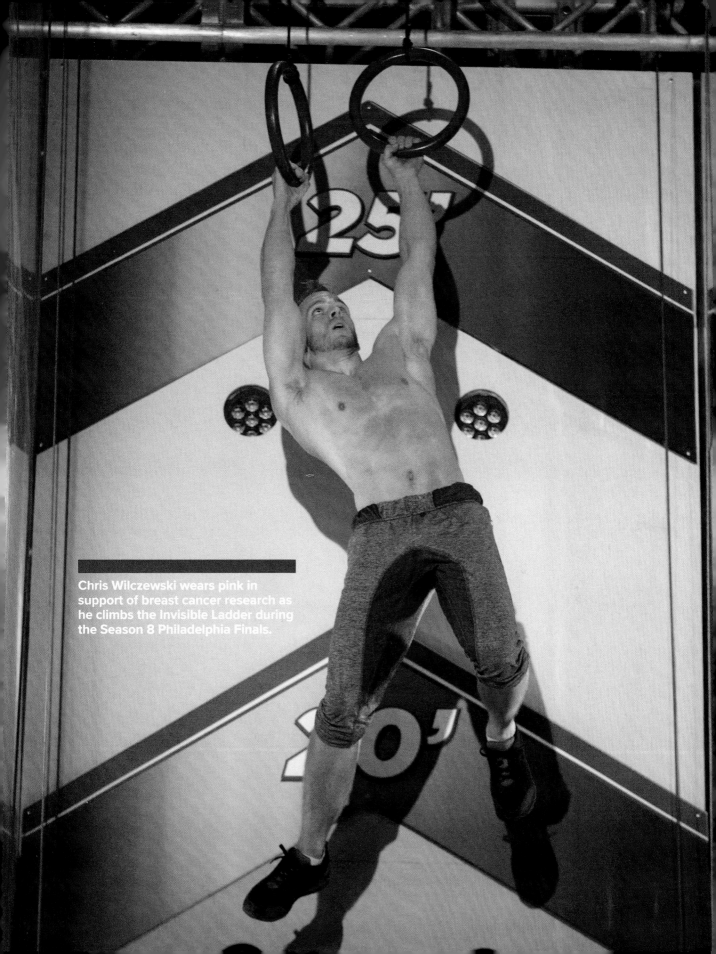

Chris Wilczewski wears pink in support of breast cancer research as he climbs the Invisible Ladder during the Season 8 Philadelphia Finals.

THE FACES OF FITNESS

Many of the ninjas who appear on *American Ninja Warrior* have gone on to become ambassadors of the sport and the faces of fitness. As a result of her appearances on *American Ninja Warrior*, Meagan Martin has started modeling with the mission to ignite a community of active, healthy, and confident women and girls. "Getting modeling jobs has probably been the best thing that's happened to me since competing on *American Ninja Warrior*," says Martin. "It's such a fun job."

"The Weatherman" Joe Moravsky, too, is making the move to fashion. Moravsky currently owns The Weather Warrior, LLC and teaches gymnastics and parkour part-time at a gym in Newtown, Connecticut, called Vasi's International Gymnastics, but he also has partnered on an endorsement deal for a men's activewear line.

> It's been a ride, and it's not over yet! I've retired from the show but now work behind the scenes. I'm involved in testing the obstacles and trying to make the difficulty just right. I plan on trying *American Ninja Warrior* at least one more time, when I turn 40. Why not?
>
> —Geoff Britten

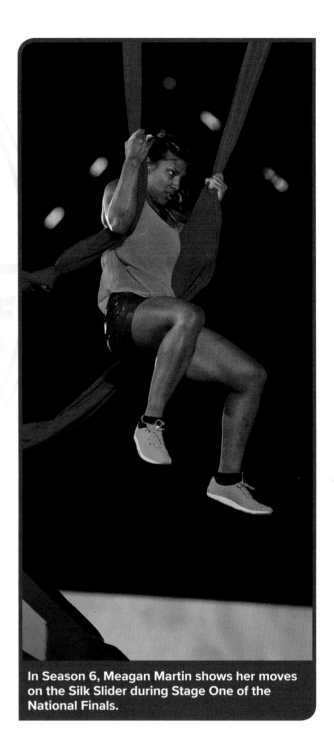

In Season 6, Meagan Martin shows her moves on the Silk Slider during Stage One of the National Finals.

THE NINJA COMMUNITY: GROWTH AROUND THE GLOBE

As *American Ninja Warrior* gains recognition and popularity year after year in the United States, so are other versions of *Ninja Warrior*, and this is creating many ninja communities in countries

> The role models that we have on this show... I don't think there are as many role models in any other show on the air right now. I really don't. The athletes that are on our show are masters of the sport. So many of them are motivational speakers and go to classes, and hospitals, and do all the right things, and teach, and pay it forward. There's so much goodwill, and it's within the community, too.
>
> —Executive Producer Arthur Smith

throughout the world. Thanks to the internet, these ninja communities often communicate with one another, despite the language barriers—ninja training is a universal language! Ninjas will train together in the United States and abroad, and American ninjas have made appearances in some of the other *Ninja Warrior* broadcasts, including Vietnamese and Indonesian versions, as well as *SASUKE*.

"The last couple of years *American Ninja Warrior* has exploded in popularity, and because of that I've had a lot of opportunities," says "Island Ninja" Grant McCartney. "I recently took six months off from my job as a flight attendant for Hawaiian Airlines and traveled on my own around the United States, going to all the different ninja gyms, seeing my buddies, doing camps, clinics, and public appearances.

People are literally paying me to show up and sign autographs! People want me to come and speak about my life or about *American Ninja Warrior*, so it's a whole new avenue of life that I didn't get to experience before and now I've had some amazing opportunities because of it."

AMERICAN NINJA WARRIOR NATION

America has indeed become a ninja nation and, as of June 2016, has an official fan site called American Ninja Warrior Nation, which is run by Vox Media's SB Nation, a sports media brand with more than 300 fan-centric team communities. Fan Nikki Lee serves as editor-in-chief of American Ninja Warrior Nation, which has thousands of registered users and a social media community in the millions.

DID YOU KNOW?

When Jessie Graff became the first woman to conquer Stage One in Season 8's National Finals, the video of her historic run was posted on the official *American Ninja Warrior* websites and shared by many media outlets around the globe. One of the videos posted on American Ninja Warrior Nation earned more than 100 million views in a mere four days—the fan site record!

NINJA SPOTLIGHT:

NIKKI LEE

EDITOR-IN-CHIEF, AMERICAN NINJA WARRIOR NATION

Tell us about the American Ninja Warrior Nation blog.

American Ninja Warrior Nation kicked off in June 2016 with the premiere of *American Ninja Warrior*'s Season 8. It's taken on a life of its own since then with thousands of registered users on the site and a social media community of more than 1.3 million.

What's it like writing about *American Ninja Warrior?*

It's a dream come true! I was selected to take on this project because I was—and am—a fan of the show. Task number one was to go behind the scenes. Literally, my first day on the job, I met my boss and we went to the set of the Los Angeles Qualifiers and City Finals on the Universal Studios backlot where I watched ninjas like Kevin Bull and Jessie Graff run the course. Pretty great way to kick things off!

I would say that it quickly shifted from working with ninjas to working with friends. Everyone always talks about what a tight-knit and supportive community the ninjas have created. Not only is that true, but it extends to those around them, even if they aren't competing. I felt almost adopted into their world. Watching the Qualifiers now is a little painful for me, because I feel like I have about 100 "favorite" ninjas and I want them all to hit the buzzer every time!

What are you asked most often by fans? What do they want to know?

Fans want to know everything. Ninja Warrior, as a concept, has such a long and storied history from *SASUKE* in Japan to what we now know as *American Ninja Warrior*. So there are fans who want to delve deep into statistics, athlete performances, and how the obstacles are designed and developed.

There are fans who are inspired to change their lives by watching the ninjas. They want to learn more about the competitors as people—what keeps them motivated, how they train. There's also a fascination with how a huge show like *American Ninja Warrior* comes together on a production level—casting logistics, pulling the whole thing together into an Emmy-nominated creation.

What is the most fun aspect of your job?

I don't think I could pick one! I get to spend about three months a year traveling to cities I've never been to. I get to watch ninjas I've always respected pull off amazing feats right in front of my face, and then I get to talk to them about it. I learn about new ninjas between seasons. Watching them train, apply, and then compete on the show is amazing. It's like I get to have an understanding of a very small part of their journey and growth.

Plus, I hang out online with fans who are just as passionate about the show as I am. I get to share my experiences with them. The entire "job" feels like just visiting with different aspects of the *American Ninja Warrior* community and reporting back. The athletes, the crew, the producers, the fans—it's like having the golden ticket to move freely through the Ninja Warrior world!

Because you attend the live events, you know lots of spoilers. Is it hard not to reveal?

Ugh, so hard! In Season 8, knowing Jessie Graff was going to beat Stage One was a killer! It's been great practice for my poker face when people ask me about spoilers. For example, when I'm writing a recap about a Qualifying episode, I already know how the City Finals end. I have to be careful to weed out anything that could give away the next move. In Season 8, the legendary Geoff Britten did great in the Philadelphia Finals, but I already knew he had that painful-to-watch exit in the National Finals. So I still needed to hype up his Philadelphia performance from the perspective of a fan thinking he's going all the way. (Sorry, Geoff!) Sometimes you want to sob into the keyboard, but other times you have to keep your mouth shut about something really exciting.

What's something about *ANW* that would surprise fans?

How good ninjas are at sleeping in odd places! They have to run the course in the dead of night. Some might not have a run time until 4 or 5 A.M. So they gotta sleep! I've seen ninjas passed out under tables, on safety mats, or just on the sidewalk in a sleeping bag.

Also, how genuine the experience is. As much as I wish there were do-overs or ways to help someone, once they're on the course, they're 100 percent on their own. They're being timed by several different people. Multiple crew members are watching to make sure they don't touch the water or disobey any of the obstacle rules. (Yes, there are rules, for everyone who comments "Why don't they just climb the truss?") It's a one-and-done situation, which definitely adds pressure and creates heartbreaking exits but also adds a simple clarity to the show that I think fans connect with.

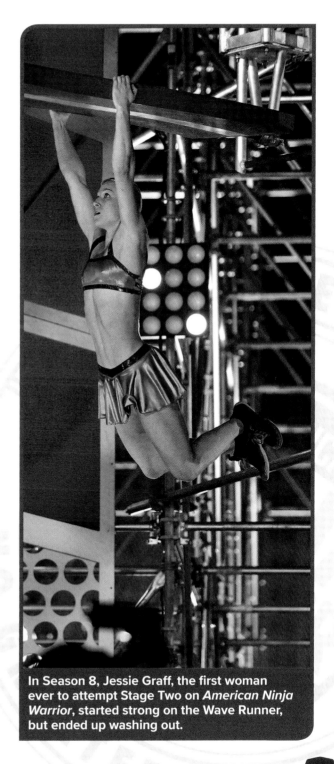

In Season 8, Jessie Graff, the first woman ever to attempt Stage Two on *American Ninja Warrior*, started strong on the Wave Runner, but ended up washing out.

WHAT'S NEXT?

As *American Ninja Warrior* embarks on another decade of sports entertainment and obstacle course competition, show executives are ready to up the ante with even more challenges and excitement—while always staying true to the show's heart and staying a step ahead of the ninjas. "The course will continue to evolve as it has over the years," says executive producer Arthur Smith. "I think we're going to see better athletic performances. We're going to see more difficult courses. We're going to see more women running it and excelling. And I think it's just going to make for better TV.

"One of the funny things that happens to us—it's happening less, but it's still happening—is that someone will come up to Kent Weed or myself and say, 'I love your new show,'" Smith says. "And I say, 'New show? Which one are you talking about?' And they say, '*American Ninja Warrior*.' After 10 years, it's still connecting with people."

> We have such a tight community, and it's not just for the cameras. We really enjoy being with each other, doing stuff together, and hanging out. Some of my closest friends are ninjas now. I wouldn't trade it for anything.
>
> —Jesse "Flex" Labreck

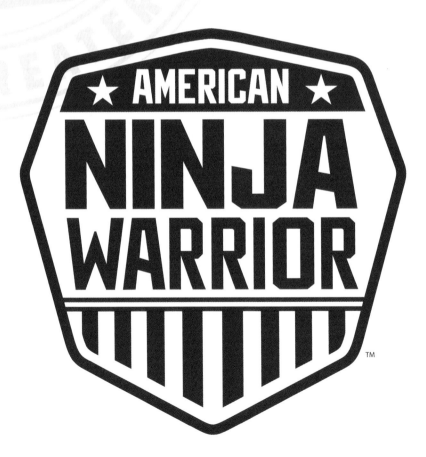

BECOME AN AMERICAN NINJA WARRIOR: THE ULTIMATE INSIDER'S GUIDE

Adam Rayl pumps his fist in the air after completing the Los Angeles Finals course in Season 9.